Xenobiotics in Foods and Feeds

John W. Finley, EDITOR
University of Iowa Hospitals

Daniel E. Schwass, EDITOR
U.S. Department of Agriculture

Based on a symposium sponsored
by the Division of Agricultural
and Food Chemistry
at the 184th Meeting
of the American Chemical Society,
Kansas City, Missouri,
September 12–17, 1982

ACS SYMPOSIUM SERIES **234**

AMERICAN CHEMICAL SOCIETY
WASHINGTON, D.C. 1983

Library of Congress Cataloging in Publication Data

Xenobiotics in foods and feeds.
(ACS symposium series, ISSN 0097–6156; 234)

"Based on a symposium sponsored by the Division
of Agricultural and Food Chemistry at the 184th
Meeting of the American Chemical Society, Kansas
City, Missouri, September 12–17, 1982."
Includes bibliographies and index.

1. Xenobiotics—Addresses, essays, lectures.
2. Food contamination—Addresses, essays, lectures.
3. Food—Analysis—Addresses, essays, lectures.
   I. Finley, John W., 1942–   . II. Schwass, Daniel
E., 1951–   . III. American Chemical Society. Division of Agricultural and Food Chemistry. IV. American Chemical Society. Meeting (184th: 1982: Kansas
City, Mo.) V. Series.

TX571.X45X45   1983   615.9′54   83–15685
ISBN 0–8412–0809–3

44,842

ACS Symposium Series

M. Joan Comstock, *Series Editor*

FOREWORD

The ACS Symposium Series was founded in 1974 to provide
a medium for publishing symposia quickly in book form. The
format of the Series parallels that of the continuing Advances
in Chemistry Series except that in order to save time the
papers are not typeset but are reproduced as they are submitted by the authors in camera-ready form. Papers are reviewed under the supervision of the Editors with the assistance
of the Series Advisory Board and are selected to maintain the
integrity of the symposia; however, verbatim reproductions of
previously published papers are not accepted. Both reviews
and reports of research are acceptable since symposia may
embrace both types of presentation.

CONTENTS

PREFACE

Xᴇɴᴏʙɪᴏᴛɪᴄs, ʙʏ ᴅᴇꜰɪɴɪᴛɪᴏɴ, ᴀʀᴇ ᴄᴏᴍᴘᴏᴜɴᴅs that are foreign, but not necessarily harmful, to a given living system. For this symposium, we have focused on biological systems that affect humans or animals. This topic represents a mild but timely departure from the traditional areas presented in symposia by the Agriculture and Food Division. Although considerable discussion of various types of xenobiotic compounds has been included in many symposia and general sessions, the current effort is the first to emphasize a variety of potentially toxic materials. In the symposium on which this book is based, the authors cover a wide variety of compounds found in the food chain. These compounds may have plant or microbiological origin or may result from changes caused by food storage, processing, or final preparation.

Currently there is high public interest in the nutritional value and safety of foods. In addition to providing a source of essential nutrients, human food consumption can represent a delightful social experience and contribute to sensory satisfaction. Organoleptic research and culinary arts have taught us to produce foods with extraordinary convenience and palatability. Microbiological research has helped us prevent age-old public health problems by ensuring sanitary handling of foods throughout production and processing. Nutritionists have established requirements and ensured the nutrient quality of foods, and we now have the opportunity to consume a nutritionally adequate diet. The overall improvement in food handling in the last 100 years now challenges us with new considerations of what constitutes a safe diet. The influence of xenobiotics on these considerations is not clearly understood. Food toxicology, particularly as related to long-term effects of low-level exposure to toxic materials, is now emerging as a branch of food science.

Most of the foods we consume are beneficial; some foods, however, may have risks. Rational assessment of these risks and benefits is an extremely difficult area of research and, too frequently, an emotional issue.

This volume presents an objective, state-of-the-art discussion of xenobiotic compounds that can exist in the diet and includes some of the approaches available to minimize the occurrence of these compounds.

We are very grateful for assistance and would like to thank the Agricultural Division of the Ciba-Geigy Corporation and Pfizer, Inc. for their generous support which enabled several speakers to attend.

JOHN W. FINLEY
University of Iowa Hospitals
Department of Pediatrics
Iowa City, Iowa

DANIEL E. SCHWASS
U.S. Department of Agriculture
Berkeley, California

June 16, 1983

Systematic Toxicity Testing for Xenobiotics in Foods

MORRIS M. JOSELOW

University of Medicine of New Jersey, Newark, NJ 07103

Substances that are not natural to a food, xenobiotics, may become a part of the food by several routes. They may be deliberately added as food or color additives; they may result indirectly from migration of additives from wrappings into the food; they may also result from the incorporation of environmental pollutants into the food while that food is growing or maturing.

All such xenobiotics inevitably raise questions of safety. This, of course, does not infer that all natural foods are safe (1). We know this to be untrue--but it does recognize that anything added to foods will be regarded with suspicion until adequate toxicity testing has established its safety--a concept that now applies to almost all foods and drugs introduced into commerce.

As might be expected, there is a large interface between toxicity testing and legal requirements. Some formal definitions, originally proposed by the National Academy of Sciences, are in order. Toxicity is defined as the capacity of a substance to cause injury, in a very broad sense, and includes injury to any mechanism or tissue of the body, as well as irritation, behavioral changes, or mental disturbances. Hazard, as used, for example, in defining a hazardous substance, involves a probability concept, like so much else in toxicology. It is an estimate of the probability or likelihood that a substance may cause injury. The converse of this is the meaning reserved for the term safety, namely, the probability (or practical certainty) that injury will not result when a substance is used in a particular manner and quantity (2).

The use aspect is a major qualification that inheres in these definitions. Any substance can cause injury if high enough concentrations are administered. The evaluation of safety or hazard must therefore take into account the conditions of use or possible predictable misuse of the substance.

Toxicity testing has become a major concern nationally because of the extensive legislation that now mandates such testing (Food, Drug, and Cosmetic Act; Hazardous Substances Act; Occupational Safety and Health Act; Toxic Substances Control Act) as well as internationally, because of the need for mutually acceptable products as a prerequisite to economic cooperation in the marketing of foods and chemicals.

0097–6156/83/0234–0001$06.00/0
© 1983 American Chemical Society

In no other area has toxicity testing assumed greater importance
than with foods, for the obvious reason that foods represent potentially the greatest population impact, and therefore the need
for greatest surveillance.

Before proceeding with consideration of some of the formal test
procedures that have been developed and are now in use, we should
recognize a fundamental flaw in the scientific basis for all
safety evaluations. All tests to evaluate safety are designed
to demonstrate a negative, the probability that injury will not
result, which, by definition and logic, cannot be proven. We
may sometimes feel, after having performed a sufficient number
of tests of a sufficient variety over a sufficient length of time,
that safety has been fully demonstrated. But it only takes a
thalidomide-type disaster, with the appearance of a new unexpected effect, to remind us that absolute safety -- the guaranteed
absence of any harm -- is an illusion that can not be unequivocal-
ly established, unless we could test all human beings over an
infinite period of time, an obviously impossible task. Faced with
this conflict between wish and reality, we have come to rely on
"scientific judgment" -- a much overused and abused phrase that
should always be suspect -- to make predictions about safety that
we then claim are beyond reasonable doubt, or that there is no unreasonable risk", as required by the Toxic Substances Control Act.

Of necessity, heavy reliance in toxicity testing must be placed
on the use of animals as surrogates or substitutes for humans.
This requirement has imposed some qualifications -- at times severe -- in the interpretation of results.

Choice of Species of Test Animal

In deciding on the animal to be used, toxicologists attempt to
follow a basic guideline: wherever possible, use a species that
biologically handles the material under study as similarly as
possible to man; and, in deciding similarity to man, considerations of metabolism, absorption, excretion, and other physiological parameters should be taken into account.

This guideline, which would seem to be so fundamental, nevertheless, poses a dilemma. The toxicologist would like to use species that is as sensitive to the injury expected for the substance under study, a species that would react physiologically
like humans, or be even more sensitive.

But the state of the art in toxicology is not sufficiently developed to permit predictions as to which species of animals are
most similar to man in their responses to chemical challenges.

In practice, the choice of a species is often dictated more by
practical considerations than by similarity of response. Con-

venience, ease of handling, availability of stock, housing facilities, cost of maintenance, and precedence of use -- all of these
enter into a judgment of the choice of species. Albino rats and
dogs have been most frequently used, because they are the most
easily available animals and have a long history of use.

The fact that rats and dogs are most widely used is also self-
perpetuating. In any study of a new chemical, the obvious first
choice would be an animal species whose reactions are well-known
and documented. Also, the practical problem of obtaining suitable animals is minimized by the use of those for which previous
demands have created adequate, dependable, and inexpensive sources
of supply.

Furthermore, some federal regulations have recommended and thereby almost mandated the use of rats and dogs, particularly, for
long-term toxicity studies of food additives and pesticides, even
though there may be important differences in metabolic capabilities and physiological responses between these species and man.
The rat is a poor choice to evaluate the liver injury potential
of a substance for man, because the rat liver is resistant, and
regenerates rapidly. The guinea pig or the rabbit would be a better choice of this. The dog does not acetylate or detoxify aromatic amines. The monkey and the guinea pig require exogenous ascorbic acid, while the rat does not, which makes the rat unsuitable for the demonstration of an ascorbic and deficiency.

For long-term studies, a species having a relatively short life
span permits determining the effects of a chemical over course
of a lifetime. The latter requirement, in a practical sense,
limits life-time studies to rats or mice or hamsters.

But here too, some basic difficulties can present themselves. For
assessing the possibility of cancer -- the main objective in long
term tests -- we rely on the use of healthy, disease-free inbred
mice, which represent characteristics that are hardly representative of a heterogeneous human population at risk. This difference only complicates known differences in metabolic responses;
e.g., mice can not decarboxylate and eliminate some carcinogenic
hydrocarbons that humans can readily "detoxify".

For preliminary studies and screening, rats, mice, rabbits, or
guinea pigs are selected for economy, ease of treatment, and, to
a large extent, according to the reported work of others who have
done similar studies.

For the chronic studies required by some Federal regulations, the
species specified by the agencies are used, usually rats and
beagle dogs. Under the Federal Hazardous Substance Act (3)
for example, the definitions of toxic, highly toxic, and non-toxic

are based in part on responses of rats to oral or inhalation ex-
posures. That recommendation has made it almost mandatory to use
rats and follow the prescribed protocols.

In summary, though we ought to use a species reacting qualitatively and quantitatively most like man, what we actually use most
often is the species for which healthy commerical stocks, reasonably priced and reasonably constant, are available.

Administration of Dose

The route chosen for administration of the substance to the test
animal and the manner of its administration should be the same as
that by which man will be exposed. In acute toxicity testing,
however, this is a practice that is intentionally violated, since
a single massive dose is usually administered by intubation or
gavage.

There will always be some differences between the effects observed in animal tests, and actual human experience. No intubated
oral dose can be relied upon to be a sound model of the effect of
a chemical in the diet, even if it is repeated day after day. The
single dose will of necessity yield a peak concentration in body
fluids higher than what would result from the slow absorption of
a chemical during slow digestion of food. Intubation also has a
greater chance of being injurious, either by the greater magnitude of the peak blood concentration or by overwhelming a metabolic pathway that could in normal circumstances handle a lower
concentration of the toxic substances.

Dose Levels and Safety Factors

A basic assumption underlying toxicity testing is that responses
are dose-related, and that, in testing, several doses should be
administered to elicit graded responses. Furthermore, there must
also be some dose below which no response will be shown (or, more
precisely, be incapable of detection). This dose has been var-
iously termed the "biologically insignificant dose" or the "NOEL"
(No Observed Effect Level), and its determination is one of the
primary objectives of toxicity testing.

The term "adverse effect" is not easily interpretable. A physiological response to a stress that is readily reversible, such as
a change in enzyme concentrations, might not necessarily be an
adverse effect, particularly if no damage is detectable.

The ability of toxicity testing to set safe levels is its most
important practical function. The procedure has been developed
most rigorously in the field of food and color additive testing
-- chemicals added to foods -- where a series of special stipula-

tions that permit estimates of "toxicologically insignificant levels" of chemicals in foods, have been proposed. In general, a "safe" level of a substance is arbitrarily set by applying a safety factor to the highest intake that is found not to injure experimental animals exposed for extended periods; i.e., over a lifetime. The "safe" level is frequently expressed as 1/100th of the experimentally determined highest No Observed Effect Level. This ratio, 1:100, is derived by applying a factor of 10 for extrapolation of the findings of animals to man, and another factor of 10 to account for variations in susceptibilities among people. A ratio of 100 is thought to provide a conservative estimate of the safety factor needed to afford adequate protection, even to persons whose dietary patterns or individual susceptibilities might be unusual. And this procedures has been so widely adopted by national and international bodies concerned with safety that the term "safe level",as applied to chemicals in food, has also become a large extent applicable to chemicals and hazardous substances that impinge on man from whatever source.

The concept that there must be some dose level below which an adverse effect will not appear has not met with universal acceptance, particularly with regard to toxic agents that have longterm, irreversible effects, such as ionizing radiation or carcinogenic substances. Some toxicologists have proposed that adequate testing can set safe limits even for carcinogenic agents; others challenge this belief, and argue that it is impossible to predict safe levels for carcinogens by taking an arbitrary fraction of the lowest No Observed Effect animal dose in any particular experimental situation. Sharp distinctions have also been made between reversible and irreversible effects. For additives that can induce reversible toxic effects, threshold levels below which human exposure would be safe can be reasonably determined. However, for chemicals inducing irreversible and possibly cumulative effects, such thresholds can not be determined; and a zero tolerance has to be set.

If a zero tolerance is mandated, then there is no need for toxicity testing. Only the techniques of analytical chemistry need be applied to determine whether a substance is present or not, and therefore, whether its use is permissible or not. Such an approach however, runs the risk of becoming a reductio ad absurdum, as analytical techniques become more refined and sensitive.

Designs and Objectives for Formal Testing

The movement toward systematic formalized toxicity testing began, as might be expected, with the problem of chemicals in foods in the 1940's. A Food and Drug Administration report published in 1943 (4) offered some general protocols. As additional toxic effects -- unsuspected at that time -- became known, these rec-

ommendations were amplified in detail and expanded in scope. The
recently published monograph (5)of the Bureau of Goods, Food
and Drug Administration, entitled, "Toxicological Principles"
can be regarded as the culmination of these efforts. It is a
considerably updated version of the original recommendations, and
is _sine qua non_ for those concerned with toxicity testing.

It provides details regarding test requirements and protocols,
and represents the consensus of judgments of the agency most concerned with the safety of xenobiotics in foods.

The original guidelines recommended only three basic types of
tests to be performed on laboratory animals to evaluate safety.
While other tests for specific toxic effects have since been
added, these basic tests still remain the backbone of current
toxicity testing procedures. These tests differ primarily in
their durations and objectives. Tests that use only single doses
of the chemical, administered on one occasion, are referred to as
"acute tests". Longer tests, in which the chemical is given at
least once daily, for periods of up to three months, are commonly
referred to as "sub-acute" or "sub-chronic" or "prolonged" tests.
Still lengthier tests, involving the administration of a chemical
to animals daily for periods of one to two years to simulate lifetime exposure, are referred to as "chronic" or "long term" or
"extended" toxicity tests.

Acute Toxicity Tests

The single test that is conducted on practically all substances
of biologic interest is the acute toxicity test. It is undoubtedly responsible for the greatest ritual mass slaughter of animals in this country.

The test requires that the animals be exposed to a relatively
large dose, on at least one occasion, to the chemical of interest.
The principal purpose is to determine the lethality or LD_{50} for
the chemical (the dose that will be fatal to 50% of the test
population.)

Almost all acute toxicity tests are done with rats or mice, largely   because of the low cost, easy availability, expendability
of these animals, and the fact that an abundant literature exists
for these two species. Initially, the chemical may be given to a
single species; at several dosage levels, to pre-conditioned
groups of animals, as prescribed by Federal recommendations.

Following administration of the doses, observations are made of
the animals for peiods ranging from a few minutes to two weeks,
to comply with the requirements of some regulations e.g.; the
Federal Hazardous Substances Act. The lethality is determined on
the basis of death occuring within the observation period (14 days).

Subchronic or Subacute Toxicity Testing

The acute test is primarily a fact-finding, exploratory experiment
to obtain some indication of toxicity. Such information is used
not only to permit comparisons among different agents (by comparing their LD_{50}'s), but also to provide a more refined basis for
the selection of dose levels for the more prolonged type of studies, extending for 3-4 months, the so-called "subchronic" or "sub-
acute animal studies.

These more prolonged studies are designed to provide additional
information on toxicity. They have three main purposes:

1) To establish more narrowly a maximum tolerated dose; i.e.,
   a dose that will produce overt adverse symptoms but not
   death.

2) To provide an estimate of the highest dose that will not
   show any effect; i.e., the "no effect" level.

3) To establish the biological nature of the damage produced
   as revealed by clinical and pathological examination of
   the sacrificed animals.

Chronic Toxicity

If the substance has been found to be satisfactory; i.e., non-
toxic, in the subchronic tests, it may then be subjected to chronic, long-term, or extended toxicity tests. These tests are meant
to simulate lifetime human experience, and the experimental protocols, therefore,call for dosing the animal with the substance
over the course of its life-time, which means, for practical purposes, that an animal with a short life span must be used; i.e.,
rats or mice. The rationale for accepting this is that in a short-
lived species, progressive injury proceeds more rapidly, and can
be detected more easily than in a long-lived species. Lifetime
dosing of a rat; i.e., for 30 months, is considered equivalent to
70 years exposure in man. The F.D.A. thus specifies and accepts
30 month exposure in rats for a lifetime study. But this rationale does not hold for dogs or other animals. Two years for a dog
is still only a fraction (20%) of its lifetime.

By the time a substance is considered for chronic toxicity studies, information will have already been obtained regarding the
nature of its toxicity and its tolerable as well as lethal doses.
The main purposes of long-term testing then are twofold:

1) To find or confirm the "No-Effect" lifetime dosage level

for the additive, i.e., the maximum that can be taken
that will not produce any observable adverse effect over
a life time.

2) To detect any more significant abnormalities that may
become apparent only over the course of a lifetime; and
the change generally sought most commonly is the development of a cancer of some kind.

This is undoubtedly the most important objective of the chronic
test -- to search for the development of a carcinogenic end result. In fact, some toxicolosits believe that if effects other
than cancer are sought, these should have become apparent in the
shorter subchronic studies -- and there would then usually be no
need to carry the test beyond the subchronic period.

As might be expected when conducting tests with animals that will
unavoidably vary to some extent in their genetic make-up, variations in results may be encountered, particularly if test conditions are not carefully controlled. Recognition of this problem
which has accounted for wide disparities reported in the literature in toxicity test findings, has led F.D.A. and others (6) to
standardize the relevant factors involved in conducting toxicity
tests. Test conditions, if not controlled, can lead to spurious
results among different laboratories, and even within the same
laboratory (7).

The standardized factors include not only the conditions under
which the tests are conducted -- and good laboratory practices are
now an added minimum requirement -- but also prescribe the clinical testing and observations that must be made on the test animals
during and after the test period (Tables I - IV).

Recent additions to the toxicity test protocols may now require
formulized examinations for genetic effects (i.e., teratogenesis,
mutagenesis, reproduction) as well as determination of the metabolic alterations of the additive and their disposition. Each of
these activities has become an important sub-branch of toxicity
testing.

A typical manner in which a decision on safety may be made, based
on sequential testing, is shown in Figure 1. Such testing obviously represents an extensive and expensive undertaking. The services
of varied professionals will be required: toxicologists, pathologists, chemists, biochemists, veterinarians, statisticians, and
attorneys (to prepare the petitions) and a host of other support-
ing personnel.

From all the toxicity data, if the study works out, will emerge a
reasonable figure for a "No Effect Level" as well as an indication

TABLE 1

OUTLINE OF GENERAL PROCEDURES*

	Animals	No. of Dose Levels	No. of Animals (minimum/group)
ACUTE (24 hrs)			
	rats, mice, guinea pigs	4 - 5	5-10 each, equal nos. of each sex
	dogs		usually total of 12
Dermal	rabbits	3	2 male & 2 female each
INTUBATION 1 - 8 hrs		3	
SUBACUTE (90 days)			
	rats	5	10 male & 10 female each
	dogs	3	2 male & 2 female each
Dermal	rabbits	4	3 male & 3 female each
CHRONIC (2 yrs)			
	rats	3	25 male & 25 female each
	dogs	3	3 male & 3 female each

* From Appraisal of Safety of Chemicals in Foods, Drugs, and Cosmetics. Association of Food and Drug Officials of U.S., 1959.

TABLE II

SUBCHRONIC ORAL TOXICITY TESTING :

STANDARDIZED FACTORS*

1. Test Duration
2. Species
3. Age of Animals
4. Number of Animals
5. Control Groups
6. Dose Groups
7. Diet
8. Route of Administration
9. Clinical Testing
        (a) Ophthalmological Examination
        (b) Hematology
        (c) Clinical Chemistry
10. Observation of Animals
11. Gross Necropsy
12. Organ Weights
13. Histopathological Examination on at least
        32 principal tissues

*   Toxicological Principles. U.S. Food and Drug
    Administration, 1982.

TABLE III

SIGNS AND SYMPTOMS FOUND IN ANIMALS UNDERGOING TOXICOLOGIC TESTS

Signs

Aggressiveness toward experimenter
Altered muscle tone
Alterations in cardiac rate and rhythm
Catatonia (phases of stupor or excitement)
Coma
Convulsions to touch
Paralysis
Change in pupillary size
Sensitivity to pain
Skin lesions
Corneal opacities
Placing reflexes
Righting reflexes
Grasping reflexes
Death

Symptoms

Abnormal excreta
Exploratory behavior
Inactivity
Convulsions, spontaneous
Dyspnea (shortness of breath)
Sedation
Nystagmus (involuntary rapid movements
    of eyeballs)
Cyanosis
Salivation
Nasal Discharge
Piloerection (erection of hair)
Phonation (utterance of vocal sounds)
Unusual physical positions
Unusual tail positions

TABLE IV

CLINICAL PROCEDURES COMMONLY EMPLOYED IN ANIMAL TOXICOLOGICAL TESTS

Blood chemistry studies
      Sodium
      Potassium
      Blood urea nitrogen
      Glucose

Urinalysis
      pH and specific gravity
      Protein
      Glucose
      Ketones
      Crystals
      Blood cells
      Bacteria

Hematology
      Hematocrit
      Total red blood cell counts
      Total and differential white blood
         cell counts

Organ function tests
      Bromsulfophthalein retention
         (liver function)
      Thymol turbidity (liver function)
      Serum alkaline phosphatase
         (liver function)
      Blood urea nitrogen (kidney function)

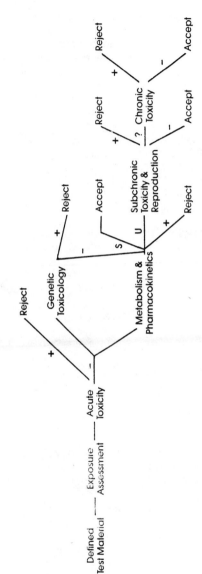

Figure 1. Safety decision tree. Key: +, presents socially unacceptable risk; −, does not present a socially unacceptable risk; S, metabolites known and safe; U, metabolites unknown or of doubtful safety; and ?, decision requires more evidence. (Reproduced with permission from Ref. 8. Copyright 1978, Food Cosmet. Toxicol.)

of the carcinogenic potential of the substance. The safety of the
substance for humans may then be estimated.
    The word "estimate" is used advisedly. After completion of
all the animal tests, only actual exposure in humans will reveal
any subtle or unforeseen toxicity. Toxicity testing cannot be considered complete until the substance has gone through extensive
use in humans. And even then, it may not be complete, unless adequate records, follow-ups, etc., have been maintained and prospec-
tive epidemiological studies are made.

Literature Cited

1. Toxicants Occurring Naturally in Foods. Report, Committee on
Food Protection, National Academy of Sciences, Washington, DC, 1973.
    2. Principles and Procedures for Evaluating the Safety of Food
Additives. Food Protection Committee, Food and Nutrition Board,
National Academy of Sciences, Publ. No. 750, December 1959.
    3. Hazardous Substances Act. Consumer Product Safety Commission,
Washington, DC, 1959.
    4. Appraisal of Safety of Chemicals in Foods, Drugs, and Cosmet-
ics. Association of Food & Drug Officials of the United States,
Washington, DC, 1959.
    5. Toxicological Principles for the Safety Assessment of Direct
Food Additives and Color Additives Used in Food. U.S. Food and
Drug Administration, 1982.
    6. O.E.C.D. Guidelines for Testing of Chemicals. O.E.C.D. Publi-
cations, Washington, DC, 1982.
    7. Weil, C.S. and Scala, R. A. Tox. Appl. Pharmacol., 1971, 19,
276.
    8. Food and Cosmetics Toxicology, 16, 9 (1978), Pergamon Press,
Oxford.

General Bibliography

Doull, J.; Klaasen, C.; Amdur, M., Eds. Toxicology, The Basic
    Science of Poisons, Macmillan Publishing Co., New York, 1980.
Hayes, A. W. Principles and Methods of Toxicology, Raven Press,
    New York, 1982.
Loomis, T. A. Essentials of Toxicology, 3rd ed., Lea & Febiger, New
    York, 1978.
Mehlman, M. A.; Blumenthal, H.; Shapiro, R., Eds. Advances in Mod-
    ern Toxicology, New Concepts in Safety Evaluation, Vol. 1, Part
    1, 2. John Wiley & Son, New York, 1979.
Paget, G. E., Ed. Methods in Toxicology. F. A. Davis & Co., Phila-
    delphia, 1970.

RECEIVED July 6, 1983

Protease and Amylase Inhibitors in Biological Materials

JOHN R. WHITAKER

Department of Food Science and Technology, University of California,
Davis, CA 95616

Proteins which specifically inhibit enzymes by forming tight inactive complexes with the enzyme are widely distributed in biological materials. With the exception of a few of the protease inhibitors and the α-amylase inhibitors, very little work has been done on the mechanism of action of the inhibitors or of their nutritional and physiological importance. The trypsin and chymotrypsin inhibitors appear to form specific complexes with the proteases because trypsin and chymotrypsin recognize the protein inhibitors as substrates. However, the normal sequence of catalytic steps cannot be completed, perhaps because of a conformational change accompanying complexation. On the other hand, the α-amylase inhibitors may not bind at the active site of α-amylase. Rather, the initial complex may undergo a conformational change which destroys the catalytic ability of the α-amylase but leaves the substrate binding ability intact. Some of the animal protease inhibitors are known to serve a protective function against proteases. There is speculation that the plant protease and amylase inhibitors may serve as a protection against insects and microorganisms, but this has not been proven.

There is a great deal of work yet to be done on the naturally-occurring protein and peptide inhibitors of enzymes. Better knowledge of their properties and their physiological, nutritional and medical roles is essential.

Any compound which decreases the activity of an enzyme is an inhibitor. Inhibitors of enzymes include: (a) small molecules which combine with an essential group of the active site (examples include heavy metal ions, acylating and alkylating reagents) or remove an essential part of the active site (an example is removal of essential cations by chelating agents) and compounds which sim-

0097–6156/83/0234–0015$09.00/0

ulate the substrates (competitive inhibitors, including products
of the reaction) and (b) large polymeric molecules which inhibit
enzymes (protein and peptide inhibitors of proteases; protein,
peptide and carbohydrate inhibitors of α-amylases). This chapter
will deal only with selected examples from the second group. pH,
temperature, denaturing agents and proteolysis, which decrease
enzyme activity, are excluded from the definition of an inhibitor
given above.

Study of naturally-occurring enzyme inhibitors is of importance for several reasons. These include: (a) the physiological
importance of an inhibitor in biological material, (b) the nutritional importance of an inhibitor when the material is consumed as
a food or feed, (c) the use of inhibitors to control enzymatic
action, such as that of polyphenol oxidase, (d) the use of inhibitors for analysis and for purification purposes and (e) a better
understanding of specific interactions among complex molecules
such as proteins (examples include antigen-antibody reactions,
subunit interactions in proteins, enzymatic actions).

Occurrence of Enzyme Inhibitors

Compounds in biological materials which inhibit proteases and
amylases were noted as early as the 1930's. Kunitz and Northrop,
during the purification of trypsinogen and trypsin from beef pancreas, found and isolated a trypsin inhibitor from the same source
(pancreatic secretory trypsin inhbitor; 1). About the same time,
Chrzaszcz and Janicki (2,3) reported that there was something in
certain plant extracts which inhibited α-amylase. Since that
time, many enzyme inhibitors have been discovered, purified and
partially characterized. Whitaker (4) has listed 54 protease
inhibitors in animal tissues, 44 protease inhibitors in plant
tissues, six protease inhibitors in microorganisms and some 25
inhibitors of non-proteolytic enzymes. While these data are
important in showing the great numbers of inhibitors present in
biological materials, the numbers are rather meaningless in most
part because many inhibitors have yet to be discovered, the
numbers reflect (in part) isoinhibitors which have been reported
and the interrelationships and homology among the inhibitors are
relatively unknown (see below).

Discovery of Enzyme Inhibitors. Discovery of enzyme inhibitors in
biological materials occurs primarily in four ways. One of the
most frequent is the observation that the percentage recovery of
an enzyme activity during purification suddenly increases at one
step in the purification (5). An example is shown in Table I.
The validity of such an observation must be collaborated by
observing a decrease in activity when some of the removed fraction
is added back to the enzyme-containing fraction. This method only
works, of course, when the activity of an enzyme of the biological
system is reduced by an inhibitor in the same preparation. In the

Table I. Effect of Presence of Inhibitor on Activity of Trypsin During Purification[a]

Preparation	Sp. Activity (relative)
1X crystallized	100
3X crystallized	120
5X crystallized	120
8X crystallized	140
3X crystallized + ppt'd with TCA	160[b]

[a]Kunitz and Northrop (1); [b]A polypeptide inhibitor was crystallized from the TCA supernatant liquid.

case of the α-amylase inhibitors described below, they do not inhibit α-amylase(s) of the same source.

A second indication of the presence of an inhibitor is when experimental animals fail to grow as well on raw as heat-treated biological materials. This was especially valuable in research on raw soybean flour.

A third method of detecting inhibitors, of rather limited utility, is the observation of multiple pH-activity optima for what is otherwise a pure enzyme. For example, Schwimmer (6) observed that potato invertase showed a double pH optima. It was discovered that the explanation of the double pH optima was due to an invertase inhibitor in the potato (7). This observation is shown schematically in Figure 1.

The fourth method of detecting the presence of naturally-occurring enzyme inhibitors in biological materials is to combine extracts with a solution of the enzyme being tested. This is the most systematic way. The procedure may be no more than a series of test tubes, containing the enzyme, to which biological tissue extracts are added. There are some hazards associated with this method and additional experiments are required.

A useful technique has been the cross-wise application of enzyme and inhibitor to an agar plate containing substrate of the enzyme. This method was originated to detect the presence of protease inhibitors in microorganisms (8); it has since been applied to the search for amylase inhibitors (9). The principle of the technique is shown in Figure 2 for protease inhibitors. The buffered agar gel contains abut 1% casein. Cellulose paper strips saturated with the biological extract to be tested are laid on the gel surface in the vertical direction. After 15-20 minutes, these strips are removed and replaced in the horizontal direction with cellulose paper strips saturated with the enzyme solution to be tested. After 15-20 minutes, these latter strips are removed and the gel plate is incubated overnight at 25-35°C. Protease

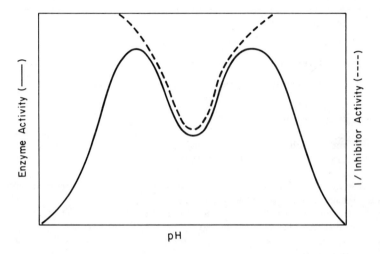

Figure 1. Schematic representation of effect of enzyme inhibitor on pH–activity curve of an enzyme.

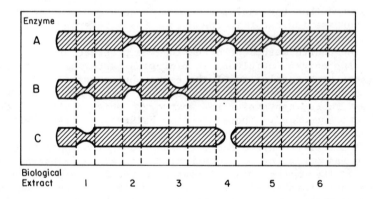

Figure 2. Schematic representation of casein–agar plate technique for detecting presence of protease inhibitors in biological extracts.

activity is indicated by a white band due to hydrolysis and precipitation of the casein. If the biological extract contains an
inhibitor, the white band will be narrow at the cross point of the
two strips (Figure 2). The system can be made more specific by
electrophoresis of the biological extract on the cellulose paper
strip prior to application to the agar-casein gel. Many samples
can be run simultaneously by this method.

Types of Protease and Amylase Inhibitors

The naturally-occurring inhibitors of proteases and amylases
can be proteins, peptides of various sizes and non-proteins.

Protease Inhibitors. The protease inhibitors can be enzyme
specific and/or group specific. Based on their mechanism of
action, the proteases are divided into four groups: (a) the serine
proteases, (b) the sulfhydryl proteases, (c) the carboxyl (acid)
proteases, and (d) the metallo proteases. Laskowski and Kato (10)
have concluded that there are no examples of individual inhibitors
which are active against proteases from two or more of the groups.
For example, human plasma α_1-trypsin inhibitor is active against
trypsin, chymotrypsin, elastase and plasmin (all serine proteases)
but it is not active against proteases from any of the other
groups (11). The thiol protease inhibitor of chicken egg white
(papain inhibitor; 12,13) is active against ficin, papain, bromelain, cathepsin B, and streptococcal protease (all sulfhydryl
proteases), but it is not active against proteases from any of the
other three groups.
     There are examples of inhibitors which are specific for only
one protease within a group. The best known examples include the
Kunitz soybean (Glycine max) inhibitor (14) and isoinhibitors I
and II of the Great Northern bean (Phaseolus vulgaris)(15). Even
these two examples are not clear cut as there is some small non-
stoichiometric combination and inhibition of α-chymotrypsin.
Chicken (16) and Japanese quail (17) egg white ovomucoids only
inhibit trypsin.
     One possible exception to the above dictum that a protease
inhibitor cannot inhibit proteases from two or more groups is α_2-
macroglobulin. This very large glycoprotein (725,000 daltons) has
a very broad specificity in that it binds to proteases from all
four groups (18-23). The possibility that this is due to non-
specific adsorption is indicated by the observation that the
enzyme-inhibitor complex retains activity on small substrates,
although activity on proteins is lost (due to steric hindrance?).
Other apparent exceptions are the small peptide protease inhibitors produced by several species of Streptomyces. For example,
the leupeptins are active against plasmin and trypsin (serine
proteases) and papain and cathepsin B (sulfhydryl proteases)(24).
Antipain (25) and the chymostatins are also active against enzymes
from both the serine and sulfhydryl groups of proteases (26).

Amylase Inhibitors. There are four types of amylases. These are:
(a) α-amylases, (b) β-amylases, (c) glucoamylases and the (d) pul-
lulanase-type (debranching) amylases. The only well-described type
of naturally-occurring protein amylase inhibitors are those
against the α-amylases from higher animals and insects. These
inhibitors, with the possible exception of the one from corn (27),
are not effective against higher plant and microbial α-amylases or
against the other three types of amylases. Quite recently, there
have been discussions of the possibility of a glycoamylase-type
inhibitor (28).

There are also small peptide inhibitors of α-amylase found in
certain Streptomyces (29). Two carbohydrate α-amylase inhibitors,
Acarbose and Amylostatin, have been described (30-32). Their
structures are shown in Figure 3. The inhibitors are very similar
in structure.

Heterogeneity of Protease and Amylase Inhibitors

There are a number of well-documented examples of heterogeneity among the protease and amylase inhibitors. This heterogeneity is a result of (a) inhibitors against multiple enzymes
from a single biological fluid, (b) isolation from different
strains (varieties) of a species, (c) isoinhibitors, (d) proteolysis, (e) chemical modification during isolation, and (f) molecular heterogeneity.

Inhibitors of Different Enzymes in a Single Biological Fluid. A
few examples will illustrate the multiplicity of inhibitors found
in biological fluids (Table II). Human plasma contains at least
eight different types of inhibitors, chicken egg white contains
three different types, the soybean contains four different types,
and the white potato six different types. These are clearly
different compounds as they inhibit quite different enzymes and
they can be separated from each other.

Isolation from Different Strains (Varieties) of a Species. Very
similar protease inhibitors have been isolated from several
different strains (varieties) of the same species or from similar
species. In some cases, the inhibitors are very similar, in
others they are quite different. Three examples will illustrate
this. Ovomucoids are probably found in all species of birds.
They are proteins of 28,000 daltons and contain ~20% carbohydrate. They are quite similar in other properties as well. However, they can be quite different in their inhibitory properties
against proteases. Chicken (16) and Japanese quail (17) ovomucoids inhibit only trypsin. Tinamou ovomucoid inhibits chymotrypsin and subtilisin (66) and turkey (67) and penguin (68) ovomucoids inhibit trypsin, chymotrypsin and subtilisin. The reason
for this difference among the ovomucoids is due to more than one
binding site for proteases in the ovomucoid molecule. As shown by

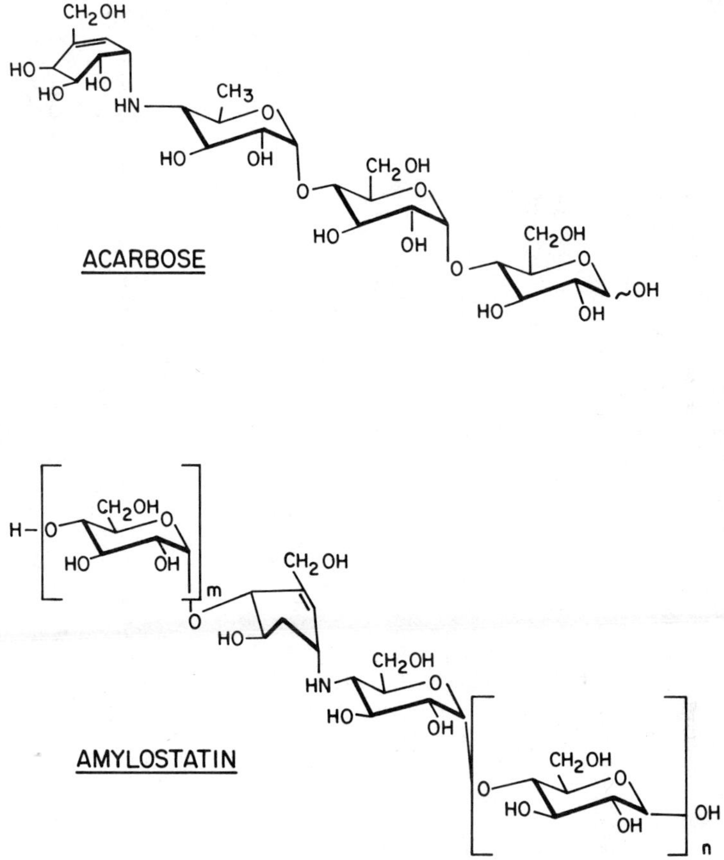

Figure 3. Structures of the carbohydrate α-amylase inhibitors acarbose (30,31) and amylostatin (32) (m = 0 to 8, n = 1 to 8, and m + n = 1 to 8).

Table II. Examples of Multiplicity of Protease Inhibitors in Biological Fluids

Source	Type	Molecular Weight	Specificity	Reference
Human plasma	α_1-Trypsin inhibitor	54,000	Trypsin, chymotrypsin, elastase, plasmin	11, 33, 34
	α_2-Macroglobulin	725,000	Very broad	18 - 23
	Antithrombin-heparin cofactor	62,000–67,000	Thrombin, other serine proteases of blood clotting sequence	35, 36
	$\overline{C_1}$ inactivator	104,000	$\overline{C_1}$ protease, plasmin, kallikrein, others	37 - 40
	Inter-α-trypsin inhibitor	160,000	Trypsin, chymotrypsin, lesser extent plasmin	41 - 44
	α_1-Antichymotrypsin		Chymotrypsin	42
	Thiol proteinase inhibitor	90,000	Ficin, papain, cathepsin B and bromelain	45, 46
	Cathepsins B and H inhibitors		Cathepsins B and H	47
Chicken egg white	Ovomucoid	28,000	Trypsin	16, 48, 49
	Ovoinhibitor	46,500	Trypsin, chymotrypsin, sub-tilisin, A. oryzae protease	50, 51
	Thiol proteinase (papain) inhibitor	12,700	Papain, ficin, cathepsin B	12, 13
Soybean	Kunitz	21,700	Trypsin	14, 52 - 54
	Bowman-Birk	8,000	Trypsin, chymotrypsin	55, 56

Table II. (continued)

Source	Type	Molecular Weight	Specificity	Reference
Soybean (continued)	Elastase		Elastase, also trypsin and chymotrypsin	57
	Components I–IV	7,000–8,000	Trypsin	58
Potato	Chymotrypsin inhibitor I	39,000	Chymotrypsin	59
	Proteinase inhibitor IIa		Chymotrypsin, nagarse, trypsin	60
	Proteinase inhibitor IIb		Chymotrypsin, nagarse	61, 62
	pKI–56, pKI–64		Kallikrein	63
	Carboxypeptidases A and B inhibitor	3,100	Carboxypeptidases A and B	64
	Papain inhibitor	80,000	Papain, chymotrypsin	65

Laskowski et al. (69), the ovomucoids contain at least three
domains each with a potential binding site for a protease. Two of
these sites are specific for trypsin and one for chymotrypsin
(subtilisin binds competitively with chymotrypsin). In chicken,
Japanese quail and tinamou ovomucoids, only one of the sites is
capable of binding a protease while in turkey and penguin ovomucoids two binding sites are expressed and in duck ovomucoid (67)
all three sites are expressed. This is shown diagramatically in
Figure 4.

    The trypsin inhibitors from several different varieties of
Phaseolus vulgaris (common bean) are quite variable in amino acid
composition (Figure 5). ASN, SER and 1/2CYS are found in the
largest amounts in most of the inhibitors. MET and TRP are quite
low in all the inhibitors and absent in a substantial number of
them. PRO is present in larger amounts than in most proteins.
PHE and TYR are in low amounts.

Isoinhibitors (Genetic Heterogeneity). The third type of heterogeneity is that of isoinhibitors. These isoinhibitors, obtained
from one organ or organism, have the same specificities for binding proteases. However, they differ in one or more properties
such as chromatographic and electrophoretic behavior, heat stability, molecular weight, or amino acid composition, as well as
quantitatively in binding with proteases.

    Snail epidermis contains at least six trypsin-kallikrein in-
hibitors with molecular weights ranging from 6431 to 6591 (70-72).
The soybean contains two basic types of protease inhibitors, the
Kunitz inhibitor of 21,500 daltons (73) and the Bowman-Birk inhibitor of 7975 daltons (74). The two are quite different proteins as shown in Figure 6. The Great Northern bean (Phaseolus
vulgaris) has at least three trypsin isoinhibitors ranging in
molecular weight from 8086 to 8884 (15). There are four and
possibly six isoinhibitors of trypsin in lima bean (Phaseolus
lunatus)(75).

    Recently, Whitaker and Sgarbieri (76) and Sgarbieri and
Whitaker (77) reported there are at least four isoinhibitors of
trypsin in Brazilian pink beans (Phaseolus vulgaris L. var.
Rosinha G2). These are separable on a DEAE-cellulose column
(Figure 7) but not by affinity chromatography (76). Properties of
three of the isoinhibitors were investigated. They are different
by disc gel electrophoresis, have slightly different amino acid
compositions but have identical molecular weights (within experimental error) and all contain one residue of mannose per mol. The
molecular weights are 20,000, about twice the size of most Bowman-
Birk type inhibitors in beans. They each bind two mol of trypsin
and one mol of chymotrypsin per mol inhibitor. One of the largest
differences among the three isoinhibitors is in the affinity for
trypsin and chymotrypsin (77). As shown in Table III, the disso-
ciation constants for trypsin range from 1.8×10^{-10} M to 8.5×10^{-10} M while those for chymotrypsin range from 2.8×10^{-8} M to

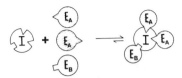

Figure 4. Schematic representation of multiple binding sites for proteases, E_A and E_B, on an inhibitor, I. In the case of duck ovomucoid, E_A is trypsin and E_B is chymotrypsin.

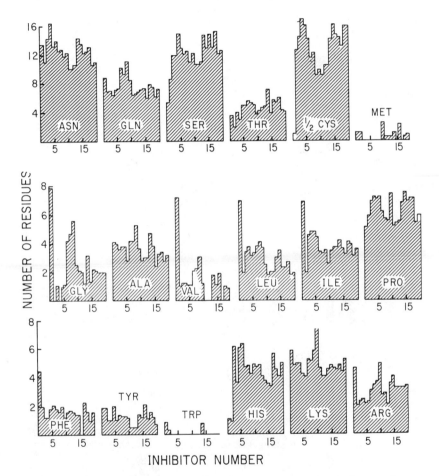

Figure 5. Amino acid composition of several protease inhibitors from soybean (Glycine max) and several species and varieties of Phaseolus. The results are expressed as amino acid residues per 10,000 grams. The inhibitors are 1, Kunitz soybean trypsin inhibitor; 2, Bowman–Birk soybean trypsin inhibitor; 3–6, lima bean (Phaseolus lunatus) isoinhibitors I, II, III, and IV; 7–9, French bean (Phaseolus coccineus) isoinhibitors 2, 3, and 4; 10, mung bean (Phaseolus aureus Roxb.) inhibitor; 11–13, Brazilian pink bean (Phaseolus vulgaris) isoinhibitors A, B, and C; 14, kidney bean (Phaseolus vulgaris) inhibitor; 15–17, Great Northern bean (Phaseolus lunatus) isoinhibitors I, II, III, and IV; 7–9, French bean (Phaseolus vulgaris) isoinhibitor; and 19 and 20, pinto bean (Phaseolus vulgaris) isoinhibitors I and II (97).

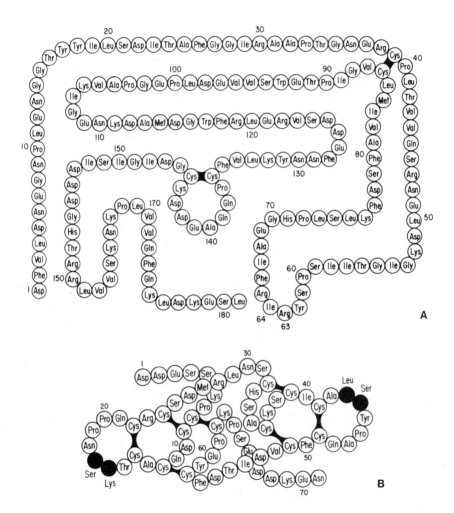

Figure 6. Primary structures of the Kunitz soybean trypsin inhibitor (A) and the Bowman–Birk soybean trypsin inhibitor (B). The solid black circles on the primary structure of the Bowman–Birk soybean trypsin inhibitor represent LYS–SER and LEU–SER and are the binding sites for trypsin and chymotrypsin, respectively. (Reproduced with permission from (A) Ref. 73, copyright 1973, E. J. of Bioch. and (B) Ref. 74, copyright 1973, J. Food Biochem.)

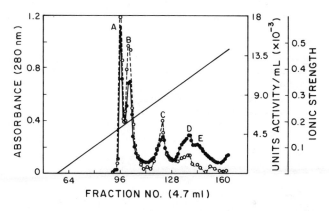

*Figure 7. DEAE–cellulose chromatography of the trypsin–chymotrypsin isoinhibitors from Brazilian pink bean (*Phaseolus vulgaris *var.* Rosinha *G2. (Reproduced with permission from Ref. 76. Copyright 1981,* J. Food Biochem.*)*

Table III. K_i Values for the Binding of α-Chymotrypsin and
            Trypsin with Brazilian Pink Bean Inhibitors A,
            B and C (77)

	K_i (M)		
Inhibitors	α-Chymotrypsin (CT)	Trypsin (T)	$K_i(CT)/K_i(T)$
A	4.4×10^{-7}	8.5×10^{-10}	520
B	2.8×10^{-8}	1.8×10^{-10}	160
C	3.0×10^{-8}	6.8×10^{-10}	44

4.4×10^{-7} M. The ratios of $K_i(CT)/K_i(T)$ are: A, 520; B, 160; C,
44. These binding properties clearly indicate that the three isoinhibitors are different and most likely are not the result of
artifacts (proteolysis or binding with phenols) produced by the
purification procedure.

Another well studied example of genetic heterogeneity is that
of the wheat α-amylase inhibitors. There appear to be at least
three different molecular weight species of inhibitors (60,000,
24,000 and 12,000) as well as distinct species within each of
these molecular weight groups. Granum and Whitaker (78) have
purified and characterized three of the α-amylase inhibitors from
Anza wheat (Triticum aestivum var. Anza). Their chemical, physical and inhibitory properties were quite different (Table IV).
They also differed in lysine, arginine, histidine, alanine (R_m

Table IV. Properties of Three α-Amylase Inhibitors of Wheat
(Triticum aestivum var. Anza)(78)

	Inhibitors[a]		
Property	R_m 0.19	R_m 0.28	R_m 0.55
Molecular weight			
Hedrick−Smith method (79)	24,000	18,500	30,000
Sedimentation equilibrium	29,000	14,500	----
pI	5.9	5.2	4.2
Specificity on α-amylases			
Human salivary	+	±	+
Hog pancreatic	+	−	−
Bacillus subtilis	−	−	−
Aspergillus oryzae	−	−	−

[a]R_m = Electrophoretic mobility relative to bromophenol blue.

0.28 only), valine (R_m 0.28 only) and phenylalanine (R_m 0.28 only)
contents. They all had relatively high contents of proline and
half-cystine. De Ponte et al. (80) have recently proposed a model
that might explain the relationship among all the known α-amylase
inhibitors in wheat (see Figure 8). How different the 12,000
dalton subunits of the three inhibitors are from the proposed
ancestral 12,000 dalton molecule is not known. Unfortunately, the
R_m 0.55 amylase inhibitor of MW 30,000 reported by Granum and
Whitaker (78) does not fit this model.

Proteolytic Artifacts. The fourth type of heterogeneity reported
is that produced by proteolysis. This must be of particular concern in the isolation of any protein since the hydrolysis of one
or two peptide bonds will give rise to a number of products. Recently, it has been reported that some of the protease inhibitors
previously isolated from winged bean are the result of proteolysis
(81). The evidence for this is quite convincing, leading to the
possibility that some of the isoinhibitors reported in the literature are the result of proteolysis. Whitaker and Sgarbieri (76)
addressed this issue in detail, providing several data to indicate
that this is probably not the case for the isoinhibitors of
Brazilian pink beans. Peptide mapping of isoinhibitors would be a
valuable tool in this respect, but it has not been previously
applied to this problem.

Chemical Modification. The fifth type of heterogeneity is due to
chemical modification, other than proteolysis, during isolation of
the inhibitors. Beans, for example, contain phenolic compounds
and various amounts of polyphenol oxidase. If polyphenol oxidase
is active during the isolation procedure there is the real possibility that some of the products (benzoquinones) formed will react
with the ε-amino group of lysine residues of the inhibitor(s),
thereby producing electrophoretically and chromatographically distinct components. Pusztai (82) purified an inhibitor from kidney
beans which contained a firmly bound pinkish-blue pigment that was
not removed by ammonium sulfate precipitation, gel filtration or
by chromatography on a DEAE-Sephadex column. For inhibitors which
are glycoproteins (ovomucoids, some of the Phaseolus vulgaris
inhibitors, the red kidney bean α-amylase inhibitors), variable
amounts of carbohydrate attached to the protein will produce isoinhibitors.

Molecular Heterogeneity. The last type of heterogeneity we shall
discuss is that of molecular heterogeneity. This type of heterogeneity was mentioned under the section on inhibitors from different varieties of a species. It is well known that many of the inhibitors have more than one binding site for proteases, either for
the same protease or for different proteases. Examples of this
molecular heterogeneity are shown in Table V. In the case of the
bird egg white ovomucoids, Laskowski et al. (69) have shown that

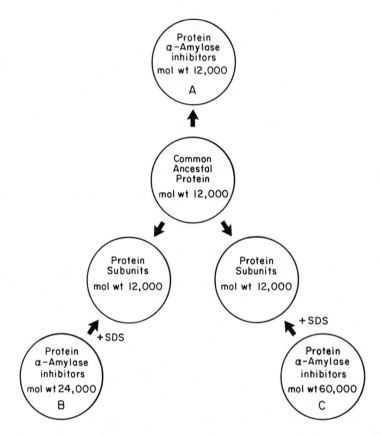

Figure 8. Possible interrelationships among the protein α-amylase isoinhibitor families from hexaploid wheats (80). All three inhibitors may have originated from a common ancestral protein of 12,000 daltons.

Table V. Some Examples of Molecular Heterogeneity of Protease Inhibitors

Inhibitor	Enzyme Inhibited		
	Trypsin	Chymotrypsin/Subtilisin	Elastase
Ovomucoid			
Chicken (16)	+	−	−
Japanese quail (17)	+	−	−
Tinamou (66)	−	+	n.d.[b]
Turkey (67)	+	+	n.d.
Penguin (68)	+	+	n.d.
Duck (67)	+(2 trypsin)	+	n.d.
Ovoinhibitor			
Japanese quail (69)	+(3 trypsin potentially)	+(3 ChTr potentially)	+(3 elastase potentially)
Bowman-Birk type			
Soybean (Glycine max) (83)	+	+	n.d.
Brazilian pink bean (Phaseolus vulgaris) (77)	+(2 trypsin)	+	n.d.
Lima bean (Phaseolus lunatus) (84)	+	+	n.d.
French bean (Phaseolus coccineus) (85)	+	+(<1)	n.d.

[a]Chymotrypsin and subtilisin probably bind at the same site on these inhibitors; [b]not determined.

there are three domains in the protein, each with a potentially
active site for binding a protease. However, not all of these
sites may be expressed (Figure 4). For example, in chicken ovomucoid, a single trypsin binding site is expressed while in duck
ovomucoid, two sites for trypsin and one site for chymotrypsin (or
subtilisin) are expressed. Ovoinhibitors from Japanese quail and
chicken egg whites contain six tandem domains (potentially or
actually active against specific proteases (69); see Table VI)).
     The distinct nature of these multiple binding sites are shown
by (a) the simultaneous binding of more than one mol/mol of a
given protease or of two or more different proteases; (b) amino
acid sequence work (69); and (c) by fragmentation of the inhibitor
molecule into separate, active parts. Cyanogen bromide has been
used effectively to cleave the inhibitor at methionine residues to
give active fragments. Examples include the Bowman-Birk soybean
inhibitor (73), turkey ovomucoid (86), the three isoinhibitors of
Brazilian pink beans (77), potato inhibitor IIa (60), and potato
inhibitor IIb (62).
     Another type of molecular heterogeneity of protease inhibi-
tors is with respect to the amino acid residue in the protease
recognition site of the inhibitor. As shown by Feeney et al.
(87), the ovomucoids can be classified as either "lysine-type" or
"arginine-type" depending on whether reductive alkylation (lysine-
type) or glyoxylation (arginine-type) destroys the ability of the
inhibitor to combine with trypsin. Either lysine or arginine has
been found to be an essential part of the active site of inhibitors from beans (see Table VII). The three isoinhibitors of
Brazilian pink bean were found to contain lysine in the binding
site for trypsin (77). While less well documented, it appears
that the chymotrypsin-binding sites of inhibitors contain either
an essential leucine residue (leucine-type inhibitors; lima bean,
soybean (Bowman-Birk type), runner bean; see Table VII; 88) or a
tyrosine or methionine (tyrosine-type or methionine-type inhibitors as found in Japanese quail ovoinhibitors; see Table VI; 69).

Similarities Among Groups of Inhibitors

     Despite the great numbers of protease and amylase inhibitors
found in biological materials, more recent data indicate there is
some homology among the inhibitors. Comparison of the complete
amino acid sequences of lima bean trypsin inhibitors I and IV
shows that the two isoinhibitors differ only in that inhibitor IV
contains an eight amino acid N-terminal segment and an additional
two Asn residues at the C-terminal end not present in inhibitor I
(75).
     There is great homology between the Bowman-Birk soybean tryp-
sin inhibitor (89), lima bean trypsin inhibitor IV (75) and the
Great Northern trypsin inhibitor II (90) as shown in Table VIII.
The tryptic peptide maps of Great Northern isoinhibitors I and
IIIb were very similar while isoinhibitors I and II had no
peptides in common (15).

Table VI. Amino Acid Sequences of the Six Reactive Sites of Japanese Quail Ovoinhibitor[a]

Reactive Site	Amino Acid Sequence	Enzyme Potentially Inhibited
	↓b	
1	...Val-Ala-Cys-Pro-Arg-Asn-Leu-Lys-Pro-Val-Cys...	Trypsin
2	...Val-Ala-Cys-Pro-Arg-Ssn-Met-Lys-Pro-Val-Cys...	Trypsin
3	...Val-Ala-Cys-Pro-Arg-Asn-Leu-Lys-Pro-Val-Cys...	Trypsin
4	...Ala-Ala-Cys-Pro-Tyr-Ile-Leu-His-Glu-Ile-Cys...	Chymotrypsin-elastase
5	...Met-Ala-Cys-Thr-Met-Ile-Tyr-Asp-Pro-Val-Cys...	Chymotrypsin-elastase
6	...Pro-Val-Cys-Thr-Met-Glu-Tyr-Ile-Pro-His-Cys...	Chymotrypsin-elastase

[a]Adapted from Laskowski et al. (69); [b]The arrow indicates the specific recognition point involving P_1 and P_1' residues.

Table VII. Homology Among the Binding Sites of Some Trypsin and Chymotrypsin Inhibitors from Leguminosae[a]

Inhibitor	Amino Acid Sequence	
	Trypsin Site	Chymotrypsin Site
	↓b	↓b
Lima Bean	...Cys-Thr-Lys$_{26}$——Ser-Ile-Pro....	...Ile-Cys-Thr-Leu$_{55}$——Ser-Ile-Pro...
Bowman-Birk (soybean)	...Cys-Thr-Lys$_{16}$——Ser-Asn-Pro....	...Ile-Cys-Thr-Leu$_{45}$——Ser-Ile-Pro
Runner Bean	...Ile-Tyr-Lys——Ser-Gln-(Pro?)....	...Asp-Val-Ala-Leu——Ser-(Pro?)
Garden Bean (Great Northern)[c]	...Cys-Thr-Arg$_{53}$——Ser-Met-Pro....	
Soybean Trypsin Inhibitor[c]	...Ser-Tyr-Arg$_{63}$——Ile-Arg-Phe....	
Ergnut[c]	...Glx-Cys-Arg$_{22}$——Ala-Pro-Pro....	

[a]Adapted from Hory and Weder (88); [b]The arrow indicates the specific recognition point involving P_1 and P_1' residues; [c]Only inhibits trypsin.

Table VIII. Amino Acid Sequence Homology Among the Bowman-Birk Soybean Trypsin Inhibitor (BB: 89), Lima Bean Trypsin Inhibitor IV (LB; 75) and Great Northern Bean Trypsin Inhibitor II (GB; 90)

```
                                        10
BB                          Asp-Asp-Glu-Ser-Ser-Lys-Pro-Cys—

LB   Ser-Gly-His-His-Glu-His-Ser-Thr-Asp-Glx-Pro-Ser-Glx-Ser-Ser-Lys-Pro-Cys—
          10


                      20                           30
BB   Cys-Asp-Gln-Cys-Ala-Cys-Thr-Lys-Ser-Asn-Pro-Pro-Gln-Cys-Arg-Cys-Ser-Asp-

GB        (Val,Cys)Thr-Ala-Ser-Ile-Pro-Pro-Gln(Cys,Ile,Cys,Thr,Asx,
              20                           30

LB   Cys-Asn-His-Cys-Ala-Cys-Thr-Lys-Ser-Ile-Pro-Pro-Gln-Cys-Arg-Cys-Thr-Asp-
          30       Leu                                          Ser


                          40                          50
BB   Met-Arg-Leu-Asn-Ser-Cys-His-Ser-Ala-Cys-Lys-Ser-Cys-Ile-Cys-Ala-Leu-Ser-

GB   Val)Arg-Leu-Asx-Ser-Cys-His-Ser-Ala-Cys-Lys-Ser-Cys-Met-Cys-Thr-Arg-Ser-
                          40                          50

LB   Leu-Arg-Leu-Asp-Ser-Cys-His-Ser-Ala-Cys-lys-Ser-Cys-Ile-Cys-Thr-Leu-Ser-
     Phe                   40
```

Continued on next page

Table VIII. Continued

						50											60	

BB   Tyr—Pro—Ala—Gln—Cys—Phe—Cys—Val—Asp—Ile—Thr—Asp—Phe—Cys—Tyr—Glu—Pro—Cys—

50   60   70

GB   Met—Pro—Gly—Lys—Cys—Arg—Cys—Leu—Asx—Thr—Thr—Asx—Tyr—Cys—Tyr—Lys—Ser—Cys—

60   70

LB   Ile—Pro—Ala—Gln—Cys—Val(Cys,Thr,Asx)Ile—Asx—Asp—Phe—Cys—Tyr—Glu—Pro—Cys—

70

BB   Lys—Pro—Ser—Glu————Asp—Asp—Lys—Glu—Asn

80

GB   Lys—Ser—Asx—Ser—Gly—Glx—Asx—Asx

80

LB   Lys—Ser—Ser—His—Ser—Asp—Asp—Asp—Asn—Asn—Asn

There appears to be sequence homology between the pineapple stem bromelain inhibitors and some of the small molecular weight inhibitors from the leguminosae (91). Human inter-α-trypsin inhibitor contains two domains with great similarity to the domains of the Kunitz-type inhibitors (44, 92-94). The ovoinhibitors from Japanese quail and chicken egg whites contain six tandem domains which are homologous to the Kazal pancreatic secretory inhibitor and to the ovomucoids (69).

Considerable homology exists within the binding sites of several of the inhibitors as shown in Table VII. It has been suggested that trypsin inhibitors require a peptide sequence of Lys-X or Arg-X located within a loop of the protein closed by a disulfide bond (95,96). Reduction of disulfide bonds are known to be quite effective in destroying the inhibitory activity (77). For example, activity of the three isoinhibitors from Brazilian pink beans against both trypsin and chymotrypsin was lost when a specific disulfide bond, of the 18-21 disulfide bonds present, was reduced (77). SER appears to be a requirement of the binding site also for lysine-type inhibitors (Table VII).

There is homology among the binding sites for chymotrypsin in the inhibitors from lima bean, soybean and runner bean (Table VII). The apparent essentiality of a serine residue in the binding site for chymotrypsin is also indicated. There appears to be much less homology among the binding sites of the arginine-type trypsin inhibitors (Table VII).

In terms of amino acid composition, there is some homology among the Bowman-Birk type inhibitors from the leguminosae as shown in Figure 5. This appears to be so, despite the fact that there are some inhibitors with molecular weights near 8000 (Bowman-Birk soybean inhibitor, lima bean inhibitors I-IV, French bean inhibitors 2, 3 and 4, mung bean inhibitor, kidney bean inhibitor, and Great Northern bean inhibitors I, II and IIIb), and others with molecular weights near 20,000 (Brazilian pink bean inhibitors A, B and C, Navy bean inhibitor and pinto bean inhibitors I and II)(see 97 for details). It certainly would be helpful to have tryptic peptide maps and amino acid sequence (ideally) data on all of these inhibitors.

Recent immunochemical data (98) have shown that the α-amylase inhibitors from several varieties of beans have great homology.

Mechanism of Action of the Protease and Amylase Inhibitors

Protease Inhibitors. There are unique and specific recognition sites on the protease inhibitors for trypsin and chymotrypsin as shown in Tables VI and VII. The best data are available for trypsin where it is known that either a specific arginine or a lysine residue in the binding site of the inhibitor is required. Modification of the arginine (by glyoxylation) or lysine (by alkylation, etc.) residue or their removal (99) results in complete loss of inhibitory activity. The binding sites for chymotrypsin appear to require leucine, tyrosine or methionine. It is probable that a serine residue attached to the lysine or tyrosine, leucine or methionine is also required (Table VI). However, this does not appear to be the case for the arginine-type trypsin inhibitors.

It appears, therefore, that trypsin and chymotrypsin recognize and bind with the same amino acid residues in the inhibitors as with any substrate. However, net hydrolysis of peptide bonds does not occur at the pH optimum of the enzymes for reasons largely unknown at this time. Specific hydrolysis of the peptide bond involving the carboxyl group of the essential amino acid residue does occur at low pH (around pH 4). However, there is little current evidence to indicate that this hydrolysis is a key step in the inhibitory process. Two types of data argue against its essentiality. (a) Complexation between inhibitor and chemically modified inactive proteases is often just as tight as with the native protease (12, 100, 101). (b) Initially, X-ray crystallographic data on the complexes between trypsin and protein inhibitors were interpreted to indicate that the complexes were probably adducts with a tetrahedral intermediate state approaching a covalent bond (102, 103). However, better refinements of the X-ray crystallographic maps indicate the distances are too great for covalent bond formation. ^{13}C-NMR studies appear to conclusively rule out formation of a tetrahedral or covalent intermediate as a step in the mechanism of inhibition (104-106).

Kinetic data indicate a conformational change may occur following formation of the initial complex (107). Such a conformational change could provide stability to the complex through preventing its ready dissociation ($k_{-2} \ll k_{-1}$) or in preventing hydrolysis of the peptide bond in the inhibitor as would occur for a regular substrate (Eqn. 1). However, Jibson et al.

$$E + I \; \underset{k_{-1}}{\overset{k_1}{\rightleftharpoons}} \; EI \; \underset{k_{-2}}{\overset{k_2}{\rightleftharpoons}} \; EI' \qquad (1)$$

(108) have recently shown that a conformational change probably does not occur in trypsin on binding with the Bowman-Birk soybean inhibitor or with the chick-pea trypsin inhibitor.

A complete explanation of why the naturally-occurring protein protease inhibitors are so effective as inhibitors is still not available.

α-Amylase Inhibitors. The protein α-amylase inhibitors form a very tight complex with salivary and pancreatic α-amylases. For example, the complex between the red kidney bean protein inhibitor and porcine pancreatic α-amylase at 30°C and pH 6.9 was calculated to be 3.5×10^{-11} M (109). The inactive complex forms slowly, requiring 60 to 120 minutes to reach complete reaction depending on pH and inhibitor and enzyme concentrations (109). The red kidney

bean protein inhibitor does not inhibit plant and microbial α-amylases; only those from higher animals and insects are inhibited.

It appears there is an initial rapid complex formed between
the enzyme and inhibitor which is still active (110). Then, a
much slower conformational change occurs (109,110) leading to loss
of activity.

Unlike the protein protease inhibitors, complexation between
the red kidney bean protein α-amylase inhibitor and α-amylase does
not appear to involve binding at the active site of the α-amylase.
Evidence for this includes ability of the complex to bind maltose
(a competitive inhibitor of α-amylase), starch, Sephadex and to
still hydrolyze small substrates.

The red kidney bean α-amylase inhibitor contains 9-10% covalently bound carbohydrate. Removal of up to 70% of the carbohydrate does not affect the activity of the inhibitor (110). The
glyco groups, removed from the protein, do not inhibit α-amylase
at 3.5×10^4 times the concentration of the inhibitor (110).
Chemical modification studies indicate that histidine and tyrosine
residues in the inhibitor may be important for its activity (110).

In summary, our present knowledge of the mechanism of action
of the red kidney bean α-amylase inhibitor indicates that an
initial complex is formed between inhibitor and enzyme which does
not involve the active site of the enzyme (complex still fully
active). Subsequently, there is a conformational change in the
complex which destroys the ability of α-amylase to hydrolyze large
substrates but does not prevent their binding to the enzyme.

Physiological and Nutritional Importance of the Protease and Amylase Inhibitors

Protease Inhibitors. In animals, the physiological roles of several of the protease inhibitors are well known. The pancreatic
protease inhibitors protect the pancreatic tissue against prema-
ture activation of the proteolytic enzyme zymogens. The inhibitors associated with the blood clotting system prevent the pre-
mature activation of the proteolytic enzyme zymogens circulating
in the blood at all times and also regulate between coagulation
and fibrinolysis. They may also be a protection against pancreatic proteases liberated into the blood, as in pancreatitis. The
protease inhibitors in the respiratory tract probably serve as a
protection against proteases liberated by granulocytes and macro-
phages brought in as a result of irritation and/or diseased conditions of the respiratory tract or through inhalation of microorganisms.

The physiological role of the protease inhibitors (especially
the small peptide derivatives) in microorganisms may, in part, be
to prevent the growth of other microorganisms . They may also be
important in the regulation of proteolysis in the cell (111-113).

The physiological role of the protease inhibitors in higher
plants is less clear even though they may account for 5-10% of the

total protein (114). The level of inhibitors varies with the
stage of growth, suggesting that the inhibitors are physiologically important (114). The thiol protease inhibitors of the
pineapple fruit have activity against the major proteolytic enzymes, bromelains, present in the fruit (115). They may also
serve as a defense against insects and microorganisms (114,116).
Infestations of potatoes with Colorado potato beetle larvae lead
to markedly increased levels of protease Inhibitor-I in the leaves
(117).

     The nutritional importance of the protease inhibitors in
major foods is reasonably clear. It is known that raw soybean
flour inhibits growth in rats, chickens and some other monogastric
animals (118) and death can result (119). It is also known that
the presence of soybean inhibitor in the small intestine increases
the secretion of a hormonal pancreozymic-like substance that
markedly stimulates external secretion by the pancreas (120). The
presence of active proteolytic enzyme inhibitors in the small
intestine increases the production and secretion of proteolytic
enzymes by the pancreas, presumably to compensate for their loss
by complexation (121-123). This results in hyperplasia of some of
the pancreatic cells and enlargement of the pancreas.

     Unambiguous interpretation of most of the data in the litera-
ture on the quantitative role of the protease inhibitors in foods
is not possible. This is because foods also contain other inhibitory substances such as hemagglutinins, amylase inhibitors, estro-
gens and phytic acid. Rackis (116) has suggested that the soybean
trypsin inhibitor appears to account for 30-50% of the growth retardation seen on feeding raw flour and probably most of the pancreatic enlargement. Other workers have suggested that a part of
the growth retardation may be due to unavailability of cystine,
due to the poor digestibility of the protease inhibitors (124).

     Most, but perhaps not all, of the protease inhibitors are
destroyed by cooking of the food. The long range consequences of
feeding humans low concentrations of active protease inhibitors
are not known.

α-Amylase Inhibitors. Proteins inhibitory of α-amylase are found
in many biological fluids (9). However, only the protein inhibitors found in legumes and in wheat have been extensively investigated. Recently, it has been shown that all insect α-amylases
tested, except one, are inhibited by the red kidney bean α-amylase
inhibitor (125). Yetter et al. (126) have suggested that the
wheat α-amylase inhibitors may be active against attack of the
wheat by insects during storage. With one exception (see below)
the plant α-amylase inhibitors do not have any activity against
higher plant or microbial amylases tested (127). The three
α-amylase inhibitors of maize have been reported to inhibit maize
α-amylase(s), indicating a possible physiological role of these
inhibitors in maize (27).

The nutritional significance of the α-amylase inhibitors is largely unknown. It is known that low levels of inhibitory activity can be detected in regularly cooked food products. When red kidney bean α-amylase inhibitor, free of protease inhibitors and hemagglutinins, was fed to rats in a casein diet at the levels of 4.5 and 75 mg/rat/day, there was no decrease in rate of growth of the rats in relation to the control (128). Jaffé and Vega Lette (129) reported fecal starch from rats fed raw white kidney beans. Lang et al. (130) reported a reduction of growth rate and increased fecal starch levels when rats were fed on a casein/starch diet containing purified wheat α-amylase inhibitors. Bo-Linn et al. (131) reported that α-amylase inhibitor, fed to humans as an impure preparation, had no effect on the caloric value of the starchy meal.

Literature Cited

1. Kunitz, M.; Northrop, J.H. J. Gen. Physiol. 1936, 19, 991–1007.
2. Chrzaszcz, T.; Janicki, J. Biochem. Z. 1933, 260, 354–68.
3. Chrzaszcz, T.; Janicki, J. Biochem. J. 1934, 28, 296–304.
4. Whitaker, J.R. "Impact of Toxicology on Food Processing"; Ayres, J.C.; Kirschman, J.C., Eds.; Avi Publishing Co., Inc., Westport, 1981; pp. 57–104.
5. Willstätter, R.; Bamann, E.; Rohdewald, M. Hoppe-Seyler's Z. Physiol. Chem. 1930, 188, 107–23.
6. Schwimmer, S. J. Theor. Biol. 1962, 3, 102–10.
7. Schwimmer, S.; Makower, R.U.; Rorem, E.S. Plant Physiol. 1961, 36, 313–16.
8. Sandvik, O. Ph.D. Thesis, Veterinary College of Norway, Oslo, 1962.
9. Fossum, K.; Whitaker, J.R. J. Nutr. 1974, 104, 930–6.
10. Laskowski, M., Jr.; Kato, I. Ann. Rev. Biochem. 1980, 49, 593–626.
11. Kress, L.F.; Laskowski, M., Sr. "Proteinase Inhibitors"; Fritz, H.; Tschesche, H.; Greene, L.J.; Truscheit, E., Eds.; Springer-Verlag, Berlin, New York, 1974; pp. 23–30.
12. Fossum, K.; Whitaker, J.R. Arch. Biochem. Biophys. 1968, 125, 367–75.
13. Sen, L.C.; Whitaker, J.R. Arch. Biochem. Biophys. 1973, 158, 623–32.
14. Birk, Y. Methods Enzymol. 1976, 45B, 700–7.
15. Wilson, K.A.; Laskowski, M., Sr. J. Biol. Chem. 1973, 248, 756–62.
16. Fredericq, E.; Deutsch, H.F. J. Biol. Chem. 1949, 181, 499–510.
17. Feeney, R.E.; Means, G.E.; Bigler, J.C. J. Biol. Chem. 1969, 244, 1957–60.
18. Schönenberger, M.; Schmidtberger, R.; Schultze, H.E. Z. Naturforsch. 1958, 13, 761–72.

19. Frénoy, J.-P.; Razafimahaleo, E.; Bourrillon, R. Biochim.
    Biophys. Acta 1972, 257, 111-21.
20. Jones, J.M.; Creeth, J.M.; Kekwick, R.A. Biochem. J. 1972,
    127, 187-97.
21. Barrett, A.J.; Starkey, P.M. Biochem. J. 1973, 133, 709-24.
22. Roberts, R.C.; Riesen, W.A.; Hall, P.K. "Proteinase Inhibi-
    tors"; Fritz, H.; Tschesche, H.; Greene, L.J.; Truscheit,
    E., Eds.; Springer-Verlag, Berlin, New York, 1974; pp. 63-
    71.
23. Harpel, P.C. Methods Enzymol. 1976, 45B, 639-52.
24. Aoyagi, T.; Miyata, S.; Nanbo, M.; Kojima, F.; Matsuzaki,
    M.; Ishizuka, M.; Takeuchi, T.; Umezawa, H. J. Antibiot.
    1969, 22, 558-68.
25. Suda, H.; Aoyagi, T.; Hamada, M.; Takeuchi, T.; Umezawa, H.
    J. Antibiot. 1972, 25, 263-6.
26. Tatsuta, K.; Mikami, N.; Fujimoto, K.; Umezawa, S.; Umezawa,
    H.; Aoyagi, T. J. Antibiot. 1973, 26, 625-46.
27. Blanco-Labra, A.; Iturbe-Chiñas, F.A. J. Food Biochem. 1981,
    5, 1-17.
28. Tanaka, A.; Ohnishi, M.; Hiromi, K.; Miyata, S.; Murao, S.
    J. Biochem. (Tokyo) 1982, 91, 1-9.
29. Ueda, S.; Koba, Y.; Chaen, H. Carbohydr. Res. 1978, 61, 253-
    64.
30. Müller, L.; Junge, B.; Frommer, W.; Schmidt, D.; Truscheit,
    E.; "Enzyme Inhibitors"; Brodbeck, U., Ed.; Verlag Chemie,
    Weinheim, 1980; pp. 109-22.
31. Junge, B.; Böshagen, H.; Stoltefuss, J.; Müller, L. "Enzyme
    Inhibitors"; Brodbeck, U., Ed.; Verlag Chemie, Weinheim,
    1980, pp. 123-37.
32. Otani, M.; Saito, T.; Satoi, S.; Mizoguchi, J.; Muto, N.
    Ger. Offen. 2855409, 1979.
33. Travis, J.; Johnson, D.; Pannell, R. "Proteinase Inhibi-
    tors"; Fritz, H.; Tschesche, H.; Greene, L.J.; Truscheit,
    E., Eds.; Springer-Verlag, Berlin, New York, 1974; pp. 31-9.
34. Hodges, L.C.; Laine, R.; Chan, S.K. J. Biol. Chem. 1979,
    254, 8208-12.
35. Rosenberg, R.D.; Damus, P.S. J. Biol. Chem. 1973, 248, 6490-
    6505.
36. Damus, P.S.; Rosenberg, R.D. Methods Enzymol. 1976, 45B,
    653-69.
37. Schultze, H.E.; Heide, K.; Haupt, H. Naturwissenschaften,
    1962, 49, 133-4.
38. Haupt, H.; Heimburger, N.; Kranz, T.; Schwick, H.G. Eur. J.
    Biochem. 1970, 17, 254-61.
39. Harpel, P.C.; Cooper, N.R. J. Clin. Invest. 1975, 55, 593-
    604.
40. Harpel, P.C. Methods Enzymol. 1976, 45B, 751-60.
41. Steinbuch, M.; Loeb, J. Nature (London) 1961, 192, 1196.
42. Heimburger, N.; Haupt, H.; Schwick, H.G. "Proteinase Inhibi-
    tors; Fritz, H.; Tschesche, H., Eds.; Walter de Gruyter,
    Berlin, 1971; pp. 1-21.

43. Steinbuch, M. Methods Enzymol. 1976, 45B, 760-72.
44. Dietl, T.; Dobrinski, W.; Hochstrasser, K. Hoppe-Seyler's Z. Physiol. Chem. 1979, 360, 1313-8.
45. Sasaki, M.; Minakata, K.; Yamamoto, H.; Niwa, M.; Kato, T.; Ito, N. Biochem. Biophys. Res. Commun. 1977, 76, 917-24.
46. Ryley, H.C. Biochem. Biophys. Res. Commun. 1979, 89, 871-8.
47. Lenney, J.F.; Tolan, J.R.; Sugai, W.J.; Lee, A.G. Eur. J. Biochem. 1979, 101, 153-61.
48. Bier, M.; Terminiello, L.; Duke, J.A.; Gibbs, R.J.; Nord, F.F. Arch. Biochem. Biophys. 1953, 47, 465-73.
49. Deutsch, H.F.; Morton, J.I. Arch. Biochem. Biophys. 1961, 93, 654-60.
50. Tomimatsu, Y.; Clary, J.J.; Bartulovich, J.J. Arch. Biochem. Biophys. 1966, 115, 536-44.
51. Liu, W.H.; Means, G.E.; Feeney, R.E. Biochim. Biophys. Acta 1971, 229, 176-85.
52. Wu, Y.V.; Scheraga, H.A. Biochemistry 1962, 1, 698-705.
53. Frattali, V.; Steiner, R.F. Biochemistry 1968, 7, 521-30.
54. Feeney, R.E.; Allison, R.G. "Evolutionary Biochemistry of Proteins: Homologous and Analogous Proteins from Avian Egg Whites, Blood Sera, Milk and Other Substances"; John Wiley & Sons, New York, 1969.
55. Odani, S.; Ikenaka, T. J. Biochem. (Tokyo) 1973, 74, 697-715.
56. Ikenaka, T.; Odani, S.; Koide, T. "Proteinase Inhibitors"; Fritz, H.; Tschesche, H.; Greene, L.J.; Truscheit, E., Eds.; Springer-Verlag, Berlin, New York, 1974; pp. 325-43.
57. Bieth, J.; Frechin, J.-C. "Proteinase Inhibitors"; Fritz, H.; Tschesche, H.; Greene, L.J.; Truscheit, E., Eds.; Springer-Verlag, Berlin, New York, 1974; pp. 291-304.
58. Hwang, D.L.R.; Davis Lin, K.-T.; Yang, W.-K.; Foard, D.E. Biochim. Biophys. Acta 1977, 495, 369-82.
59. Melville, J.C.; Ryan, C.A. J. Biol. Chem. 1972, 247, 3445-53.
60. Iwasaki, T.; Iguchi, I.; Kiyohara, T.; Yoshikawa, M. J. Biochem. (Tokyo) 1974, 75, 1387-90.
61. Iwasaki, T.; Kiyohara, T.; Yoshikawa, M. J. Biochem. (Tokyo) 1974, 75, 843-51.
62. Iwasaki, T.; Wada, J.; Kiyohara, T.; Yoshikawa, M. J. Biochem. (Tokyo) 1975, 78, 1267-74.
63. Hojima, Y.; Moriwaki, C.; Moriya, H. J. Biochem. (Tokyo) 1973, 73, 933-43.
64. Ryan, C.A.; Hass, G.M.; Kuhn, R.W. J. Biol. Chem. 1974, 249, 5495-9.
65. Rodis, P. Ph.D. Thesis, Purdue University, Lafayette, 1974.
66. Osuga, D.T.; Feeney, R.E. Arch. Biochem. Biophys. 1968, 124, 560-74.
67. Rhodes, M.B.; Bennett, N.; Feeney, R.E. J. Biol. Chem. 1960, 235, 1686-93.

68. Osuga, D.T.; Bigler, J.C.; Uy, R.L.; Sjöberg, L.; Feeney, R.E. Comp. Biochem. Physiol. 1974, 48B, 519-33.
69. Laskowski, M., Jr.; Kato, I.; Kohr, W.J. "Versatility of Proteins"; Li, C.H., Ed.; Academic Press, New York, 1978; pp. 307-18.
70. Dietl, T.; Tschesche, H. Eur. J. Biochem. 1975, 58, 453-60.
71. Tschesche, H.; Dietl, T. Eur. J. Biochem. 1975, 58, 439-51.
72. Tschesche, H.; Dietl, T. Methods Enzymol. 1976, 45B, 772-85.
73. Koide, T.; Ikenaka, T. Eur. J. Biochem. 1973, 32, 417-31.
74. Odani, S.; Ikenaka, T. J. Biochem. (Tokyo) 1973, 74, 857-60.
75. Stevens, F.C.; Wuerz, S.; Krahn, J. "Proteinase Inhibitors"; Springer-Verlag, Berlin, New York, 1974; pp. 344-54.
76. Whitaker, J.R.; Sgarbieri, V.C. J. Food Biochem. 1981, 5, 197-213.
77. Sgarbieri, V.C.; Whitaker, J.R. J. Food Biochem. 1981, 5, 215-32.
78. Granum, P.E.; Whitaker, J.R. J. Food Biochem. 1977, 1, 385-401.
79. Hedrick, J.L.; Smith, A.J. Arch. Biochem. Biophys. 1968, 126, 155-64.
80. DePonte, R.; Parlamenti, R.; Petrucci, T.; Silano, V.; Tomasi, M. Cereal Chem. 1976, 53, 805-20.
81. Lorensen, E.L.; Prevosto, R.; Wilson, K.A. Plant Physiol. 1981, 68, 88-92.
82. Pusztai, A. Biochem. J. 1966, 101, 379-84.
83. Yamamoto, M.; Ikenaka, T. J. Biochem. (Tokyo) 1967, 62, 141-9.
84. Jones, G.; Moore, S.; Stein, W.H. Biochemistry 1963, 2, 66-71.
85. Belitz, H.-D.; Fuchs, A.; Nitsche, G.; Al-Sultan, T. Z. Lebensm. Unters.-Forsch. 1972, 150, 216-20.
86. Feinstein, G.; Feeney, R.E. Biochim. Biophys. Acta 1967, 140, 55-61.
87. Haynes, R.; Osuga, D.T.; Feeney, R.E. Biochemistry 1967, 6, 541-7.
88. Hory, H.-D.; Weder, J.K.P. Z. Lebensm. Unters.-Forsch. 1976, 162, 349-56.
89. Odani, S.; Ikenaka, T. J. Biochem. (Tokyo) 1972, 71, 839-48.
90. Wilson, K.A.; Laskowski, M., Sr. "Proteinase Inhibitors"; Fritz, H.; Tschesche, H.; Greene, L.J.; Truscheit, E., Eds.; Springer-Verlag, Berlin, New York, 1974; pp. 286-90.
91. Szilagyi, S.; Szilagyi, E. Acta Biochim. Biophys. 1978, 13, 165-70.
92. Hochstrasser, K.; Wachter, E. Hoppe-Seyler's Z. Physiol. Chem. 1979, 360, 1285-96.
93. Wachter, E.; Hochstrasser, K.; Bretzel, G.; Heindl, S. Hoppe-Seyler's Z. Physiol. Chem. 1979, 360, 1297-303.
94. Wachter, E.; Hochstrasser, K. Hoppe-Seyler's Z. Physiol. Chem. 1979, 360, 1305-11.
95. Ozawa, K.; Laskowski, M., Jr. J. Biol. Chem. 1966, 241, 3955-61.

96. Laskowski, M., Jr.; Sealock, R.W. The Enzymes 1971, 3, 375-473.
97. Sgarbieri, V.C.; Whitaker, J.R. Adv. Food Res. 1982, 28, 93-166.
98. Pick, K.-H.; Wöber, G. Hoppe-Seyler's Z. Physiol. Chem. 1978, 359, 1379-84.
99. Finkenstadt, W.R.; Laskowski, M., Jr. J. Biol. Chem. 1965, 240, PC962-3.
100. Feinstein, G.; Feeney, R.E. J. Biol. Chem. 1966, 241, 5183-9.
101. Ako, H.; Foster, R.J.; Ryan, C.A. Biochemistry 1974, 13, 132-9.
102. Sweet, R.M.; Wright, H.T.; Janin, J.; Chothia, C.H.; Blow, D.M. Biochemistry 1974, 13, 4212-28.
103. Tschesche, H. Angew. Chem., Int. Ed. Engl. 1973, 12, 510-1.
104. Hunkapiller, M.W.; Forgac, M.D.; Yu, E.H.; Richards, J.H. Biochem. Biophys. Res. Commun. 1979, 87, 25-31.
105. Baillargeon, M.W.; Laskowski, M., Jr.; Neves, D.E.; Porubcan, M.A.; Santini, R.E.; Markley, J.L. Biochemistry 1980, 19, 5703-10.
106. Richarz, R.; Tschesche, H.; Wüthrich, K. Biochemistry 1980, 19, 5711-5.
107. Haynes, R.; Feeney, R.E. Biochemistry 1968, 7, 2879-85.
108. Jibson, M.D.; Birk, Y.; Bewley, T.A. Int. J. Pept. Protein Res. 1981, 18, 26-32.
109. Powers, J.R.; Whitaker, J.R. J. Food Biochem. 1977, 1, 239-60.
110. Wilcox, E.; Whitaker, J.R., unpublished data.
111. Saheki, T.; Matsuda, Y.; Holzer, H. Eur. J. Biochem. 1974, 47, 325-32.
112. Lenney, J.F. J. Bacteriol. 1975, 122, 1265-73.
113. Bünning, P.; Holzer, H. J. Biol. Chem. 1977, 252, 5316-23.
114. Richardson, M. Phytochemistry 1977, 16, 159-69.
115. Heinrikson, R.L.; Kézdy, F.J. Methods Enzymol. 1976, 45B, 740-51.
116. Ryan, C.A. Ann. Rev. Plant Physiol. 1973, 24, 173-96.
117. Green, T.R.; Ryan, C.A. Science 1972, 175, 776-7.
118. Rackis, J.J. J. Am. Oil Chemists' Soc. 1974, 51, 161A-74A.
119. Antunes, P.L.; Sgarbieri, V.C. J. Agric. Food Chem. 1980, 28, 935-8.
120. Khayambashi, H.; Lyman, R.L. Am. J. Physiol. 1969, 217, 646-51.
121. Green, G.M.; Lyman, R.L. Proc. Soc. Expt'l. Biol. Med. 1972, 140, 6-12.
122. Lyman, R.L.; Olds, B.A.; Green, G.M. J. Nutr. 1974, 104, 105-10.
123. Schneeman, B.O.; Lyman, R.L. Proc. Soc. Expt'l. Biol. Med. 1975, 148, 897-903.
124. Kakade, M.L.; Arnold, R.L.; Liener, I.E.; Waibel, P.E. J. Nutr. 1969, 99, 34-42.

125. Powers, J.R.; Culbertson, J.D. J. Food Prot. 1982, 45, 655–7.
126. Yetter, M.A.; Saunders, R.M.; Boles, H.P. Cereal Chem. 1979, 56, 243–4.
127. Powers, J.R.; Whitaker, J.R. J. Food Biochem. 1977, 1, 217–38.
128. Savaiano, D.A.; Powers, J.R.; Costello, M.J.; Whitaker, J.R.; Clifford, A.J. Nutr. Reports Int. 1977, 15, 443–9.
129. Jaffé, W.G.; Vega Lette, C.L. J. Nutr. 1968, 94, 203–10.
130. Lang, J.A.; Chang-Hum, L.E.; Reyes, P.S.; Briggs, G.M. Fed. Proc. 1974; 33, 718.
131. Bo-Linn, G.W.; Santa Ana, C.A.; Morawski, S.G.; Fordtran, J.S. N. Engl. J. Med. 1982, 307, 1413–6.

RECEIVED June 17, 1983

Antibiotics in Foods

BEVERLY A. FRIEND and KHEM M. SHAHANI

Department of Food Science and Technology, University of Nebraska,
Lincoln, NE 68583-0919

Antibiotic residues may occur in foods in several
ways. Antibiotics can be added either directly to
foods to retard spoilage and extend shelf life, or
can be added indirectly through contamination from
the immediate environment, through animals treated
with antibiotics for medical and prophylactic purposes or animals given antibiotic treated feeds for
growth. Conversely, during fermentation, certain
lactic cultures synthesize "natural" antibiotics
which may remain in the food. These compounds include Nisin produced by Streptococcus lactis,
Diplococcin from S. cremoris, "Antibacterials" from
S. thermophilus, S. diacetylactis and Leuconostoc
cremoris, Bulgarican from Lactobacillus bulgaricus,
Lactobrevin from L. brevis, Lactolin from L.
plantarum and Acidophilin, Lactocidin and Acidolin
from L. acidophilus. The increase in the incidence
of antibiotic residues in the food supply poses
certain public health risks including the emergence
of antibiotic resistant microorganisms and possible
sensitivity reactions in certain individuals. The
presence of antibiotics in dairy products causes
technical problems because of starter culture
inhibition. On the other hand, the natural antibiotics present in fermented food products may be
considered beneficial since they can increase the
shelf life, and possibly inhibit the growth and
toxin production of pathogenic organisms and afford
protection against disease organisms to the consumer.

Antibiotics are a chemically diverse group of drugs whose therapeutic properties can be related to structural and metabolic
differences between microbial and mammalian cells. Because
of their potent antimicrobial activity, simplicity of use and
relatively low cost, antibiotics have been used widely for

0097–6156/83/0234–0047$06.00/0

disease control, food and feed preservation and growth promotion, resulting in significant economic benefits to the producer and consumer.

Table I.   Origin of Antibiotics in Foods

  I.   Direct addition to foods
       Technological reasons

 II.   Indirect addition to foods
       Contamination from environment
       Medical and prophylactic treatment of animals
       Natural constituent of feeds
       Feed additives for growth promotion or other purpose
       Unintentional feed additives

III.   Natural constituents of food
       Synthesis by lactic cultures

Source: WHO/FAO Expert Committee on Food Additives (1).

As shown in Table I, antibiotics may be added to foods directly for technological reasons, indirectly through treated animals and feeds or naturally through lactic starter culture biosynthesis. Recent increases in antibiotic use for food production as well as for disease control poses certain risks. These include the emergence of potentially dangerous antibiotic resistant microorganisms, the possibility of toxic or allergic reactions in sensitive individuals and/or technological problems of starter culture inhibition associated with antibiotic residues in food products. This paper summarizes the risks, as well as some of the benefits, of antibiotics in foods and feeds.

Risks of Antibiotics in Foods and Feeds

On the average, 40% of the antibiotics sold in the United States, or more than 1.0 million kilograms, have been used as animal feed additives (2). According to Aschbacher (3), the following levels of antibiotic supplementation are recommended for growth promotion: Bacitracin at 10-50 g/ton feed, Bambermycins at 1-2 mg/ton, Carbadox at 10-25 mg/ton, Chlorotetracycline at 10-50 mg/ton, Erythromycin at 4-70 g/ton, Lincomycin at 1-11 g/ton, Oxytetracycline at 5-50 g/ton, Penicillin at 2-50 g/ton, Tylosin at 4-100 g/ton and Virginiamycin at 10 g/ton. Higher levels have been recommended for prophylactic purposes. As medical and non-medical use of antibiotics increases, the risks associated with antibiotics in foods and feeds also increase.

Microbial resistance. Microbial resistance to antibiotics in
feeds is not harmful per se, but may create a public health
hazard if the resistance interferes with the control of a given
microorganism, especially a pathogen, in animals or humans.

The Food and Drug Administration (4) has declared that
antibiotics cannot be used in animal feeds if: (a) administration of antibiotics to animals significantly increases the animal reservoir of pathogenic gram-negative bacilli which could be
transferred to humans via the food chain; (b) antibiotic use
significantly increases gram-negative bacilli in animals
resistant to antibiotics used in human medicine; or (c)
ingestion of antibiotic residues in foods leads to an increase
of antibiotic-resistant pathogenic organisms in human flora.
One important consideration, therefore, is the effect of feed
antibiotics on the Salmonella reservoir in animals, since these
gram-negative bacilli may contaminate food products and cause
illness and death in humans. In addition, a large proportion of
the Salmonella typhimurium organisms isolated from humans carry
R factors, the DNA-containing plasmids responsible for the
transfer of antibiotic resistance.

Table II. Antibiotic Resistance of Salmonella in Humans

| Serotype | % Resistant | | |
	1965	1969	1974
S. typhimurium	18.5	36.7	57.6
S. enteritidis	4.2	4.9	5.8
S. heidelberg	28.6	10.5	30.0
S. saint paul	12.5	21	15.9
S. newport	16.7	20	36.3

Source: Winshell et al. (9) and Neu et al. (10).

The effect of antibiotics on the Salmonella reservoir
varies with the antibiotic susceptibility of the organisms. In
previous studies the Salmonella reservoir decreased when animals
were infected with an antibiotic-sensitive organism (5-7), but
increased when infected with an antibiotic-resistant organism
(8). Neu and coworkers (9-10) have confirmed that antibiotic
resistance is increasing in Salmonella isolated from humans
(Table II.). Resistance of S. typhimurium to Ampicillin increased
from 23.4% in 1969 to 36.9% in 1974, resistance to Streptomycin
increased from 27.3% to 45.6% and resistance to Tetracycline
increased from 12.5% to 44.8%.

Table III.   Effect of Antibiotic Supplemented Feeds on the
Incidence of Resistant E. coli

Antibacterial drugs	% Resistant			
	Illinois Swine	Illinois Poultry	Illinois Beef	Montana Range Cattle[*]
Oxytetracycline	89.8	59	49.1	0
Dihydrostreptomycin	93.2	72	50.0	0.6
Ampicillin	52.5	17	13.2	1.3
Neomycin	20.5	0	12.3	0
Sulfamerazine	82.9	21	29.2	0.6

Source: Siegel et al. (15).

[*]Range cattle, minimally exposed to antibiotics, served as the
control.

      It has also been well documented that antibiotics in animal
feeds lead to a high level of antibiotic-resistant coliforms
(11-15).   As illustrated in Table III, Siegel et al. (15) found
that Illinois farm animals fed rations containing antibiotics
had more antibiotic-resistant E. coli than Montana range cattle
minimally exposed to antibiotics.
      A recent study by Hankin et al. (16) showed that raw milk
contains substantial numbers of antibiotic-resistant microorganisms and that some organisms resistant to Streptomycin, Tetracycline and Polymyxin can survive pasteurization.   Several
gram-negative isolates also were capable of transferring their
resistance to E. coli.

Toxic and Allergic Reactions.   While the medical use of antibiotics involves voluntary treatment for short periods of time
under controlled supervision, the exposure to traces of antibiotics in food products is involuntary and uncontrolled.
Although these trace levels are below the limit required to
cause acute toxic reactions, it is not known whether these traces are sufficient to cause chronic toxicity problems (17).
      Certain antibiotics notably Penicillin, Streptomycin,
Chloramphenicol and Novobiocin are strongly allergenic in sensitized individuals.   The majority of the hypersensitivity reactions have occurred with Penicillin most probably because of its
widespread usage.   Sensitization occurs most often during therapeutic treatment.   Once an individual is sensitized to Penicillin,
for example, as little as 40 IU (0.024 mg) administered orally
may elicit allergic reactions.   While the only food-related epi-

sodes of hypersensitivity reported in the literature involved Penicillin-sensitive individuals who consumed milk containing Penicillin (18-21), it is possible that allergic reactions caused by other antibiotic residues in food have gone unrecognized.

In order to control chronic toxicity and allergic reactions, safety standards for antibiotic residues in food have been established. The WHO/FAO guidelines for antibiotic residues in milk, meat and egg used for human consumption are given in Table IV. Chloramphenicol is highly toxic and, as shown, its use is forbidden for any purpose which might yield residues in food (1).

Although not approved in the United States, in other countries Nisin may be added directly to food at 20 units/gram (1, 64). Pimaricin (Natamycin) dips to control mold growth on the surface of cheese received recent approval from the U.S. Food and Drug Administration (58).

Inhibition of Starter Cultures. The primary cause of antibiotic residues in milk and milk products is the failure of producers to withhold milk from the market for a sufficient time period following veterinary therapy for mastitis or other diseases in dairy cattle. Consumption of antibiotic-supplemented feed may also lead to residues in the milk. These antibiotics are quite stable and remain in the milk even after manufacturing processses including pasteurization, drying or freezing. Marth and Ellickson (22), Marth (23) and Mol (17) have reviewed extensively problems in the dairy industry associated with antibiotic residues in the fluid milk supply.

The major problem has been the partial or complete inhibition of acid production by dairy starter cultures used in the manufacture of cheese, buttermilk, sour cream or yogurt (23). Shahani and Harper (24) determined the minimum amount of antibiotic needed to inhibit growth of 19 stock cheese cultures. They reported from 0.05 - 1.0 IU/ml Penicillin and from 0.05 - 10.0 µg/ml Auremycin were required. Whitehead and Lane (25) also noted that during cheese manufacture, as little as 0.05 IU of Penicillin per milliliter of milk delayed acid production, while 0.5 IU/ml completely inhibited acid production. Low levels of antibiotic also affect the flavor and texture of the final product (17, 26), as well as increase the probability of growth of undesirable antibiotic-resistant coliforms (17, 27).

Several workers (28-29) reported an increase in the methylene blue reduction time when 0.05-0.5 IU Penicillin were present per milliliter of milk. Similarly, Manokidis et al. (30) noted that Penicillin and Oxytetracycline were responsible for a false positive phosphatase test in pasteurized or partially pasteurized milk while Streptomycin, Erythromycin and Neomycin inhibited the phosphatase test to some extent in partially pasteurized milk, but not in raw milk. Although raw milk containing antibiotic residues was never mistakenly identified as pasteurized, these authors suggested that as a "precaution" antibiotic assays be run in conjunction with the phosphatase test.

Table IV. Acceptable Levels of Antibiotics in Food[1]

Antibiotic	Milk (ppm)	Meat (ppm)	Egg (ppm)
1. Penicillins	0-0.006	0-0.06	0-0.18
2. Oligosaccharides			
Streptomycin	0-0.2	0-1.0	0-0.5
Neomycin	0-0.15	0-0.5	0-0.2
3. Chloramphenicol	0	0	0
4. Tetracyclines			
Tetracycline	0-0.1	0-0.5	0-0.3
Chlorotetracycline	0-0.02	0-0.05	0-0.05
Oxytetracycline	0-0.1	0-0.25	0-0.3
5. Macrolides			
Erythromycin	0-0.04	0-0.3	0-0.3
Tylosin	0	0-0.2	0
6. Polyenes			
Nystatin [2]	0-1.1	0-7.1	0-4.3
Pimaricin	0	0	0
7. Siderochromes			
8. Polypeptides			
Nisin	-[3]	-	-
Polymyxin	0-0.2	0-0.5	0-0.5
Bacitracin	0-28	0-16	0-110
9. Griseofuivin			
10. Novobiocin	0-0.15	0-0.5	0-0.1

[1] Source: WHO/FAO Report (1).

[2] Acceptable only for cheese surfaces at a level of 15 ppm.

[3] No residue level has been established. Nisin maybe used as a direct food additive at a level less than 20 units/gram.

Benefits of Antibiotics in Foods and Feeds

Improved livestock production. For more than 25 years, anti-biotic supplementation of feeds has been used routinely to de-crease production costs and ultimately consumer costs. A five year feeding study with swine given 100g of Chlorotetracycline, 100g Sulfmethazine and 50g Pencillin per ton of feed demonstrated that antibiotic supplementation markedly increases the average daily gain and feed efficiency (Table V). Although growth responses have been observed to increase up to a limit of 250g antibiotic/ton, lower levels are used to maximize benefits and minimize costs.

The annual savings of U.S. pork consumers was estimated as $200 million in 1982 (31). Previously, Henry (32) reported an annual savings of $241 million in production costs for broilers, and $73 million for market turkeys when antibiotic supplemen-tation was used.

Table V. Effect of Antibiotics on Weight Gains of Swine

Year	Avg. Daily Gain (g)		Imp. (%)	Feed Efficiency (g/g)		Imp. (%)
	Ctrl	Antibiotic		Ctrl	Antibiotic	
1960	263	413	57	2.13	2.11	1.0
1961	222	395	78	2.08	1.85	11.1
1962	186	359	93	2.15	1.81	15.8
1963	191	336	76	2.99	2.18	27.1
1964	200	322	61	2.71	2.36	12.9
1965	250	331	62	2.77	2.28	17.7

Source: Hays (2).

Inhibition of pathogens and toxin production. Bacus and Brown (33) noted that staphylococcal food poisoning has been asso-ciated with defectively fermented sausage in at least six instances since 1967. As shown in Table VI, lactic starter cultures used for fermented sausage produce antimicrobial com-pounds which inhibit both the growth of Staphylococci and the production of enterotoxin (34). When these cultures are used in combination with glucose or sucrose, they are also effective in preventing the formation of toxin by Clostridium botulinum, even in the absence of nitrite (35-36).

Table VI. Lactic Culture Inhibition of Staphylococci in
Dry Sausage

Sausage formulation	Storage, 3 da			Storage, 7 da		
	Log CFU	pH	Toxin	Log CFU	pH	Toxin
Without lactic starter	8.84	5.9	+	8.88	5.7	+
With lactic starter	6.78	5.6	–	7.53	5.3	–

Source: Niskanen and Nurmi (34)

Shahani and associates (37) studied the effects of the
antifungal antibiotic Natamycin (Pimaricin) on the growth of
several mycotoxigenic molds (Table VII). They found that at 1.0
ppm, Natamycin inhibited mycelial growth from 16.0 to 23.6%
depending on the mold tested. Ochratoxin production was inhibited 93.2%, penicillic acid 70.6% and patulin 97.8% at the same
concentration.

Table VII. Inhibitory Effect of Natamycin on Mold Growth and
Toxin Production of A. ochraceus NRRL 3174, P.
cyclopium NRRL 1888 and P. patulum NRRL 989

Natamycin (ppm)	A. ochraceus		P. cyclopium		P. patulum	
	Growth	Ocratoxin	Growth	Penicillic acid	Growth	Patulin
	(% Inhibition)					
0	---	---	---	---	---	---
1.0	16.0	93.2	16.4	70.6	23.6	97.8
10.0	46.0	100.0	61.5	98.8	71.7	100.0
50.0	52.2	100.0	65.0	100.0	77.5	100.0

Source: Shahani et al. (37).

Lactobacillus acidophilus significantly inhibited
Staphylococcus aureus, Salmonella typhimurium and enteropathic
E. coli when grown in associative culture in a milk thio medium
(Table VIII). Shahani et al. (39) also noted that L. acidophilus
and L. bulgaricus inhibited a number of food borne pathogens
when tested by antibiotic disc assay procedures.

Table VIII. Inhibition of Pathogens by L. acidophilus in
Associative Culture

Test Culture	Treatment	Pathogen (CFU/ml)	Inhibition (%)
Staph. aureus	Control	1.5×10^7	98.2
	L. acidophilus	2.7×10^5	
S. typhimurium	Control	1.7×10^6	86.5
	L. acidophilus	2.3×10^5	
E. coli	Control	3.3×10^7	87.0
	L. acidophilus	4.3×10^6	

Source: Gilliland and Speck (38)

The production of natural antibiotics by lactic starter cultures has been well documented (40). Some of these compounds have been isolated and identified as noted in Table IX.

Shahani and associates (39, 49, 56-57) have studied the production of Acidophilin and Bulgarican by L. acidophilus DDS 1 and L. bulgaricus DDS 14, respectively. These antibiotics were isolated from fermented milk using a combination of methanol and acetone extraction coupled with silica gel and Sephadex chromatography. Different culture strains were found to vary greatly in their production of antibacterial compounds and factors such as incubation medium, pH, temperature and had a pronounced effect on antibiotic production. Milk was an essential medium, since these organisms failed to produce antibiotics when grown on other synthetic or semi-synthetic media. Approximately 30-60 µg or 0.2 to 0.4 units of Acidophilin per ml of aqueous solution caused a 50% inhibition in vitro of a wide variety of gram-positive and gram negative organisms (56-57).

Extended shelf life. Several antibiotics including Tetracyclines, Penicillin, Streptomycin, Bacitracin, Neomycin and Subtilin inhibit food spoilage microorganisms (23). Until 1967,

Table IX. Natural Antibiotics Produced by Lactic Cultures

Culture	Compound	Reference
Lactobacillus acidophilus	Acidolin	(41)
	Acidophilin	(39)
	Lactocidin	(42)
	"Antibiotic	
	Substance"	(43-44)
	"Bacteriocin"	(45)
Lactobacillus brevis	Lactobacillin	
	(H_2O_2)	(46-47)
	Lactobrevin	(48)
Lactobacillus bulgaricus	Bulgarican	(49)
Lactobacillus plantarum	Lactolin	(50)
Streptococcus cremoris	Diplococcin	(51)
Streptococcus diacetylactis	"Antimicrobial	
	Substance"	(52)
Streptococcus lactis	Nisin	(53-54)
Streptococcus thermophilus	"Antimicrobial	
	Compounds"	(55)

Chlorotetracycline was approved by the FDA for limited use in poultry and fish chill water. The purpose was to extend the shelf life of these raw products and it was assumed that all residues were destroyed during the normal cooking process. The FDA subsequently rescinded their approval primarily because of the emergence of resistant microorganisms.

Until recently, no antibiotic could be added directly to food for human consumption in the U.S. Natamycin (Pimaricin) has now been approved for use on the surface of cheese and cheese slices to extend shelf life (58). Shahani and associates (59) noted that Natamycin treatment prolonged the shelf life of Cottage cheese, Cheddar cheese and Parmesan cheese samples inoculated with toxigenic molds. Natamycin has also been found effective in controlling surface mold in Italian cheeses (60).

Table X. Effect of Nisin on Low Fat Dairy Spread Stored at 40°C

Storage Time (wk)	Microbial Count (CFU/g)		Flavor Score[*]	
	HG Stablilizer	HG + Nisin	HG Stabilizer	HG + Nisin
0	15×10^4	3.7×10^2	3.1	3.0
1	47×10^4	11×10^3	2.6	2.6
3	14×10^5	33×10^3	2.5	2.6
5	35×10^6	60×10^4	2.7	2.4

Source: Goel et al. (62)

[*]Flavor Score: 1 - excellent, 2 - good, 3 - fair, 4 - poor, 5 - unacceptable.

The antibiotic Nisin is inhibitory against several gram-positive Streptococci, Lactobacilli, Clostridia, Staphylococci and Bacilli (61-62). Goel et al. (63) noted that the addition of Nisin increased the shelf life of low fat dairy spread (Table X). In 20 countries outside the United States, Nisin is permitted as a direct food additive (64), and one major application has been to prevent the growth and subsequent gas production by Clostridia in hard cheese and processed cheese products. In France, for example, Nisin-producing Streptococci have been employed in the manufacture of processed cheese. Nisin has also been studied as a possible alternative to nitrite in the preservation of meats (65).

Mather and Babel (66) observed that the addition of Leuconostoc cremoris to a Cottage cheese creaming mixture inhibited coliforms and prevented slime formation by Pseudomonas spp. This procedure has been used commercially to extend the shelf life of Cottage cheese (40).

Possible protection against disease. The natural antibiotic effects of L. acidophilus and L. bulgaricus against human disease have received increased interest, especially in Eastern Europe, Russia and Japan. In 1978, for example, a Russian conference reported the use of Koumiss, a fermented mare's milk product containing L. acidophilus, L. bulgaricus and Saccharomyces lactis, in the treatment of a number of diseases including non-specific and chronic lung disease, digestive tract disease, myocardial infarction, chronic cholesocystitis and chronic enterocolitis.
Beck and Necheles (67) reported that L. acidophilus was effective in treatment of different types of diarrhea. Aci-

dophilus milk has been used to treat E. coli-mediated diarrhea
in infants in Yugoslavia (68), and Shigella-and-Salmonella-
mediated dysentery in children in Poland (69-70). The Polish
researchers suggested that the production of antibiotic substances by L. acidophilus may in part be responsible for the
observed effect.

Hamada et al. (71) fed a Lactobacilli-fermented milk known
as Yakult to a group of 500 servicemen in Japan and noted that
none was infected with dysentery or became carriers of
Salmonella/ Shigella organisms during a 6 month period. A
control group had 55 patients with dysentery and 50 carriers of
dysentery organisms during the final month of the investigation.

In contrast, Pearce and Hamilton (72), Merson et al. (73)
and DeDios Pozo-Olano et al. (74) among others have reported no
significant effect on diarrhea when Lactobacilli were fed.
Controlled clinical studies using double blind treatment protocols with viable cultures are required to assess whether disease
protection can be achieved in persons consuming cultures or
culture-containing products.

There is considerable strain-to-strain variation among the
lactic starter cultures and any therapeutic effects linked to
the production of antibiotic by one specific strain may not
necessarily apply to all other strains of the same organism.
Screening studies in our laboratory (39) showed that although L.
acidophilus DDS 1 produced Acidophilin and L. bulgaricus DDS 14
produced Bulgarican, none of the other strains of these organisms produced significant quantities of antibiotic. Commercial
preparations containing starter cultures which produce antibiotics in the laboratory also may not contain sufficient numbers of viable organisms and/or antibiotic to be of any benefit.
Finally, these cultures are quite fastidious in their growth and
metabolic requirements and therefore must not be grown or
ingested in the presence of incompatible foods or food ingredients.

In summary, antibiotic residues in foods pose certain
potential risks as well as potential benefits. The emergence of
possibly dangerous antibiotic resistance organisms has led to
the consideration that antibiotics commonly used in humans or
those which are cross resistant with important antibiotics used
in humans, be eliminated from the food supply by banning their
use in livestock production. Additional research in this area
and that of toxic and/or allergic sensitivity reactions is
required to make assessment of their public health risks. Only
then can critical risk/benefit decisions be made for antibiotics.

Acknowledgments

Published as Paper Number 7008, Journal Series, Nebraska
Agricultural Experiment Station. Research supported, in part,
by the National Dairy Council.

Literature Cited

1. WHO/FAO Expert Committee on Food Additives. Report Series No. 430, Geneva, 1969, p. 5.
2. Hays, V. W. In "Nutrition and Drug Interrelations," Hathcock, J. N. and Coon, J., Eds.; Academic:New York, 1978, p.545.
3. Aschbacher, P. W. In "Nutrition and Drug Interrelations," Hathcock, J. N. and Coon, J., Eds.; Academic:New York, 1978, p. 630.
4. Gardner, S. Fed. Regis. 1973, 38, 9811-14.
5. Evangelisti, D. G.; English, A. R.; Girard, A. E.; Lynch, J. E.; Solomons, I. A. Antimicrob. Agents and Chemother. 1975, 8, 664-72.
6. Gutzmann, F.; Layton, H.; Simkins, K.; Jarolmen, H. Am. J. Vet. Res. 1976, 37, 649-55.
7. Jarolmen, H.; Sairk, R. J.; Langworth, B. F. J. Appl. Bacteriol. 1976, 40, 153-61.
8. Silver, R. P.; Mercer, H. D. In "Nutrition and Drug Interrelations," Hathcock, J. N. and Coon, J., Eds.; Academic:New York, 1978, p. 649.
9. Winshell, E. B.; Cherubin, C.; Winter, J.; Neu, H. C. 1969. In "Antimicrob. Agents and Chemother.", pp. 86-89.
10. Neu, H. C.; Cherubin, C. E.; Longo, E. D.; Flouton, B.; Winter, J. 1975. J. Infec. Dis. 132, 617-22.
11. Smith, H. W.; Crabb, W. E. Vet. Rec. 1957, 69, 24-30.
12. Smith, H. W. N. Z. Vet. J. 1967, 15, 153-66.
13. Loken, K. I.; Wagner, L. W.; Henke, C. L. Am. J. Vet. Res. 1971, 32, 1207-12.
14. Mercer, H. D.; Pocurull, D.; Gaines, S.; Wilson, S.; Bennett, J. V. Appl. Microbiol. 1971, 22, 700-5.
15. Siegel, D.; Huber, W. G.; Enloe, F. Antimicrob. Agents and Chemother. 1974, 6, 697-701.
16. Hankin, L.; Lacy, G. H.; Stephens, G. R.; Dillman, W. F. J. Food Protect. 1979, 42, 950-3.
17. Mol, H. "Antibiotics and Milk", A. A. Balkema:Rotterdam, 1975.
18. Vickers, H. R.; Bagratuni, L.; Alexander, S. Lancet 1958, 1, 351-2.
19. Erskine, D. Lancet 1958, 1, 431-2.
20. Zimmerman, M. C. Arch. Dermatol. (N.Y.) 1959, 79, 1.
21. Borrie, P.; Barret, J. Brit. Med. J. 1961, 11, 1267.
22. Marth, E. H.; Ellickson, B. E. J. Milk Food Technol. 1959, 22, 266-72.
23. Marth, E. H. Residue Revs. 1966, 12, 65-161.
24. Shahani, K. M.; Harper, W. J. Milk Prod. J. 1958, 49, 15-16, 53-54.
25. Whitehead, H. R.; Lane, D. J. J. Dairy Res. 1956, 23, 355-60.
26. Hunter, G. J. E. J. Dairy Res. 1949, 16, 235-41.

27. Kastli, P. Schweiz. Arch. Tierheilk. 1948, 90, 685-95.
28. Hunter, G. J. E. J. Dairy Res. 1949, 16, 149-51.
29. Johns, C. K.; Desmaris, J. G. Can. J. Agr. Sci. 1953, 33, 91-7.
30. Manokidis, K. S.; Alichanidis, E. S.; Varvoglis, A. G. J. Dairy Sci. 1971, 54, 335-8.
31. "Feed Additives" Council for Agricultural Science and Technology, 1982, No. 82.
32. Henry, W. R. "Proceedings of the Antibiotics Presentations to the U.S. Food and Drug Administration Task Force on the Use of Antibiotics in Feeds". Washington, D.C., 1970.
33. Bacus, J. N.; Brown, W. L. Food Technol. 1981, 35, 74-8.
34. Niskanen, A.; Nurmi, E. Appl. Microbiol. 1976, 34, 11-20.
35. Christiansen, L. N.; Tompkin, R. B.; Shaparis, A. B.; Johnston, R. W.; Kautler, D. A. J. Food Sci. 1975, 40, 488-90.
36. Tanaka, N.; Traisman, E.; Lee, M. H.; Cassens, R. G.; Foster, E. M. J. Food Protection 1980, 43, 450-7.
37. Shahani, K. M.; Bullerman, L. B.; Barnhardt, H. M.; Hartung, T. E. Proc. 1st Intl. Cong. Bact. 1973, 2, 41.
38. Gilliland, S. E.; Speck, M. L. J. Food Protection 1977, 40, 820-3.
39. Shahani, K. M.; Vakil, J. R.; Kilara, A. Cult. Dairy Prod. J. 1977, 11(4), 14-7.
40. Babel, F. J. J. Dairy Sci. 1977, 60, 815-21.
41. Hamdan, I. Y.; Mikolajcik, E. M. J. Antibiotics 1974, 27, 631-6.
42. Vincent, J. G.; Veomett, R. C.; Riley, R. I. J. Bacteriol. 1959, 78, 477-84.
43. DeKlerk, H. C.; Coetzee, J. H. Nature 1959, 192, 340-1.
44. Hosono, H.; Yastuki, K. Milchwissenschaft 1977, 31, 727-30.
45. Barefoot, S. F.; Klaenhammer, T. R. J. Dairy Sci. 1981, 64 (Supplement 1), 51.
46. Wheater, D. M.; Hirsch, A.; Mattick, A. T. R. Nature 1951, 168, 659.
47. Wheater, D. M.; Hirsch, A.; Mattick, A. T. R. Nature 1952, 170, 623-4.
48. Kavasnikov, E. I.; Sodenko, V. I. Mikrobiol. Zh. Kyviv. 1967, 29, 146; Dairy Science Abstracts 1967, 29, 3972.
49. Reddy, G. V.; Shahani, K. M.; Friend, B. A.; Chandan, R. C. Cult. Dairy Prod. J. 1983, 18(2), 15-9.
50. Kodama, R. J. Antibiotics 1952, 5, 72-4.
51. Davey, G. P.; Richardson, B. C. Appl. Environ. Microbiol. 1981, 41, 84-9.
52. Branen, A. L., Go, H. C.; Genske, R. P. J. Food Sci. 1975, 40, 446-50.
53. Mattick, A. T. R.; Hirsch, A. Nature 1944, 154, 551-4.
54. Mattick, A. T. R.; Hirsch A. Lancet 1947, 253, 5-8.

55. Pulusani, S. R.; Rao, D. R.; Sunki, G. R. J. Food Sci.
    1979, 44, 575-8.
56. Shahani, K. M.; Vakil, J. R.; Kilara, A. Cult. Dairy Prod.
    J. 1977, 12(2), 8-11.
57. Kilara, A.; Shahani, K. M. J. Dairy Sci. 1978, 61,
    1793-1800.
58. Federal Register, June 22, 1982.
59. Shahani, K. M.; Bullerman, L. B.; Evans, T. A.; Arnold, R.
    G. Archives de L'Institut Pasteur de Tunis 1977,
    3-4, 511-20.
60. Neviani, E.; Enaldi, G. C.; Carini, S. Il Latte 1981,
    6:1-9.
61. Hawley, H. B. Food Manuf. 1957, 32, 370-6.
62. Shahani, K. M. J. Dairy Sci. 1962, 45, 827-32.
63. Goel, M. C.; Calbert, H. E.; Marth, E. H. J. Milk Food
    Technol. 1969, 32, 312-8.
64. Lipinska, E. In "Antibiotics and Antibiosis in
    Agriculture", Woodbine, M., Ed.; Butterworths: Boston,
    1977, 103-30.
65. Rayman, M. K.; Aris, B.; Hurst, A. 1981. Appl. Environ.
    Microbiol. 1981, 375-80.
66. Mather, D. W.; Babel, F. J. J. Dairy Sci. 1959, 42,
    1917-26.
67. Beck, C.; Necheles, H. Am. J. Gastroenterology 1961, 35,
    522-30.
68. Tomic-Karovic, K.; Fanjek, J. J. Annals Pediatrics 1962,
    199, 625-34.
69. Zychowicz, C.; Kowallzyk, S.; Cieplinska, T. Pediatria
    Polska 1977, 50(4), 429-35; Dairy Science Abstracts 38,
    2382.
70. Zychowicz, C.; Suranzynska, A.; Siewierska, B.; Cieplinska,
    T. Pediatria Polska 1974, 49(8), 997-1003, Dairy Science
    Abstracts 38, 395.
71. Hamada, K.; Waki, Y.; Kitagawa, T.; Uchida, K.; Chiba, H.
    et al. in "The Summary of Reports on Yakult". Yakult
    Honsha, Co., Ltd. Tokyo, Japan, 1971, pp. 54-6.
72. Pearce, J. L.; Hamilton, J. R. J. Pediatrics 1974, 84,
    261-2.
73. Merson, M. H.; Morris, G. K.; Sack, D. A. et al. N.
    England J. Medicine 1976, 294, 1299-1305.
74. De Dios Pozo-Oland, J.; Warram, J. H.; Gomez, R. G. et al.
    Gastroenterology, 1976, 74, 829-30.

RECEIVED June 28, 1983

Effects of Lipid Hydroperoxides on Food Components

H. W. GARDNER

Northern Regional Research Center, Agricultural Research Service, U.S. Department of Agriculture, Peoria, IL 61604

Undesirable changes in nutritional quality of foods are initiated by the autoxidation or enzymic oxidation of unsaturated lipids to lipid hydroperoxides. Lipid hydroperoxides and their products of decomposition can react with food components, such as amino acids, proteins and certain other biochemicals. These reactions and the potential role of hydroperoxides in causing mutagenicity are reviewed.

Food fabrication requires many ingenious methods to prevent the development of rancidity, and the food industry largely has been successful in this endeavor. However, the problem continues to receive serious attention by researchers. Obviously, a food that has become rancid through either enzymic oxidation or autoxidation will diminish in both nutritional value and palatability. Because rancid foods usually are rejected before consumption, it has been debated that lipid oxidation in foods has little impact on health. It is a concern that radical reactions in food can cause alterations below the threshold of detection by the human senses.

Considering the complexity of lipid peroxidation per se, the parameters added by numerous ingredients in food pose a nearly insurmountable problem to the experimentalist. As a result, nearly all we know about specific molecular reactions between food biochemicals and lipid hydroperoxides has come from studies of model reactions employing simple systems. Data from the models must be extrapolated to the composite, and this approach is not necessarily wholly inadequate. Obviously, certain biochemicals are more susceptible than others to radical attack and/or reaction with secondary products.

With sufficient kinetic data one could predict the predominating reactions expected in a complex mixture of potential reactants.

It is the purpose of this review to: (a) briefly outline the various radical reactions occurring during the course of autoxidation, (b) discuss the use of model systems in the study of the effects of lipid autoxidation on food ingredients, particularly proteins, and (c) assess the potential mutagenicity of autoxidation products.

Reactions of Autoxidation

An unsaturated fatty acid will not oxidize in the presence of ordinary ground-state O_2 unless a hydrogen is first abstracted from the fatty acid by a radical. This abstraction initiates the radical chain needed to overcome the lag or initiation phase required before autoxidation can accelerate. Since the C-H bond of an allylic carbon has a relatively weak bond dissociation energy, the abstraction of this hydrogen is favored, as illustrated in Figure 1. The resultant allylic radical (pentadiene radical in the example given in Figure 1) then combines with O_2 to produce a peroxy radical. The peroxy radical in turn propagates the same sequence by further H-abstraction. The lipid hydroperoxide, thus formed, is also susceptible to homolytic dissociation via Reactions A and B.

$$ROOH + X \cdot \rightleftharpoons ROO \cdot + XH \qquad (A)$$

$$X = R, RS, RO, ROO, \text{etc.}$$

$$ROOH \longrightarrow RO \cdot + \cdot OH \qquad (B)$$

It should be noted that Reaction A is an H-abstraction, and thus it is usually reversible. In contrast, Reaction B is not readily reversible after the $RO \cdot$ and $\cdot OH$ radicals escape from the solvent cage. The net result of both Reactions A and B is the formation of secondary products and the generation of additional radicals. Figure 2 outlines the progress of a hypothetical autoxidation of a lipid. The initiation phase is followed by rapid accumulation of radicals that promote both the formation and destruction of hydroperoxides. Finally, radical combination (termination) leads to nonradical secondary products. As discussed later, both secondary products and radical reactions per se are involved in food deterioration.

The main pathways to secondary products of lipid oxidation are described in the following text, but the reader should refer to more comprehensive reviews on this subject (1, 2).

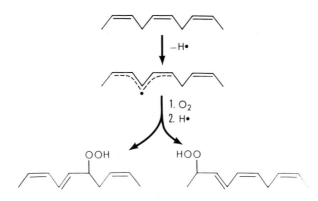

Figure 1. *Autoxidation of linolenic acid. Structures are abbreviated to show only polyunsaturation. H-Abstraction is signified by H·.*

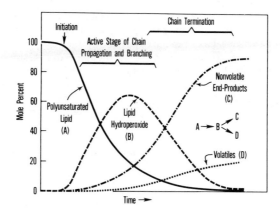

Figure 2. *Hypothetical autoxidation of a polyunsaturated lipid as a function of time.*

<u>Peroxy radicals</u>. Lipid peroxy radicals generated by Reaction A are important in propagating other radicals by H-abstraction (reverse of Reaction A). Weakly bonded hydrogens are particularly susceptible to abstraction by the peroxy radical. The radical generated in this way can become oxidized via Reaction C.

$$X\cdot + O_2 \longrightarrow XOO\cdot \qquad\qquad (C)$$

Because XH is often a nonlipid, which becomes oxidized in the presence of peroxidizing lipids, this process is sometimes called "cooxidation."

In addition to H-abstraction, other reactions compete for peroxy radicals, such as β-scission and intramolecular rearrangement (3). β-Scission occurs by the reverse of Reaction C, but it is difficult to surmise how this reaction would have an impact on food ingredients. On the other hand, peroxy radical rearrangement may have more relevance to food systems. Rearrangement occurs if a double bond is positioned β to the carbon bearing the peroxy group. This can lead to formation of cyclic peroxides (4, 5) and prostaglandin-like endoperoxides (6) by the pathways shown in Figure 3. These compounds are believed to be important in the genesis of malondialdehyde (7), radical propagation and formation of other secondary products.

Peroxy radicals can react by yet other competing routes. For example, evidence for lipid peroxy radical combination through a tetraoxide has been reported recently (8). Such tetraoxides could generate singlet oxygen and nonradical products by the Russell mechanism (9) as shown in Reaction D.

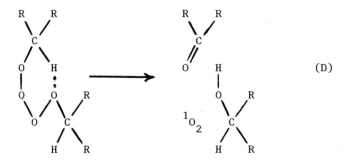

Intermolecular addition of the peroxy radical to a double bond also is possible but has not been documented in detail for lipids. It has been presumed that the polymerization of polyunsaturates may proceed in this manner.

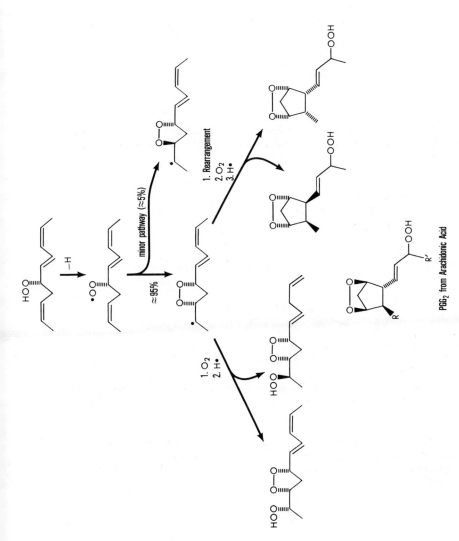

Figure 3. The formation of hydroperoxy cyclic peroxides and prostaglandin-like endoperoxides from the 13S-hydroperoxide of linolenic acid by peroxy radical rearrangement. Structures are abbreviated (6).

Oxy radicals. Heat and single electron reduction by transition
metal ions are among the more important ways lipid oxy radicals
are formed from homolytic cleavage of hydroperoxides.

The reactive oxy radical is known to participate in
several competitive radical processes. Like peroxy radicals,
oxy radicals have a propensity for H-abstraction (Reaction E).

$$\underset{R^1}{\overset{R}{\diagdown}}CH\text{-}O\cdot + XH \longrightarrow \underset{R^1}{\overset{R}{\diagdown}}CH\text{-}OH + X\cdot \tag{E}$$

Commonly, a self-induced H-abstraction, called disproportionation,
is observed (Reaction F), and indeed, fatty ketones and alcohols
are found among secondary products.

$$2\ \underset{R^1}{\overset{R}{\diagdown}}CH\text{-}O\cdot \longrightarrow \underset{R^1}{\overset{R}{\diagdown}}CH\text{-}OH + \underset{R^1}{\overset{R}{\diagdown}}C = O \tag{F}$$

β-Scission (Reaction G) generates volatile aldehydes and
hydrocarbons.

$$2\ \underset{R^1}{\overset{R}{\diagdown}}CH\text{-}O\cdot \underset{\searrow}{\overset{\nearrow}{}} \begin{array}{l} R\text{-}CH = O + R^1\cdot \\[4pt] R^1\text{-}CH = O + R\cdot \end{array} \tag{G}$$

Although volatiles usually do not exceed 10-15% of the oxidized
lipid, the aldehyde portion of the volatiles receives
disproportionate attention because of its contribution to
rancid odors.

Oxy radicals add to olefins by both intermolecular and
intramolecular mechanisms. Experimental evidence has indicated
that intramolecular addition (Reaction H) may be much more
important than its intermolecular counterpart (10, 11).

(H)

Since O_2 is an excellent scavenger of radicals, the expoxyallylic radical is oxidized further via Reaction I.

(I)

The hydroperoxy group of these compounds may undergo further homolysis in the cascade to secondary products (11).

In theory, combination of oxy radicals is possible (Reaction J); however, there is little detailed evidence to support this type of reaction at present.

$$RO\cdot + X\cdot \longrightarrow ROX \qquad (J)$$

Effect of Lipid Oxidation on Protein

The interaction of peroxidizing lipids with protein recently has been reviewed by several investigators (12-17). This review will emphasize the molecular basis for the changes in protein caused by exposure to peroxidized lipid. First, it must be understood that protein can be affected by lipid hydroperoxides in three general ways: (a) through formation of noncovalent complexes with either lipid hydroperoxide or its secondary products, (b) by radical reactions, and (c) through reactions with nonradical secondary products. The formation of noncovalent complexes will be ignored here, but complexation is probably important in causing flavor entrainment, changes in protein physical properties and promotion of chemical reactions.

Radical reactions of protein. Radical reactions of proteins promoted by lipid hydroperoxides fall into three general categories: (a) protein-protein or lipid-protein crosslinking, (b) protein scission, and (c) protein oxidation.

As illustrated by a number of recent reports, peroxidizing lipid affects protein in a variety of ways. For example, Jacks et al. (18) observed that rancid oil (P.V. = 144) had no effect on the storage protein of peanut. Other studies with lysozyme (19, 20), γ-globulins and albumin (21) demonstrated considerable damage to protein. Lysozyme exposed to either peroxidizing linoleic acid or methyl linoleate resulted in mainly the formation of lysozyme dimers and trimers (19, 20),

as well as denatured lysozyme (20). While Funes and Karel
(19) observed very little lipid bound covalently to lysozyme,
Nielsen (21) found that peroxidized phospholipid exposed to
either albumin or γ-globulin under N_2 caused mainly phospholipid-
protein covalent bonds. However, Nielsen (21) also did observe
some dimer and higher oligomers of protein. Several variables
in these investigations may have been the cause of the differing
results, illustrating the complexity of the problem.
       Although the study of peroxidizing lipid-protein interaction
is necessary to determine the overall effects, studies of
model systems employing peroxidized lipid and individual amino
acids also are necessary to understand the molecular basis of
the damage.
       The radical processes that appear to be important with
amino acids are H-abstraction, radical combination (Reaction K),
β-scission of amino acid oxy radicals (Reaction G) and possibly
radical addition (Reaction L).

$$X\cdot + X\cdot \longrightarrow X\text{-}X \qquad\qquad (K)$$

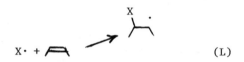

$$\qquad\qquad\qquad\qquad\qquad\qquad (L)$$

The first process, H-abstraction, may initiate an important
generic reaction of amino acids (Fig. 4). Radicals attributed
to the α-carbon have been identified by electron spin resonance
(ESR) of peroxidized proteins (22). Further reaction with O_2
(hypothetical) would lead to amino acid hydroperoxides. A
different pathway to amino acid hydroperoxide has been proposed
by Yong and Karel (23), but their proposal involves an indirect
pathway to the α-carbon radical. Homolysis of the hydroperoxy
group would afford an amino acid oxy radical susceptible to
β-scission via Reaction G. Thus, β-scission between the
α-carbon and the amino group may explain the increase in amide
content of protein that has been peroxidized in dry systems,
as well as the coincident protein chain scission observed
(24). In addition, moieties vicinal to the α-carbon may be
susceptible to radical attack, and the products of these
reactions may give the false impression that they were derived
from attack directly on the α-carbon. For example, the amino
group could be oxidized by a free radical mechanism, and
subsequently could cause the loss of the α-amino group. The
conversion of proline to proline nitroxide (25) can be cited
as an example of such an oxidation.
       Besides the attack at the α-carbon, the side chains are
susceptible to radical damage. Undoubtedly, the varying

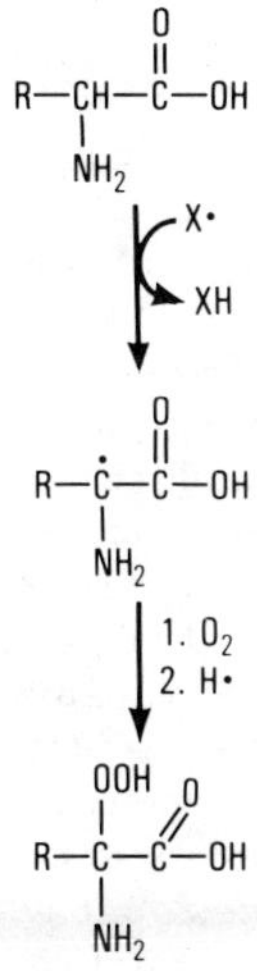

Figure 4. Postulated mechanism of amino acid oxidation by radical attack of α-carbon.

sensitivity of side chains is the reason for selectivity in
the peroxidation of certain amino acids. Generally, the most
labile amino acids are histidine, cysteine/cystine, methionine,
lysine, tyrosine and tryptophan (14).

The degradation of cysteine probably proceeds through the
thiyl radical by H-abstraction from the thiol group. Strong
sulfur signals were observed by ESR in a mixture of cysteine
plus   peroxidized   methyl   linoleate   demonstrating   the
susceptibility of thiol to radicals (22). As shown in Figure 5,
cystine, various oxides of cysteine/cystine (26-28), alanine
and H_2S (27) are products. Glutathione peroxidized by lipid
hydroperoxide also afforded the disulfide and oxides of
glutathione (29).

The absence of O_2 from a reaction of linoleic acid
hydroperoxide plus cysteine caused an interesting shift in
products. Instead of cystine and cysteine/cystine oxides,
cystine and lipid-cysteine adducts were identified from the
reaction mixture (30). The RS· plus RS· and RS· plus R·
combinations were favored because O_2 was not present to scavenge
both the lipid radicals (R·) and thiyl radicals (Fig. 5). The
detailed mechanism proposed for the combination reaction is
given in Figure 6. The epoxyallylic radical shown at the top
of Figure 6 arises from lipid oxy radical rearrangement
(Reaction H). We have recently isolated the epoxyene-cysteine
adduct by using a reaction system devoid of protic solvents
(31). In protic solvent the epoxide readily solvolyzes by
anchimeric assistance of the thiyl ether into the final products
shown in the figure. This new data refutes a mechanism I
proposed earlier (14). Such a reaction possibly could account
for a lipid to protein crosslink; however, proof of this
particular lipid-protein bond remains to be demonstrated.

As shown in Figure 7, the degradation of tryptophan by
peroxidizing methyl linoleate has been reported by Yong et al.
(32). They postulated that the initiating event was a radical
addition of a hydroxyl (or lipid oxy) radical to the indole
ring; however, others (33, 34) have demonstrated that formation
of a hydroperoxy group at carbon-3 of the indole ring was
intermediate in the oxidation of indole derivatives by various
oxidants. This latter pathway seems a more plausible route to
the products observed by Yong et al. (32). Schaich and Karel
(22) postulated that an unspecified tryptophan radical was a
major contributor to protein ESR because the ESR signal of
peroxidized nonsulfhydryl protein strongly resembled the
signal of peroxidized tryptophan. Their observation may
indicate that a resonance-stabilized indole radical is also
possible.

Histidine with peroxidizing lipid was altered both at the
α-carbon and the imidazole side chain (23, 35). Histamine,
imidazole acetic acid and imidazole lactic acid evidently

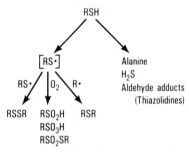

RSH
[RS·]
RS·
O2
R·
RSSR
RSO2H
RSO3H
RSO2SR
RSR
Alanine
H2S
Aldehyde adducts
(Thiazolidines)

Figure 5. Pathways of cysteine (RSH) degradation by exposure to peroxidizing lipid.

O
RS•
H+
OH
SR
(1) R'OH
(2) −H+
R'O

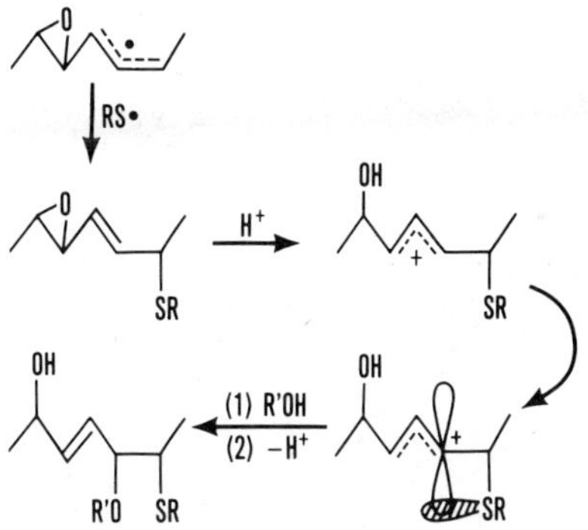

Figure 6. Mechanism of cysteine–fatty acid adduct formation from the reaction of 13-hydroperoxylinoleic acid and cysteine in the absence of O_2. The epoxyallylic radical at the top originates from the oxydiene radical of 13-hydroperoxylinoleic acid (abbreviated structure) and RS · is the cysteine thiyl radical. (Reproduced with permission from Ref. 28.)

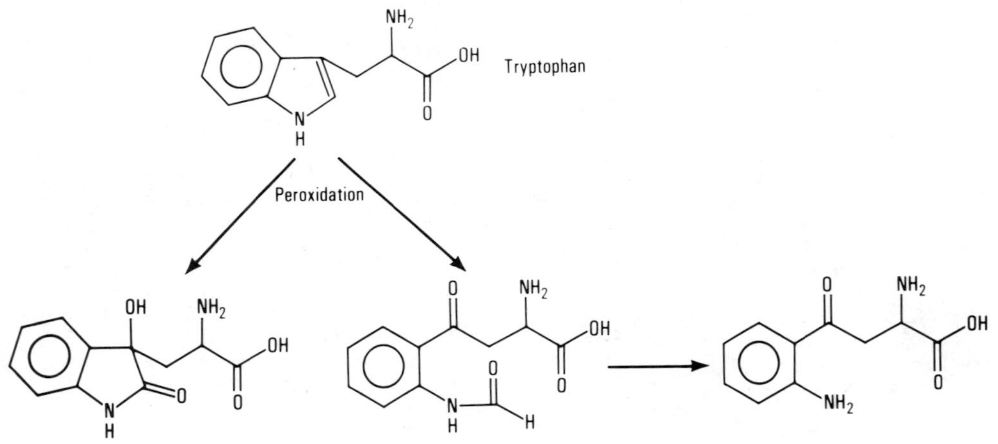

Figure 7. Products of tryptophan exposed to peroxidizing methyl linoleate (32).

arose from attack on or vicinal to the α-carbon. Degeneration of the imidazole ring was intimated by the formation of valine and aspartic acid. Additional research with the histidine derivatives, hippurylhystidylleucine and N-benzoylhistidine, accentuated the degradation of the imidazole group (36). These derivatives were designed to model the structural environment of histidyl residues in protein, thus attack on the side chain may be more important in proteins than with free histidine. Accordingly, the main products from peroxidation of N-benzoylhistidine were N-benzoylasparagine and N-benzoylaspartic acid.

The products from degeneration of lysine caused by peroxidizing methyl linoleate (13) are shown in Figure 8. The structures of the products are indicative of radical reaction at both the α-carbon and the side chain. Of particular interest is 1,10-diamino-1,10-dicarboxydecane, which potentially could provide a crosslink between lysinyl residues in proteins. Presumably, a C-6 radical of 2-aminohexanoic acid originated from scission of lysine ε-amino group, and self-combination of the C-6 radical generated the dimer. The ε-amino group also provides the site for crosslinking by malondialdehyde as explained in the following section.

Finally, methionine and tyrosine are known to be sensitive to peroxidation. Methionine was oxidized to methionine sulfoxide in the presence of peroxidizing methyl linoleate (13) or peroxidizing oil (37), illustrating the ease of radical initiation on sulfur substituents. The radical destruction of tyrosine is known (38), but I am not aware of any studies that specifically subject tyrosine to peroxidized lipid. Extrapolation from other radical reactions of tyrosine indicates that the initial event is H-abstraction of the phenol to afford a phenoxy radical.

Effect of nonradical oxidation products on protein. The aldehydes formed from lipid autoxidation by Reaction G have a propensity to react with amino groups to form a Schiff base (Reaction M).

$$R^1-CH = O + R-NH_2 \longrightarrow R^1-CH = N-R \qquad (M)$$

The implications of Schiff base formation in biological systems have been reviewed in more detail elsewhere (12, 14, 17); thus, this aspect of lipid oxidation will be brief.

With proteins, Schiff base formation will occur only with amino acid residues possessing a side chain amino group, including, of course, the amino terminus. The ε-amino group of lysine is important in this regard, and the loss of bioavailability of lysine by Schiff base formation is a nutritional concern.

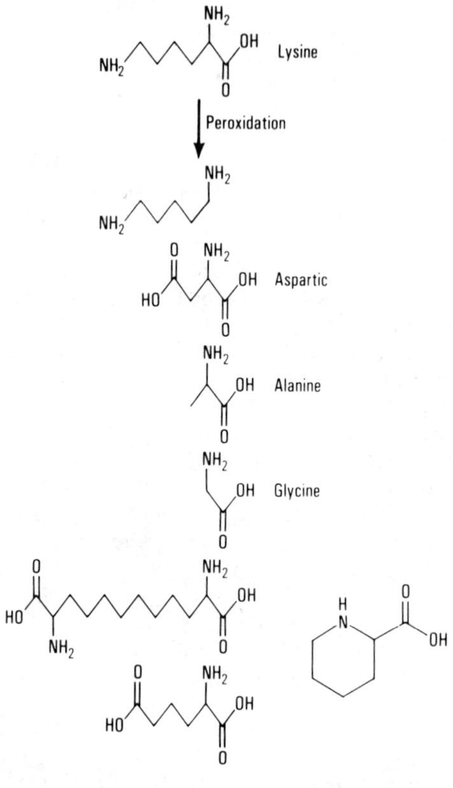

Figure 8. Products of lysine exposed to peroxidizing methyl linoleate (13).

The bifunctional malondialdehyde has caused protein crosslinking as illustrated by Reaction N.

$$O = CH-CH_2-CH = O \rightleftharpoons HO-CH = CH-CH = O$$

$$2R-NH_2 \qquad (N)$$

$$R-NH-CH = CH-CH = NR$$

Other derivatives from reaction of malondialdehyde and amino acids have been described (39).

Radical Reactions of Nonproteins

Radicals initiated by lipid peroxidation affect a number of nonprotein biochemicals. In general, most of the labile compounds are characterized as possessing an easily abstractable hydrogen. Accordingly, antioxidants and H-donors, such as α-tocopherol, ascorbic acid and glutathione, fall into this category.

Lipid hydroperoxide caused the oxidation of α-tocopherol to α-tocopherolquinone through an unidentified intermediate (40). Porter et al. (41) proposed a mechanism of oxidation that includes an intermediate from combination of α-tocopherol semiquinone with a peroxy radical (Reaction O).

The absence of O_2 causes a shift in products to the formation of α-tocopherol-lipid adducts (42, 43) via the combination of a lipid oxy radical with α-tocopherol semiquinone (Reaction P).

(P)

Reaction P is very similar to the combination reaction of
lipid oxy radical with the cysteine thiyl radical (Fig. 6).
Both combination reactions proceed only in the absence of O_2,
implying the O_2 effectively competes for the radicals involved.
    Under certain conditions ascorbic acid is an antioxidant
probably because it readily loses H to abstraction. Attention
also has been given to the prooxidative effect of ascorbic
acid in the presence of transition metal ions (44). It is
thought that ascorbic acid reduces metal ions which in turn
are more effective in catalyzing lipid oxidation. Consequently,
ascorbic acid becomes oxidized to dehydroascorbic acid.
    The destruction of β-carotene during lipid peroxidation
is readily observed by bleaching of the carotene color (44).
Presumably, β-carotene oxidation is initiated by H-abstraction,
and such a mechanism has been proposed for the cooxidation of
carotenoids during the lipoxygenase catalyzed oxidation of
polyunsaturated fatty acids (45), as shown by Reaction Q.

Mutagenicity Induced by Lipid Oxidation

    Free radical oxidation in vivo has been much touted as a
detriment to both health and life. Indeed, aberrant free
radical reactions have been cited as contributors to aging
(46, 47) and cancer (47, 48), but unequivocal evidence for
these claims often is lacking. The connection between free
radicals and the promotion of cancer has received the most
attention. As discussed later, the evidence is compelling
that lipid hydroperoxide activates certain carcinogens by
cooxidation.
    A direct mutagenic effect of lipid hydroperoxides has
been sought for some time with varying success. Recently, the
Ames test has been utilized to demonstrate weak mutagenicity
of both peroxidized fatty acid (49) and isolated hydroperoxides

of methyl linoleate (50). Because cumene hydroperoxide and
t-butyl hydroperoxide were also found to be mutagenic, while
peroxides, peracids and H_2O_2 were not, the mutagenicity was
attributed to the hydroperoxide group (50). As shown in
Table I, we have also observed weak mutagenicity for methyl
13-hydroperoxylinoleate by the Ames test (51). A third
laboratory has failed to find mutagenicity for linoleic acid
hydroperoxide (52). The reason for weak mutagenicity of
hydroperoxide is not clear. It is known that free radical
damage to nucleic acids can be induced by radiation (53), and
DNA radicals have been detected after exposure of DNA to lipid
peroxidation (54). However, it may be erroneous to extrapolate
the ESR signals in model systems into relevance concerning in
vivo DNA damage with concomitant mutagenicity.

It has been implied that secondary products of lipid
autoxidation are mutagenic. Interest in this area of research
was stimulated when Mukai and Goldstein (55), as well as
others, reported that malondialdehyde elicited a mutagenic
response by the Ames test. Since some evidence for DNA
crosslinking by malondialdehyde has been shown in chemical
models (56), it might be presumed that this reaction is the
molecular basis of the mutagenicity. However, the importance
of the observed response was questioned by Marnett and Tuttle
(57), who found very weak mutagenicity with highly purified
malondialdehyde. According to them, impurities from the use
of tetraethoxypropane to generate malondialdehyde probably
were responsible for the greater mutagenicity observed by
others.

As pointed out in the text above, lipid epoxides are
common secondary products of autoxidation. For a number of
potent mutagens, like benzo[α]pyrene, the ultimate mutagen has
been found to be an epoxide of the parent compound, which in
turn undergoes nucleophilic substitution by the amino group of
a DNA base pair, such as guanine (58-60). It has been postulated
by some workers that lipid epoxides also may be mutagenic by a
similar mechanism. A convincing mutagenic response was not
obtained when either cis- or trans-9,10-epoxyoctadecanoic acid
was injected into mice (61). However, many mutagenic epoxides
have been characterized as having electron-withdrawing substituent
groups that cause the epoxide to be more susceptible to
nucleophilic attack (62). For this reason, we tested by the
Ames method (63) the mutagenicity of a number of fatty epoxides
with vicinal functionality as shown in Figure 9. These fatty
epoxides were isolated from a mixture of products obtained
after the free radical decomposition of 13-hydroperoxylinoleic
acid (11). Methyl esters were synthesized from fatty acids
with diazomethane. Despite the presence of electron-withdrawing
groups vicinal to the epoxide, mutagenicity was not observed
even at the 2000 μg level per plate (51). Apparently, the

Table I

Ames Test[a] for Mutagenicity of 13-Hydroperoxylinoleate (Methyl Ester)

Test compound, μg/plate	TA 100 No. S-9		TA 100 S-9 Added		TA 98 No. S-9		TA 98 S-9 Added	
1000		538[c]		235[b]	0			94[b]
500	233[c]	300[c]	171	176	37	55	58	41
100	164	164	158	130	26	35	58	44
50	158	158		130		39		41
Control	114	132	144	129	27	38	46	44

[a] Each column indicates a separate experiment.

[b] Exceeds 'control' by more than $\text{LSD}_{0.01}$.

[c] Exceeds 'control' by more than $\text{LSD}_{0.001}$.

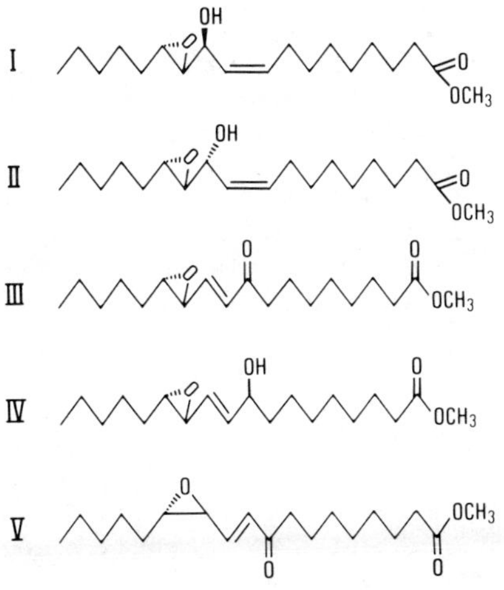

Figure 9. Structures of fatty ester epoxides tested for mutagenicity by the method of Ames et al. (63). (Reproduced with permission from Ref. 51.)

lack of response stems from the 1,2-disubstitution of the epoxide, which usually diminishes the response (62, 64). The size of the hydrocarbon side chains also may have an effect. Systematic studies of a series of glycidyl ethers indicated that mutagenicity was considerably reduced when the side chain exceeded 4-6 carbons (65).

The role of lipid hydroperoxides in activating chemical mutagens is more convincing. A number of studies have demonstrated that lipid hydroperoxides can initiate the free radical oxidation of the carcinogen to the ultimate active form. For example, benzo[α]pyrene was oxidized to the highly mutagenic   7,8-dihydroxy-9,10-epoxy-7,8,9,10-tetrahydrobenzo[α]pyrene   in   the   presence   of 13-hydroperoxylinoleic acid and the catalyst, hematin (66). Similarly, Floyd et al. (67) used 13-hydroperoxylinoleic acid and hematin to activate N-hydroxy-N-acetyl-2-amino-fluorene into the carcinogens, nitrosofluorene and N-acetoxyacetylamino-fluorene. Thus, lipid hydroperoxides may serve as efficient oxidants of a variety of chemical carcinogens that require oxidation to an active form. This area of research appears to be promising for future work.

Literature Cited
1.   Gardner, H. W. "Autoxidation of Unsaturated Lipids," Chan, H. W.-S., Ed.; Academic:London, in press.
2.   Frankel, E. N. Prog. Lipid Res. 1980, 19, 1.
3.   Porter, N. A.; Lehman, L. S.; Weber, B. A.; Smith, K. J. J. Am. Chem. Soc. 1981, 103, 6447.
4.   Chan, H. W.-S.; Matthew, J. A.; Coxon, D. T. J. Chem. Soc. Chem. Commun. 1980, 235.
5.   Mihelich, E. D. J. Am. Chem. Soc. 1980, 102, 7141.
6.   O'Connor, D. E.; Mihelich, E. D.; Coleman, M. C. J. Am. Chem. Soc. 1981, 103, 223.
7.   Pryor, W. A.; Stanley, J. P. J. Org. Chem. 1975, 40, 3615.
8.   Scheiberle, P.; Grosch, W.; Kexel, H.; Schmidt, H. L. Biochim. Biophys. Acta 1981, 666, 322.
9.   Nakano, M.; Takayama, K.; Shimizu, Y.; Tsuji, Y.; Inaba, H.; Migita, T. J. Am. Chem. Soc. 1976, 98, 1974.
10. Hamberg, M. Lipids 1975, 10, 87.
11. Gardner, H. W.; Kleiman, R. Biochim. Biophys. Acta 1981, 665, 113.
12. Tappel, A. L. Fed. Proc. Fed. Am. Soc. Exp. Biol. 1973, 32, 1870.
13. Karel, M.; Schaich, K.; Roy, R. B. J. Agric. Food Chem. 1975, 23, 159.
14. Gardner, H. W. J. Agric. Food Chem. 1979, 27, 220.
15. Porkorny, J.; Janicek, G. Nahrung 1975, 19, 911.

16. Miquel, J.; Oro, J.; Bensch, K. G.; Johnson, J. E., Jr., "Free Radicals in Biology," Pryor, W. A., Ed.; Academic:New York, 1977, Vol. III, p. 132.
17. Tappel, A. L., "Free Radicals in Biology," Pryor, W. A., Ed.; Academic:New York, 1980, Vol. IV, p. 1.
18. Jacks, T. J.; Hensarling, T. P.; Muller, L. L.; St. Angelo, A. J.; Neucere, N. J. Int. J. Pept. Protein Res. 1982, 20, 149.
19. Funes, J.; Karel, M. Lipids 1981, 16, 347.
20. Leake, L.; Karel, M. J. Food Sci. 1982, 47, 737.
21. Nielsen, H. Lipids 1981, 16, 215.
22. Schaich, K.; Karel, M. Lipids 1976, 11, 392.
23. Yong, S. H.; Karel, M. J. Am. Oil. Chem. Soc. 1978, 55, 352.
24. Zirlin, A.; Karel, M. J. Food Sci. 1969, 34, 160.
25. Lin, J. S.; Olcott, H. S. J. Agric. Food Chem. 1974, 22, 526.
26. Lewis, S. E.; Wills, E. D. Biochem. Pharmacol. 1962, 11, 901.
27. Roubal, W. T.; Tappel, A. L. Arch. Biochem. Biophys. 1966, 113, 5.
28. Gardner, H. W.; Jursinic, P. A. Biochim. Biophys. Acta 1981, 665, 100.
29. Finley, J. W.; Wheeler, E. L.; Witt, S. C. J. Agric. Food Chem. 1981, 29, 404.
30. Gardner, H. W.; Kleiman, R.; Weisleder, D.; Inglett, G. E. Lipids, 1977, 12, 655.
31. Gardner, H. W., unpublished data.
32. Yong, S. H.; Lau, S.; Hsieh, Y.; Karel, M., "Autoxidation in Food and Biological Systems," Simic, M. G.; Karel M., Eds.; Plenum:New York, 1980, p. 237.
33. Sundberg, R. J., "Chemistry of Indoles," Academic Press:New York, 1970, p. 282-315.
34. Saito, I.; Imuta, M.; Nakada, A.; Matsugo, S.; Matsuura, T. Photochem. Photobiol., 1978, 28, 531.
35. Roy, R. B.; Karel, M. J. Food Sci. 1973, 38, 896.
36. Yong, S. H.; Karel, M. J. Food Sci. 1979, 44, 568.
37. Njaa, L. R.; Utne, F.; Braekkan, O. R. Nature 1968, 218, 571.
38. Neukom, H., "Autoxidation in Food and Biological Systems," Simic, M. G.; Karel, M., Eds.; Plenum:New York, 1980, p. 249.
39. Kikugawa, K.; Machida, Y.; Kida, M.; Kurechi, T. Chem. Pharm. Bull., 1981, 29, 3003.
40. Gruger, E. H., Jr.; Tappel, A. L. Lipids 1970, 5, 326.
41. Porter, N. A.; Lehman, L. S.; Khan, J. A. 184th ACS National Meeting, Organic Section 3, Kansas City, September 12-17, 1982.
42. Gardner, H. W.; Eskins, K.; Grams, G. W.; Inglett, G. E. Lipids 1972, 7, 324.
43. Gardner, H. W., unpublished data.

44. Kanner, J.; Mendel, H.; Budowski, P. J. Food Sci. 1977, 42, 60.
45. Weber, F.; Grosch, W. Z. Lebensm. Unters.-Forsch. 1976, 161, 223.
46. Harman, D. Proc. Natl. Acad. Sci. USA 1981, 78, 7124.
47. Pryor, W. A. Ann. N.Y. Acad. Sci. 1982, 393, 1.
48. McBrien, D. C. H.; Slater, T. F., Eds., "Free Radicals, Lipid Peroxidation and Cancer," Academic:London, 1982.
49. Yamaguchi, T.; Yamashita, Y. Agric. Biol. Chem. 1979, 43, 2225.
50. Yamaguchi, T.; Yamashita, Y. Agric. Biol. Chem. 1980, 44, 1675.
51. Gardner, H. W.; Crawford, C. G.; MacGregor, J. T. Food Chem. Toxicol., in press.
52. Scheutwinkel-Reich, M.; Ingerowski, G.; Stan, H.-J. Lipids 1980, 15, 849.
53. Myers, L. S., Jr., "Free Radicals in Biology," Pryor, W. A., Ed., Academic:New York, 1980, Vol. IV, p. 94.
54. Fukuzumi, K. Mem. Fac. Eng. Nagoya Univ. 1978, 30, 200.
55. Mukai, F. H.; Goldstein, B. D. Science 1976, 191, 868.
56. Brooks, B. R.; Kalmerth, O. L. Eur. J. Biochem. 1968, 5, 178.
57. Marnett, L. J.; Tuttle, M. A. Cancer Res. 1980, 40, 276.
58. Jeffrey, A. M.; Blobstein, S. H.; Weinstein, I. B.; Beland, F. A.; Harvey, R. G.; Kasai, H.; Nakanishi, K. Proc. Natl. Acad. Sci. USA 1976, 73, 2311.
59. Jeffrey, A. M.; Jennette, K. W.; Blobstein, S. H.; Weinstein, I. B.; Beland, F. A.; Harvey, R. G.; Kasai, H.; Miura, I.; Nakanishi, K. J. Am. Chem. Soc. 1976, 98, 5714.
60. Essigmann, J. M.; Croy, R. G.; Nadzan, A. M.; Busby, W. F., Jr.; Reinhold, V. N.; Büchi, G.; Wogan, G. N. Proc. Natl. Acad. Sci. USA 1977, 74, 1870.
61. Swern, D.; Wieder, R.; McDonough, M.; Meranze, D. R.; Shimkin, M. B. Cancer Res. 1970, 30, 1037.
62. Voogd, C. E.; van der Stel, J. J.; Jacobs, J. J. J. A. A. Mutat. Res. 1981, 89, 269.
63. Ames, B. N.; McCann, J.; Yamasaki, E. Mutat. Res. 1975, 31, 347.
64. Wade, D. R.; Airy, S. C.; Sinsheimer, J. E. Mutat. Res. 1978, 58, 217.
65. Thompson, E. D.; Coppinger, W. J.; Piper, C. E.; McCarroll, N.; Oberly, T. J.; Robinson, D. Mutat. Res. 1981, 90, 213.
66. Dix, T. A.; Marnett, L. J. J. Am. Chem. Soc. 1981, 103, 6744.
67. Floyd, R. A.; Soong, L. M.; Walker, R. N.; Stuart, M. Cancer Res. 1976, 36, 2761.

RECEIVED June 28, 1983

Some Lipid Oxidation Products as Xenobiotics

P. B. ADDIS, A. SAARI CSALLANY, and S. E. KINDOM

Department of Food Science and Nutrition, University of Minnesota, St. Paul, MN 55108

Lipid oxidation is important in the quality and acceptability of foods and can influence wholesomeness by forming toxins. One such compound, malonaldehyde (MA), has been shown to be toxic, mutagenic, and possibly carcinogenic. Traditionally, MA has been determined by thiobarbituric acid (TBA) test (1-5). However, since TBA reacts with numerous compounds, it should not be used to quantify MA. Recently, a liquid chromatographic method developed in our laboratory to quantify free MA clearly demonstrated extensive overestimation of MA by TBA. Recent studies suggested that atherogenic and perhaps carcinogenic properties previously attributed to cholesterol were the result of contaminating cholesterol oxidation products; their existence in foods is of concern.

Malonaldehyde

MA, a three carbon dialdehyde, can experience a number of configurational modifications as discussed by Kwon and Watts (6). Enolization of the diketo form may take place. The enolic tautomer may further undergo molecular rearrangement into its open cis-, open trans-, or chelated forms. At pH 3 or lower, MA is chelated and exists as β-hydroxy-acrolein; above pH 6.5 MA is completely dissociated and exists as an enolate anion. Between pH 3 and 6.5, MA is an equilibrium mixture of enolate anion and chelated forms. MA (also malondialdehyde), is one of the main secondary products of lipid oxidation. It forms a pink color by condensing with 2 moles of TBA (7).

Biological Significance of Malonaldehyde

The biological significance of MA stems from the fact that it may be formed in vivo or in food products which are then consumed. Kwon and Brown (8) demonstrated that MA can cross-link

0097–6156/83/0234–0085$06.00/0

bovine serum albumin to form a stable complex. Manzel (9)
provided evidence that MA can react with ribonuclease resulting
in polymerization and loss of enzymatic activity. Brooks and
Klamerth (10) reported that glyoxal, a structural analogue, was
toxic to human fibroblasts in cell culture, by inhibiting DNA
replication. Klamerth and Levinsky (11) examined rats which
were fed MA and observed damaged liver DNA and loss of template
activity.

Studies on lipid oxidation in vivo have been closely linked
with aging and MA appears to have a role. Chio and Tappel (12)
reported that MA takes part in formation of lipofuscin "age"
pigment production.

Bird and Draper (13) recently studied biological effects of
MA on growth, morphology and macromolecular biosynthesis in a
neonatal rat skin fibroblast cell culture. Acetaldehyde was used
as a reference compound. Cells exposed to 10^{-3} M MA for 120
hours exhibited altered morphology, cytoplasmic vacuolization,
karyorrhexis, micro- and multi-nucleation, and a marked reduction
in mitotic index, and DNA-, RNA-, and protein-synthesizing capacity. At 10^{-4} M, MA caused mitotic aberrations, nuclear morphological irregularities, a reduced mitotic index and inhibition of
RNA and DNA synthesis. At 10^{-5} and 10^{-6} M, MA induced only formation of small and irregular nuclei. MA was approximately 10
times more toxic to rat skin fibroblasts than acetaldehyde.
Neither MA or acetaldehyde exerted any noticeable effects on
cellular metabolism, indicating that skin fibroblasts are either
able to catabolize the two aldehydes efficiently at these concentrations or are capable of repairing any damage induced at the
molecular level. Subsequently, Bird et al. (14) continued their
toxicological study of MA and acetaldehyde using the fibroblast
system and noted dose-dependent production of micronuclei for
concentrations of MA between 10^{-4} and 10^{-3} M. Twelve hours of
treatment with MA resulted in chromosomal aberrations. MA was
again about ten times as potent as acetaldehyde with respect
to micronuclei formation. MA probably exerts its chromosome-
damaging effects by cross-linking strands of DNA, thus producing
inactivating alterations in DNA structure which inhibit DNA
replication (unless eliminated by repair).

Shamberger et al. (15) observed that MA was carcinogenic
to mouse skin. Mukai and Goldstein (16) reported that MA was
mutagenic in histidine-requiring strains of Salmonella typhimurium. Yau (17) found that MA was highly mutagenic and cytotoxic in mammalian cells and therefore may be a potent carcinogen
in humans. Exposure to as little as 20 μM MA was cytotoxic and
increased mutation frequency among survivors of murine L5178Y
lymphoma cell cultures as well.

From the foregoing studies, it is possible to conclude that
MA is highly mutagenic, carcinogenic and cytotoxic. However,
Marnett and Tuttle (18) suggested that perhaps the causative
agent for the mutagenic and carcinogenic properties of MA is an

intermediate formed in production of MA from 1,1,3,3-tetraethoxy-propane (TEP), an intermediate which does not arise during lipid peroxidation. Marnett and Tuttle (18) noted that β-ethoxyacrolein, an incomplete hydrolysis product of TEP, was 20 times more mutagenic than MA. When producing MA by hydrolysis of 1,1,3,3-tetramethoxypropane (TMP), both intermediates formed, 3,3-dimethoxy-propanaldehyde and β-methoxyacrolein, were more mutagenic than MA and they appeared to be more mutagenic than β-ethoxyacrolein as well. Since these intermediates are much stronger mutagens than MA, they could be responsible for a portion of the mutagenicity and carcinogenicity attributed to MA by Shamberger (15) and by Mukai and Goldstein (16). However, this question is not yet completely resolved.

Malonaldehyde Measurements in Food Products

The first extensive investigation into the use of TEP and TMP as MA standards for the TBA method was conducted by Gutteridge (19). His findings were as follows: (1) TEP was hydrolyzed completely in 90 minutes at 56°C. (2) TMP required four hours for complete hydrolysis. By that time a 60 nmole TMP solution had lost 50% of its TBA reactivity. (3) Thin-layer chromatography showed at least nine compounds can be recovered from TEP and TMP, all of which react with TBA to give a red pigment with maximum absorbance at 532 nanometers. Gutteridge (19) concluded from thin-layer chromatography data that bands in extracts from autoxidized polyunsaturated fatty acids which react with TBA are not merely polymers of MA; they are "probably larger molecular weight precursors of MA that are broken down to MA when heated with the TBA reagent." He further suggested that the best method for preparing a standard curve from TEP would be to heat TBA directly with TEP without any prehydrolysis, so that polymerization of MA and loss of TBA reactivity could be minimized.

As early as 1951 (20), and numerous times since then, TBA has been used to measure MA levels in foods. However, TBA should be used to measure extent of lipid oxidation in general, not to quantify MA specifically. At the present time there are numerous substances known to interfere with the TBA reaction. Dugan (21) showed that sucrose and some compounds in wood smoke react with TBA to produce a red color. A yellow pigment found by Yu and Sinnhuber (22) was able to significantly affect the TBA method; however, it could be separated by chromatography. Saslaw et al. (23) reported that other unidentified carbonyl compounds will react with TBA. Additionally it was possible (24) by irradiation to produce TBA reactive substances, none of which were MA. Kwon and Olcott (25) concluded that the TBA method was a quantitative measure of lipid oxidation, but only during initial stages of oxidation since highly polymerized MA (unreactive) forms in advanced stages of oxidation. Schneir et al. (26) indicated that N-acetyl-neuraminic acid has a high absorbance at 549 nm in the TBA test. Marcuse and Johansson (27) identified

other aldehydes which produced a positive TBA reaction, including
2,4-alkadienals and 2-alkenals. Baumgartner et al. (28) noticed
that acetaldehyde in the presence of sucrose and acid was capable
of reacting with TBA. Pryor et al. (29) determined that MA may
be generated from its prostaglandin-like endoperoxide precursors
by the conditions (acid and heat) of the TBA procedure. Ohkawa
et al. (30) noted that glucose, sucrose and N-acetyl-neuraminic
acid could interfere with MA determination by TBA.

In recent studies (unpublished) in our laboratory, copper
was found to diminish color development in the TBA test. The
foregoing studies led Witte et al. (5) and later Rethwill et al.
(31) to modify the TBA procedure of Tarladgis et al. (4) in order
to eliminate heating and distillation. In most cases TBA-inter-
ferences resulting from other compounds have lead to elevated
levels quoted for MA. The need for a direct method of MA
determination is obvious. Recently, Csallany and coworkers
(32) developed a high performance liquid chromatographic (HPLC)
method for quantification of free MA in tissues or meat. HPLC
separation was performed with a TSK G1000 PW column using a
mobile phase of 0.1 M Na_3PO_4, pH 8.0 buffer at a flow rate of
0.6 ml per minute. The eluant was monitored at 267 nm. Free
MA in a tissue sample can be separated and quantified in approximately 50 minutes at levels as low as one nanogram per injection. Table I outlines some results that were obtained on MA
content of food.

TABLE I. Comparison of MA content of meat by HPLC and TBA

Sample	MA content ($\mu g/g$)		TBA/HPLC ratio
	HPLC	TBA	
Beef (N = 9)	0.14	0.44	3.1
SD	0.085	0.19	2.2
Pork (N = 9)	0.11	0.39	3.5
SD	0.06	0.12	2.0

[a] $\mu g/g$ wet tissue

Comparisons were made with TBA. As can be seen, TBA greatly
overestimates the true amount of free MA which is present,
leading the authors (32) to conclude that it is not an acceptable means of determining MA levels in food products or tissues.
A more accurate description of what the test measures would be
"TBA-reactive substances." In spite of this fact, numerous
authors have reported levels of MA using the TBA procedure in
the literature (c.f. 33,34). The variability of the TBA
procedure is also much greater than that for the HPLC determination of MA (Table I).

Cholesterol Oxidation Products

As is the case for MA, there is little agreement concerning existence and significance of cholesterol oxidation products in foods. The role of cholesterol containing foods in the American diet has been the subject of many investigations in recent years, largely due to hypothesized links between cholesterol and coronary heart disease (CHD) in humans. It is not the purpose of this paper to review all of the pros and cons concerning lipid involvement in CHD. However, a few of the highlights as they pertain to cholesterol are worth reviewing. The original studies linking cholesterol to CHD were performed on vegetarian animals which were fed extremely high dietary levels of cholesterol. These types of studies were criticized for their choice of animal and levels of cholesterol fed. From another standpoint, Taylor and coworkers (35) have seriously questioned the validity of many early experiments based on the supposition that the cholesterol used was most likely contaminated with oxidation products of cholesterol and that these oxidation products, not cholesterol, were the cause of atherosclerosis. Therefore, cholesterol may be much safer than believed by organizations such as the American Heart Association which recommends reducing the amount of cholesterol in our diets. On the other hand, reports indicating that cholesterol oxidation products are present in certain types of foods raises questions about their safety.

In 1963, cholesterol hydroperoxides were reported (36) in egg-containing foods irradiated by sunlight. Chicoye et al. (37) observed the following 5 photoxidation derivatives of cholesterol in spray-dried yolk exposed to either 40-watt fluorescent lamp (approx. 280 hours) or summer sunlight (5 hours): 3β-hydroxy-cholest-5-en-7-one (7-keto); cholest-5-ene-3β,7α-diol (7α-diol); cholest-5-ene-3β,7β-diol (7β-diol); 5,6β-epoxy-5α-cholestan-3β-ol (β-epoxide) and 5α-cholestane-3β,5α,6β-triol (triol). Subsequently, Tsai et al. (38) developed methodology to demonstrate the presence of 5,6α-epoxy-5α-cholestan-3β-ol (α-epoxide) in dried egg products which were spiked with the epoxides.

Refined edible beef tallow used as a deep-fat frying medium by fast-food restaurants can be subjected to conditions which are suitable for oxidation of cholesterol. Ryan et al. (39) identified several cholesterol oxidation products in tallow heated at 180°C intermittently (8 hours/day) during storage times of 75 and 150 hours. The extent to which these oxides are absorbed by foods during frying is unknown. The inhibition of cholesterol oxidation and ultimate improvement of food safety may now be an interesting area of study.

Atherogenicity

Oxidation products derived from cholesterol appear to have the greatest potential for health impairment of all classes of compounds isolated from rancid foods up to the present time. Potent angiotoxic effects have been noted (40-44) for several of these compounds leading researchers to hypothesize a likely role

for them in CHD. The early work of Seifter and Baeder (43)
provides clues which suggest that the atherogenic effects
attributed to cholesterol may have been due to its contaminating
oxidation products. The study involved inducing hypercholesterolemia by dietary and endogenous (hormonal) mechanisms. Hormonal
treatment led to severe hypercholesterolemia and yet less athero-
genicity compared to the milder hypercholesterolemia produced by
diet. In retrospect, it seems logical that dietary induction of
hypercholesterolemia included the introduction of cholesterol
oxidation products into experimental animals. In contrast, one
would expect endogenous hypercholesterolemia to be limited to
native cholesterol, free of oxidation products.

In 1971, it was suggested (44) that the level of α-epoxide
in human serum may be related to the severity of atherosclerosis.
This hypothesis was based on the measurement of very high concentrations (250-3,250 µg/100 ml serum) of α-epoxide in Type II
hypercholesterolemia patients, whereas controls contained less
than 5 µg/100 ml serum. Imai et al. (40) demonstrated angiotoxic
effects from contaminants of USP-grade cholesterol. By the use
of methanolic extraction, USP-grade cholesterol was purified and
the oxidation products concentrated. Both newly purchased and
5 year old cholesterol were extracted. Purified cholesterol was
obtained by the dibromination procedure according to Fieser (45).

Rabbits were administered concentrate of oxidation products
or purified cholesterol by gavage, sacrificed, and their aortas
examined microscopically for angiotoxic effects. The concentrate, containing products of spontaneous oxidation of cholesterol, increased the frequency of dead aortic smooth muscle
cells and induced focal intimal edema in rabbits 24 hours after
gavage. Both new and old cholesterol extracts were found to be
angiotoxic. Old cholesterol, new cholesterol and controls
(gelatin) showed the following frequency of aggregate debris and
degenerated cells per 100 nucleated cells: 0.7, 0.2, 0.03 and
7.6, 4.4 and 0.61. Purified cholesterol appeared to have no such
effect. In a longer term study, cholesterol oxidation product
"concentrate" was administered 1 g/kg body weight per 7 week
period. Intimal diffuse fibrous lesions without foam cells or
hypercholesterolemia were induced. Purified cholesterol at the
same dose had no effect.

In a sequel, Peng et al. (41) purified known oxidation
products of cholesterol and studied their toxicity in cultured
rabbit aortic smooth muscle cells. Using thin layer chromatography for separation followed by UV detection in 50% aqueous
sulfuric acid spray, the oxidation products separated into 6
fractions according to their mobilities and were used in the cell
culture. Potent cytoxic effects were noted for a number of the
identified cholesterol oxidation products. In contrast, purified
cholesterol at the same concentration produced no toxic effects.
The results demonstrated that 25-hydroxycholesterol and triol
were the most toxic agents. Peng et al. (42) confirmed and

extended their earlier work on angiotoxicity of cholesterol
oxidation products. Commercially obtained cholesterol oxidation
products were introduced into rabbit aortic smooth muscle cell
cultures. Degree of cytoxicity was estimated as a percentage of
dying and dead cells in cultures within 24 hours of application.
The results indicated that 25-hydroxycholesterol and triol were
the most toxic compounds tested. Additional studies indicated
that when these oxidation derivatives were added to cultured
cells they significantly depressed the activity of 3-hydroxy-3-
methylglutaryl coenzyme A reductase, a regulatory enzyme of
cholesterol biosynthesis. The degree of inhibition by 25-hy-
droxycholesterol was remarkable: 3 µg/ml in culture resulted
in an 83% inhibition. Purified cholesterol showed no cytotoxic
effects and minimal inhibition of cholesterol biosynthesis. Most
recently, Peng et al. (46) has demonstrated that in monkeys, 24
hours after ingestion of [14]C-25-hydroxycholesterol, 55.1%, 34.7%
and 10.2% of the radioactivity was located in low density lipoproteins (LDL), very low density lipoproteins (VLDL) and high
density lipoproteins (HDL), respectively. This is in contrast
to ^{14}C-cholesterol fed controls after the same time period which
revealed the following distribution of label: LDL (47.6%), VLDL
(3.1%) and HDL (49.3%). Since the ultimate metabolic fate of
VLDL is conversion to LDL which is then transported to peripheral
tissues, it was speculated that proportionally more 25-hydroxy-
cholesterol would be incorporated into vascular tissue where it
could inhibit cholesterol biosynthesis, cause membrane dysfunc-
tion and induce arterial injury.

Smith (47) and Simic and Karel (48) have contributed useful
monographs on the subjects of lipid (including cholesterol)
oxidation in food and biological systems.

Carcinogenicity of Cholesterol Oxides: Historical Background

Speculation into the carcinogenic potential of cholesterol
and its derivatives began once their structural relationship to
polycyclic hydrocarbons was realized. In 1933, Roffo (49)
suggested that photo-induced oxidation products of cholesterol
might be responsible for UV-induced carcinogenesis of the skin.
About this same time, it was recognized (50) that artifacts
(cholesterol oxidation products) may arise during the bromina-
tion-debromination reaction (51) used in purification of cholesterol. Also, when Haslewood (52) showed triol to be present in
ox-liver residue, it was not possible to decide whether these
compounds are natural constituents or autoxidation products
formed during isolation (53). Bischoff and Rupp (54) found a
32% local incidence of cancer in ovariectomized mice administered
a crude progesterone preparation (containing 20 mg/mouse of
unidentified cholesterol oxidation products) subcutaneously in
sesame oil verses 0% for pure progesterone. Fieser (55) postulated that a carcinogenic conversion product of cholesterol was
the offender. The foregoing findings coupled by the ease with
which cholesterol is oxidized in aqueous colloidal solutions by

air (56,57), a condition that conceivably could be duplicated in
vivo, prompted a further investigation (58).
Problem of Oily Vehicle
    Purified cholesterol, all known initial and subsequent
oxidation products of cholesterol and some related compounds
were tested: cholest-5-en-3-one; 7α-diol; 7β-diol; 7-keto;
cholesta-3,5-dien-7-one; α-epoxide; triol; cholest-4-en-3-one;
6β-hydroperoxycholest-4-en-3-one; 6β-hydroxycholest-4-en-3-one;
cholest-4-ene-3,6-dione; cholest-5-ene-3β,4β-diol; 5α-cholest-6-
ene-3β,5α-diol; 5β-cholestan-3β-ol; cholesta-1,4-dien-3-one;
5α-cholest-7-en-3β-ol; cholesta-7,9-dien-3β-ol acetate; 7,8,9,11-
diepoxy-22-isoallospirostan-3β-ol acetate; cholesteryl acetoace-
tate; and cholesteryl isoheptylate. Many were carcinogenic when
administered subcutaneously into Marsh-Buffalo mice with sesame
oil as the vehicle; α-epoxide, 6β-hydroperoxycholest-4-en-3-one
and cholest-4-en-3,6-dione were most potent (34-66% incidence
of fibrosarcoma verses 1.4% for vehicle control). All share
the property of oxygen linkage at carbon 6. 6β-hydroxycholest-
4-en-3-one was mildly (15%) carcinogenic. Sesame oil was
described (58) a cocarcinogen because negative results were
obtained if certain of these carcinogens were given as aqueous
colloids. Some steroids that are normal body constituents were
carcinogenic if injected in sesame oil and heated or oxidized
oil had positive tumorigenic results when administered alone.
    Hieger (59,60), on the other hand, conclusively stated a
carcinogenic effect for cholesterol subcutaneously injected in
an oily vehicle. Bischoff and Bryson (61) were able to show that
the critical difference between these results was the physical
state of cholesterol at the injection site. Hieger's method had
produced crystals at the dose site and was an example of smooth-
surface carcinogenesis. To prevent this, cholesterol concentration in an oil must be below 4%.
    Cholesterol oxidation product evaluation has continued.
However, a myriad of problems have plagued these investigations
including insufficient survival time among experimental animals,
spontaneous occurrence of fibrosarcoma and membrane encapsulation
(oleoma) of injected material, probably due to physical (surface
or texture) effects (62-65). Frequently studies were complicated
by the use of an oily vehicle, as discussed previously for sesame
oil. It was suggested that oils not be used as carriers due to
their variability, capacity to react metabolically with steroids,
ability to promote crystallization of cholesterol derivatives,
potential for containing other carcinogen contaminants and
ability to induce tissue inflammation (66).
    The only product of cholesterol oxidation known to be car-
cinogenic in the absence of oil is α-epoxide, which was shown to
be carcinogenic in rats and mice (62,63).
Ultraviolet-Induced Skin Carcinogenesis
    Formation of polar cholesterol derivatives was demonstrated
(67,68) in human and hairless mouse skin specimens irradiated in

ultraviolet (UV) light. It was clearly established that
α-epoxide originated from naturally occurring sterols (68).

Skin of hairless mice subjected to chronic low levels of UV
displayed increased epoxide at 4 weeks and maximum levels at 10
weeks (69,70). Subsequently, it was shown α-epoxide hydrase
increased starting at 8 and peaking at 15 weeks and that its
elevation coincided with a decline in epoxide but also a rapid
increase in tumor incidence (70,71). Dietary intake of ascorbate, butylated hydroxytoluene (BHT), dl-α-tocopherol and reduced
glutathione decreased levels of α-epoxide by 50% and suppressed
tumor formation induced by UV light (72,73).

Although the cited evidence argues for α-epoxide as a carcinogen, no data exists demonstrating it as a topical carcinogen
(74).

Colon Carcinogenesis

The colon is the most common site for development of cancer
in the U.S. population. A specific carcinogen has not been
identified, but a potent mutagen has recently been isolated from
feces of high-risk patients (75). Epidemiological studies
suggest that diets high in animal fat and protein, especially
beef, and low in natural carbohydrate, including fiber, may be
involved in the etiology (76,77) and it has been reported that
fecal mutagenic activity is higher in subjects consuming such
diets (78). The fact that ascorbate or tocopherol supplementation reduced fecal mutagenic activity suggests need for studies
on the possible role of lipid oxidation products (79).

A possible role in colon cancer for cholesterol and its oxidation products is suggested by several studies (76,80-83). Hill
and coworkers (81,84) observed that a high fat diet reduced
intestinal redox potential and increased levels of fecal cholesterol and bile acid metabolites. Patients with adenomatous
polyps and ulcerative colitis, both at increased risk from colon
cancer (86,87), or with active bowel cancer, excreted greater
levels of cholesterol, coprostanol and triol than controls
(80,85).

Reddy and coworkers (88-90) evaluated carcinogenic or tumor-
promoting activity of cholesterol, α-epoxide, triol and primary
and secondary bile acids, with and without induction by
N-methyl-N'-nitro-N-nitrosoguanidine (MNNG). Tumor development
required MNNG, and bile acids acted as promoters. Cholesterol
and its metabolites were not found to have promoting activity.

Other Cancers

Cholesterol, α- and β-epoxides were present in 45% of breast
fluid specimens examined with α-isomer predominating. Epoxide
levels tended to be higher in fluids with high cholesterol levels
and in those taken from older women prompting researchers to
speculate that benign breast disease and cancer could result
(91). The nonlactating breast concentrates its secretions and
thereby exposes the mammary epithelium to α-epoxide.

Schaffner et al. (92) noted high levels of cholesterol

epoxides in prostatic secretions and postulated a role for them in prostatic cancer.

Recently, Smith et al. (93) demonstrated that air-aged commercial samples of USP- or reagent-grade cholesterol contain compounds which are mutagenic toward three strains of Salmonella typhimurum.

Future Research Needs. It is obvious that studies on toxicity and carcinogenicity of lipid oxidation products, as they occur in food, are in their infancy. It is still not established that any of these compounds constitute a threat to public health. It is certain that, at the levels normally encountered in foods, acute effects on humans would not be seen. The chronic area remains an enigma. It is known that levels of MA in foods have been overstated by the TBA test. Extensive studies are urgently needed to quantify free MA directly by HPLC (32). Further investigations are also necessary to determine more fully the toxicity of MA.

Even less well understood than MA is the possible occurrence of cholesterol oxidation products in foods and their health significance. It seems clear that some of the products of cholesterol autoxidation are atherogenic. Much more research will be required to establish or refute their proposed carcinogenic properties. Methods for the determination of cholesterol oxidation products in foods and studies to establish levels of occurrence, if any, are most urgently needed. Further studies on antioxidants and procedures for the inhibition of oxidation are also needed. It is difficult to overstate the potential importance to the animal products industry of studies on quantification of cholesterol oxides in food products. Concern about this area of research is becoming widespread (47,48).

Acknowledgments

Scientific Journal Series Paper No. 13,492, Minnesota Agricultural Experiment Station.

Literature Cited

1. Turner, E. W.; Paynter, W. D.; Montie, E. J.;
    Bessert, M. W.; Struck, G. M; Olson, F. C.
    Food Technol. 1954, 8, 326-9.
2. Sidwell, C. G.; Salwin, H.; Mitchell, J. H., Jr.
    J. Am. Oil Chem. Soc. 1955, 32, 13-6.
3. Yu, T. C.; Sinnhuber, R. O. Food Technol. 1957, 11,
    104-8.
4. Tarladgis, B. G.; Watts, B. M.; Younathan, M. T.;
    Dugan, L., Jr. J. Am. Oil Chem. Soc. 1960, 37, 44-8.
5. Witte, V. C.; Krause, G. F.; Bailey, M. E. J. Food Sci.
    1970, 35, 582-5.

6. Kwon, T. W.; Watts, B. M. J. Food Sci. 1963, 28, 627-30.
7. Sinnhuber, R. O.; Yu, T. C.; Yu, Te Chang. Food Res. 1958, 23, 626-34.
8. Kwon, T. W.; Brown, W. D. Fed. Proc. 1965, 24, 592.
9. Manzel, D. B. Lipids 1967, 2, 83-4.
10. Brooks, B. R.; Klamerth, O. L. Europ. J. Biochem. 1968, 5, 178-82.
11. Klamerth, O. L.; Levinsky, H. FEBS Letters 1969, 3, 205-7.
12. Chio, K. S.; Tappel, A. L. Biochemistry 1969, 8, 2827-32.
13. Bird, R. P.; Draper, H. H. J. Toxicol. Environ. Health 1980, 6, 811-23.
14. Bird, R. P.; Draper, H. H.; Basrur, P. K. Mutation Res. 1982, 101, 237-46.
15. Shamberger, R. J.; Andreone, T. L.; Willis, C.E. J. National Cancer Inst. 1974, 53, 1771-3.
16. Mukai, F. H.; Goldstein, B. D. Science 1976, 191, 868-9.
17. Yau, T. M. Mechan. Aging Develop. 1979, 11, 137-44.
18. Marnett, L. J.; Tuttle, M. A. Cancer Res. 1980, 40, 276-82.
19. Gutteridge, J. M. C. Anal. Biochem. 1975, 69, 518-26.
20. Patton, S.; Kurtz, G. W. J. Dairy Sci. 1951, 34, 669-74.
21. Dugan, Jr. L. R. J. Am. Oil Chem. Soc. 1955, 32, 605-8.
22. Yu, T. C.; Sinnhuber, R. O. Food Technol. 1962, 16, 115-7.
23. Saslaw, L. D.; Anderson, A. J.; Waravdekar, V. S. Nature 1963, 200, 1098-9.
24. Saslaw, L. D.; Waravdekar, V. S. Rad. Res. 1965, 24, 375-89.
25. Kwon, T. W.; Olcott, H. S. J. Food Sci. 1966, 31, 552-8.
26. Schneir, M.; Benya, P.; Buch, L. Anal. Biochem. 1970, 35, 46-53.
27. Marcuse, R.; Johansson, L. J. Am. Oil Chem. Soc. 1973, 50, 387-91.
28. Baumgartner, W. A.; Baker, N.; Hill, V.A.; Wright, E. T. Lipids 1975, 10, 309-11.
29. Pryor, W. A.; Stanley, J. P.; Blair, E. Lipids 1976, 11, 370-79.
30. Ohkawa, H.; Ohishi, N.; Yagi, K. Anal. Biochem. 1979, 95, 351-8.
31. Rethwill, C. E.; Bruin, T. K.; Waibel, P. E.; Addis, P. B. Poultry Sci. 1981, 60, 2466-74.
32. Csallany, A. S.; Guan, M. D.; Manwaring, J. D.; Addis, P. B. J. Chromatography 1983 (submitted).
33. Shamberger, R. J.; Shamberger, B. A.; Willis, C. E. J. Nutr. 1977, 107, 1404-9.
34. Siu, G. M.; Draper, H. H. J. Food Sci. 1978, 43, 1147-9.

35. Taylor, C. B.; Peng, S-K.; Werthessen, N. T.; Tham, P.;
     Lee, K. T. Am. J. Clin. Nutr. 1979, 32, 40-57.
36. Acker, L.; Greve, H. Fette Seif. Anstrich. 1963, 1009.
37. Chicoye, E.; Powrie, W. D.; Fennema, O. J. Food Sci.
     1968, 33, 581-7.
38. Tsai, L. S.; Ijichi, K.; Hudson, C. A.; Meehan, J. J.
     Lipids 1980, 15, 124-8.
39. Ryan, T. C.; Gary, J. I.; Morton, I. D. J. Sci. Food
     Agric. 1981, 32, 305-8.
40. Imai, H.; Werthessen, N. T.; Taylor, C. B.; Lee, K. T.
     Arch. Path. Lab. Med. 1976, 100, 565-72.
41. Peng, S. K.; Taylor, C. B.; Tham, P.; Werthessen, N. T.;
     Mikkelson, B. Arch. Path. Lab. Med. 1978, 102, 57-61.
42. Peng, S. K.; Tham, P.; Taylor, C. B.; Mikkelson, B. Am.
     J. Clin. Nutr. 1033-42.
43. Seifter, J.; Baeder, D. H. Proc. Soc. Exptl. Biol. Med.
     1956, 91, 42.
44. Gray, M. F.; Laurie, T. D. V. Lipids 1971, 6, 836-43.
45. Fieser, L. F. J. Am. Chem. Soc. 1953, 75, 5421.
46. Peng, S-K.; Taylor, C. B.; Mosbach, E. H.; Huang, W. Y.;
     Hill, J.; Mikkelson, B. Atherosclerosis 1982, 41,
     395-402.
47. Smith, L. L. "Cholesterol Autoxidation"; Plenum, New York.
48. Simic, M. G.; Karel, M. "Autoxidation in Food and Biological
     Systems"; Plenum, New York.
49. Roffo, A. H. Am. J. Cancer. 1933, 17, 42-57.
50. Rosenheim, O.; Starling. W. W. Chem. & Ind. (London)
     1933, 52, 1056
51. Windaus, A.; Luders, H. Z. Physiol. Chem. 1920, 109,
     183.
52. Haslewood, G. A. D. Biochem. J. 1941, 35, 708.
53. Bergstrom, S.; Samuelson, B. Chp. 6, 233-48 (1961),
     "Autoxidation And Antioxidants Volume I." Ed. Lundberg,
     W.O.; Interscience Publishers, New York and London.
54. Bischoff, F.; Rupp, J. J. Cancer Res. 1946, 6, 403-9.
55. Fieser, L. F. Science 1954, 119, 710-6.
56. Bergstrom, S.; Wintersteiner, O. J. Biol. Chem. (1941)
     141, 597-610.
57. Mosbach, E. H.; Neirenberg, M.; Kendall, F. E.
     (Abstract) Am. Chem. Soc. 10 C, Sept. (1952).
58. Bischoff, F. J. Nat. Cancer Inst. (1957) 19, 977-8 .
59. Hieger, I. Brit. J. Cancer 1949, 3, 123-39.
60. Hieger, I. Brit. Med. Bull. 1958, 14, 159-60.
61. Bischoff, F.; Bryson, G. (Abst.) Am. Chem Soc. 62 C,
     Sept. (1960).
62. Bischoff, F. Progr. Exp. Tumor Res. 1963, 3, 412-44.
63. Bischoff, F. Adv. Lipid Res. 1969, 7, 165-244.
64. Bischoff, F.; Bryson, G. Adv. Lipid Res. 1977, 15,
     61-155.
65. Dunn, T. B.; Heston, W. E.; Deringer, M. K. J. Nat. Cancer
     Inst. 1956, 17, 639-47.

66. Bryson, G.; Bischoff, F. Progr. Exptl. Tumor Res. 1969, 11, 100.
67. Lo, Wan-Bang; Black, H. S. J. Invest. Derm. 1972, 58, 278-83.
68. Black, H. S.; Douglas, D. R. Cancer Res. 1972, 32, 2630-2.
69. Black, H. S.; Douglas, D. R. Cancer Res. 1973, 33, 2094-6.
70. Chan, J. T.; Black, H. S. Science 1974, 186, 1216-7.
71. Lo, Wan-Bang; Black, H. S.; Knox, J. M. Clin. Res. 1974, 22, 618A.
72. Lo, Wan-Bang; Black, H. S. Nature 1973, 246, 489-91.
73. Black, H. S.; Chan, J. T. J. Invest. Derm. 1975, 65, 412-4.
74. Black, H. S.; Chan, J. T. Oncology 1976, 33, 119-22.
75. Anon. "Mutagen Implicated in Human Colon Cancer"; Chem. Eng. News. 1982, 60, 22-3.
76. Reddy, B. S. Cancer Res. 1981, 41, 3766-8.
77. Drasar, B. S.; Irving, D. Brit. J. Cancer 1973, 27, 167-72.
78. Reddy, B. S.; Sharma, C.; Darby, L.; Laakso, K.; Wynder, E. L. Mutation Res. 1980, 72, 511.
79. Bruce, W. R.; Varghese, A. J.; Furrer, R.; Land, P. C. "A mutagen in the feces of normal humans." In: H. H. Hiatt; J. D. Watson; J. A. Winsten (eds.,). Origins of human cancer, 1641-6 Cold Spring Harbor, N.Y.: Cold Spring Harbor Laboratory (1977).
80. Reddy, B. S.; Wynder, E. L. Cancer 1977, 39, 2533-9.
81. Hill, M. J. Digestion 1974, 11, 289-306.
82. Wynder, E. L.; Kajitani, T.; Iskikawa, S.; Dodo, H.; Takano, A. Cancer, (Philad.) 1969, 23, 1210-20.
83. Hill, M. J.; H. H. Hiatt; J. Watson; J. A. Winstein (eds.) pp. 1627-40. Cold Spring Harbor, N.Y.: Cold Spring Harbor Laboratory (1977).
84. Hill, M. J.; Drasar, B. S.; Aries, V. C.; Crowther, J. S.; Hawlsworth, G. B.; Williams, R. E. O. Lancet 1971, 1 95-100.
85. Reddy, B. S.; Martin, C. W.; Wynder, E. L. Cancer Res. 1977, 37, 1697-1701.
86. Buntain, W. L.; ReMine, W. H.; Farrow, G. M. Surg. Gynecol. Obstet. 1972, 134, 499-508.
87. Lipkin, M. Cancer 1974, 34, 878-88.
88. Reddy, B. S.; Narisawa, T.; Weisburger, J. H.; Wynder, E. L. Natl. Cancer Inst. 1976, 56, 441-2.
89. Reddy, B. S.; Wantanabe, K.; Weisburger, J. H.; Wynder, E. L. Cancer Res. 1977, 37, 3238-42.
90. Reddy, B. S.; Watanabe, K. Cancer Res. 1979, 39, 1521-4.
91. Petrakis, N. L.; Gruenke, L. D.; Craig, J. C. Cancer Res. 1981, 41, 2563-6.

92.   Schaffner, C. P.; Bril, D. R.; Singhall, A. K.   Presence
      epoxy-cholesterols in the aging human prostrate gland as a
      risk factor in cancer.   In: Proceedings Fourth Interna-
      tional Symposium on the Prevention and Detection of Cancer,
      London.   July (1980).
93.   Smith, L. S.; Smart, V. B.; Ansari, G. A. S.   Mutation Res.
      1979, 68, 23-30.

RECEIVED July 11, 1983

Metabolism of Comutagens and Mutagens Produced from Tryptophan Pyrolysis

PAUL P. LAU

Department of Biochemistry and Molecular Biology, University of Texas Medical School at Houston, Houston, TX 77025

YUHSHI LUH[1]

Gulf Research and Development Company, Pittsburgh, PA 15230

Trp-P-2 and Norharman are the mutagen and comutagen shown to be metabolized by the reconstituted, puri-fied rat-liver microsomal cytochrome P-448 system. The comutagenic action of Norharman upon aryl hydro-carbon hydroxylase activity is shown to be cytochrome P-448 dependent by immunochemical analysis. The hydroxylated products of Norharman and Harman may play an important role in their comutagenic action by fluidizing the microsomal or nuclear membranes. The enhancement or inhibitory effect of the comuta-gens on mutagenicity may be a net result of sub-strate inhibition and membrane fluidization in the microsomal or nuclear mixed-function-oxidase system. A schematic pathway is hypothesized for the chemical mutagenesis and comutagenesis of these tryptophan pyrolysis products.

Two potent mutagenic principles, 3-amino-1,4-dimethyl-5H-pyrido(4,3-b)indole, Trp-P-1 and 3-amino-1-methyl-5H-pyrido(4,3-b) indole, Trp-P-2 and two comutagens, Harman and Norharman were found in the pyrolysis of the amino acid, D,L-tryptophan(1).

The same pyrolysis products were also found in charred meat, smoke condensate, cigarette tar and naturally occurring food(2-4). Numerous studies of these pyrolysis products of tryptophan and other amino acids(1) have been reported by Sugimura and coworkers (1,3). Pyrolysates of tryptophan, glutamic acid, lysine, serine and ornithine were shown to have high mutagenicity in the Ames test(5). The chemical structures of these mutagenic principles have been identified(8) and they are all N-containing heterocyclic compounds of three or more rings(8).

During the isolation of these pyrolysis products of the amino acids and proteins from the charred pyrolysates, Sugimura et al.

[1] Current address: Callery Chemical Company, Division of Mine Safety Appliances Co., Callery, PA 16024

(1,2) found that the total mutagenicity decreased after the removal of the fractions containing Harman and Norharman. Norharman
and Harman have found to enhance the mutagenicity of Trp-P-2 and
Trp-P-1, Benzo(a)pyrene and other mutagens. However, other workers
(9,10)found that both Norharman and Harman inhibited the mutagenesis of Trp-P-1 and Trp-P-2 and covalent DNA binding of Benzo(a)
pyrene in vitro. Later, Nagao et al.(5) reported that the action
of Norharman on comutagenesis depended on the chemical structure
of the chemical mutagens and the amount of S-9 (the cytosol
fraction of rat-liver microsomes preparation) that was added
in the Ames test(11,12).

   It has been shown that the expression of mutagenicity and
covalent DNA binding of Trp-P-1 and Trp-P-2 required microsomal
activation in the revertant mutation assay or the forward mutation
assay(13,19). Nebert et al.(14) showed that these pyrolysis products from amino acids and proteins required the cytochrome P-450$_I$
which was defined as the groups of the multiple forms of cytochrome P-450 inducible by polycyclic aromatic compounds. The role
of cytochrome P-450 in the metabolic activation of mutagens and
carcinogens and the existence of the multiple forms of cytochrome
P-450 in hepatic and extrahepatic tissues of rats, rabbits, human
and various living organisms including bacteria, yeast, and
fruit flies(15,16)have been reviewed.

   Hayashi et al.(17) have shown that Norharman and Harman bound
to DNA noncovalently by intercalation causing 17°unwinding of the
supercoiled DNA duplex. We have shown that Trp-P-1 and Trp-P-2
bound to DNA noncovalently(18) in addition to their covalent DNA
binding. The noncovalent DNA binding constants were found to cor-
relate with the mutagenicity in the forward mutation assay(19)
when six other synthetic analogs were studied. The correlation of
noncovalent binding to DNA in the absence of metabolic activation
with mutagenicity in which metabolic activation was required, was
considered as an unique characteristic of these N-containing
heterocyclic compounds. It was also suggested that the mechanism
of mutagenesis involves metabolic activation followed by physio-
chemical interaction with DNA and for these compounds, the latter
step might be limiting for the expression of mutagenicity(19).

   Umezewa et al.(28) showed that there was a comutagenic action
of Norharman on N-acetoxy-aminofluorene(AAF), which does not
require metabolic activation for covalent DNA binding. Therefore
they proposed that the comutagens altered the conformation of DNA
which in turn increased the covalent DNA binding. This meant to
be analogous to the finding of Krugh and Young(21) that Dauno-
rubicin and Adriamycin which intercalate DNA covalently, facilitate the binding of Actinomycin D to DNA. We, however, have shown
that the alteration of the DNA helix by intercalation of Harman
or Norharman did not affect the affinity of Trp-P-1 and Trp-P-2
for DNA. The covalent DNA binding in which metabolic activation
by cytochrome P-448 was required, was shown to be inhibited by
the addition of Harman and Norharman(18).

The confusion on the mechanism of the comutagenesis and mutagenesis of these pyrolysis products, especially pertaining to the
enhancement and inhibition effects of Harman and Norharman,centers
around the problem of the lack of certain fixed variables in the
experimentation, particularly, the availability of the purified
enzymes involved in the metabolic activation, which constitute
the cytochrome P-450 mixed function oxidase system. We, therefore,
undertake this problem to elucidate the mechanism of microsomal
metabolism of these pyrolysis products with the purified mixed
function oxidase(MFO) system.

Materials and Methods

Materials: Harman and Norharman were purchased from Aldrich Co.
(Milwaukee, WIS). All chemicals were reagent-graded. HPLC solvents
were HPLC graded.

Synthesis of Chemical Mutagens: Akimoto et al(20) reported the
first syntheses of potent mutagens, Trp-P-1 and Trp-P-2 in 1977.
The synthetic schemes for Trp-P-1, [1], and Trp-P-2, [2] were
shown in figure 1.
2,5-Dimethyl-4 -nitropicolinic acid [4] was readily(21)
prepared from commercially available 2,5-lutidine [3]. The reactive nitro group of picolinic acid [4] was smoothly substituted
with O-phenylenediamine to give m-aminopicolinic acid[5]. Treatment of [5] with nitrous acid resulted a benzotriazolylpicolinic
[6] in quantitative yield. The carboxylic acid group on [6] was
easily transformed to an amino group via Curtius rearrangement by
DPPA method(22), producing [7]. Thermal decomposition of [7] to
evolve nitrogen in the usual way(23)yielded the desired compound,
3-amino-1,4-dimethyl-5H-pyrido(4,3-b)indole[1]; m/e 211(M^+);νmax
(KBr): 1620,1600 cm^{-1}; δ (CD$_3$OD): 3.32(3H,S), 2.73(3H,S), 7.13-7.33
(3H,m), 7.86(1H,m).
The synthesis of Trp-P-2[2] started with an intermediate,
indole-2-acetonitrile[9](24), prepared from commercially available
indole-2-carboxylic acid[8]. Vilsmeier reaction(25) of [9], with
dimethylacetamideand phosphoryl chloride, gave 3-acetylindole-2-
acetonitrile[10]. Cyclization of [10] on treatment with methanolic
ammonia and aromatization involving a hydrogen transfer of the
α-methylene group yielded the desired 3-amino-1-methyl-5H-pyrido
(4,3b)indole[2]; m/e 197(M+); νmax(KBr) :1635,1605 cm^{-1}; δ (CD$_3$OD):
2.3(3H,s), 5.92(1H,s), 6.53-7.00(3H,m), 7.35(1H,d).
Takeda et al(26) prepared mutagen Trp-P-2 in an alternative
way as shown in figure 2.
Indole-2-acetonitrile[9] prepared from the Reissert compound
(27). Ethyl 2-cyano-1,2dihydroquinoline-1-carboxylate[11] was
chosen as an intermediate for the synthesis of Trp-P-2. The photo-
product from irradiation of [11] in ether at 0-5ºC is the allene
[12]. Treatment of [12] with alumina or silica gel gave[13]. This
step is considered to proceed by base or acid catalyzed intra-

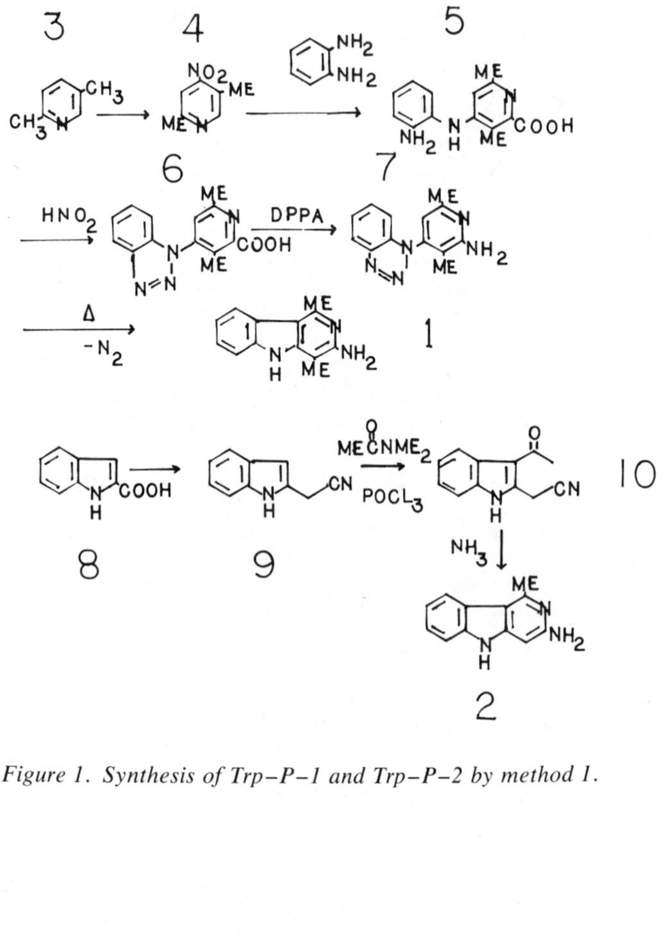

Figure 1. Synthesis of Trp–P–1 and Trp–P–2 by method 1.

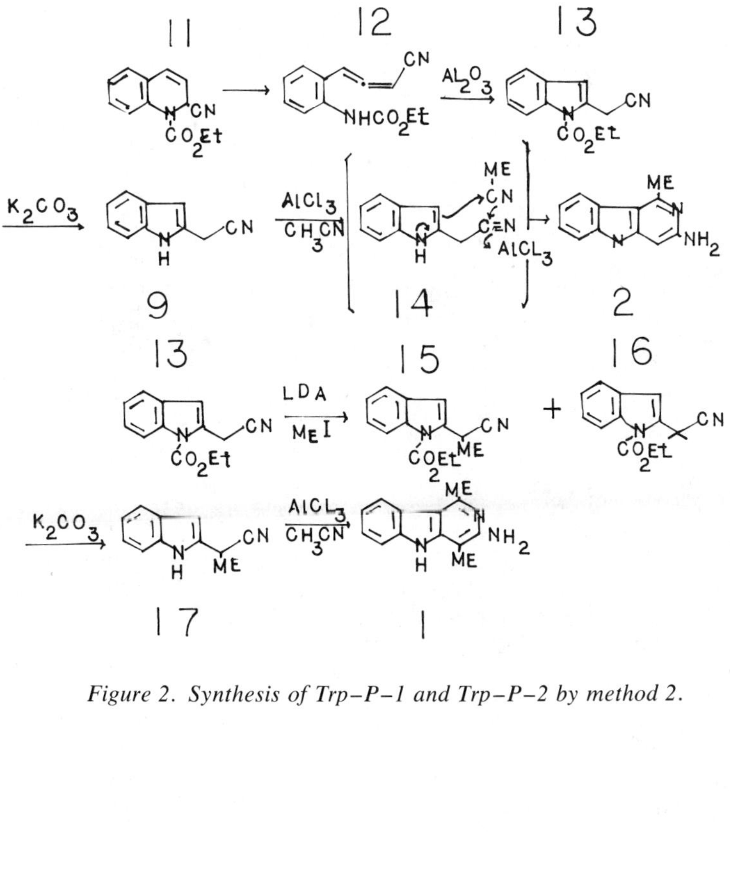

Figure 2. Synthesis of Trp–P–1 and Trp–P–2 by method 2.

molecular cyclization(29). Removal of the N-1 substituent in
Indole-1-carboxylate(13) by mild hydrolysis with potassium carbonate in ethanol afforded 2-cyanomethyl indole[9]. Subsequent
Lewis acid($AlCl_3$)catalyzed cyclization of [9] in the presence of
acetonitrile yielded Trp-P-2. The formation of [2] from [9] is
proceeded by Friedel-Crafts intermediary of [14] followed by
aromatization via hydrogen migration.

The successful synthesis of Trp-P-2 from 2-cyanomethylindole
[9] allowed us to envisage similar sequences to afford Trp-P-1
from 2-(1-cyano)ethylindole[17]. Due to the nucleophilic properties of the indole ring at C-3 position, an electron-withdrawing
group(eg. carboxylate) is required to eliminate alkylation at
both N-1 and C-3 positions in favor of C-2atom to the desired
configuration. The readily available N-substituted 2-cyanomethyl-
indole[13] was selected as starting material for our new procedure
for the synthesis of Trp-P-1 as shown in Figure 2.

Akylation of [13] with methyliodide gave a mixture of mono-
[15] and di-alkylated products [16] with sodium hydride as the
base. By employing lithium diisopropylimide(LDA) in dry THF at
-78°C, a sole product of ethyl 2-(1-cyano)ethyl-indole-1-carbo-
xylate[15] was obtained. The selective alkylation in this step
is due to the steric effect of bulky LDA molecule to suppress
second alkylation. Mild hydrolysis of [15] in the same fashion
with dry ethanolic potassium carbonate gave [17] in good yield.

Preparation of Enzymes: Preparation of rat-liver microsomes was
performed as described(30). Purification of cytochrome P-450 and
separation of the multiple forms were done as described previously
by Lau and Strobel(30). Antibody, IgG fraction was prepared as
described(30). P-450 reductase was prepared according to the
procedure of Dignam and Strobel(31). The reconstitution of the
MFO system with the purified cytochrome P-450, cytochrome P-450
reductase and phospholipid vesicles was performed according to
Lu and Coon(32). Cytochrome P-448 was prepared from 3-MC microsomes of mature Sprague-Dawley rats. The hepatic cytochrome P-448
prepared from these microsomes induced by 3-methylcholanthrene
are indentical immunologically and structurally to those by
β Naphthoflavone as shown by Lau et al(33).The same form of cytochrome P-448 has been purified from other induced microsomes such
as those by PCB and TCDD(34).

Microsomal Metabolism: A typical reaction of microsomal metabolism or metabolism by the purified and reconstituted MFO system
contained 1 ml of aqueous solution:0.075 vol. of drug in methanol,
0.1 mol potassium phosphate(pH7.4), 10μmol $MgCl_2$, 0.75μmol NADPH
and 0.15 vol of the enzyme system. Incubation at 37°C for ten
min was terminated by the addition of 1 ml of acetone on ice and
the metabolites were extracted twice with ethyl acetate. Dry
M_gSO_4 was added and the liquid portion was dried with a stream
of nitrogen gas. All of these reactions were carried out under
the yellow light.

When the antibody to cytochrome P-450 was involved in the experiment, the P-450 IgG fraction was added to the crude microsomes before the addition of the drug and NADPH. The HPLC analyses were performed as described.(35)

Results and Discussion

Microsomal Metabolism of Trp-P-2: Trp-P-2 and AAF were metabolized by the 3-MC rat-liver microsomes in vitro. The extracts with benzene, diethyl ether, ethyl acetate and ethylene chloride were dried before injection onto a reverse-phase µBondapak C-18 column. The HPLC profiles of the metabolites of Trp-P-2 and AAF are very similar(figure 3). These metabolites of Trp-P-2 have the same fluorescence spectra with emission maximum at 332 nm. The UV spectra are identical to that of Trp-P-2, that is, with a maximum at 260 nm.

The peak, which has the same retention time as that of the N-OH product in the AAF profile, may be the N-OH metabolite of Trp-P-2. Detailed chemical characterization of each peak is underway. The similarity of the metabolic profiles of these two carcinogens is not unexpected as they have similar chemical structures. Cytochrome P-450s are known to perform N-hydroxylation, arene oxidation and demethylation(15,16). These functions should not be interfered with by the internal nitrogens in the polycyclic ring such as those in the Trp-P-2. It is not surprising to see similar metabolic profiles for Trp-P-2 and AAF.

Microsomal Metabolism of Norharman: Crude 3-MC microsomes metabolized norharman in vitro, as shown in Figure 4. The major metabolites of norharman were eluted at earlier retention times than the parent compound. They could be some hydroxylated products as they showed more polar potential in the reverse-phase chromatography.

The significance of microsomal metabolism of norharman is based on our earlier hypothesis that norharman might utilize the same microsomal enzymes as Trp-P-2(18). Peura et al(36) has shown an increased membrane fluidity caused by tetrahydro-β-carbolines(tetrahydroharman) in a recent publication. This suggests that norharman, after it is hydroxylated, acts as a fluidizing agent for the microsomal membrane which in turn could increase the activity of cytochrome P-450 and the membrane embedded cytochrome P-450-reductase. The change of activity due to fluidization of the microsomal membrane may be dependent upon the concentration of the microsomal proteins as well as the amount of the comutagens and mutagens added. Whether it results in a total net increase or decrease may well depend on the balancing of the effect of substrate inhibition and that of enhancement due to fluidization of the microsomal membrane.

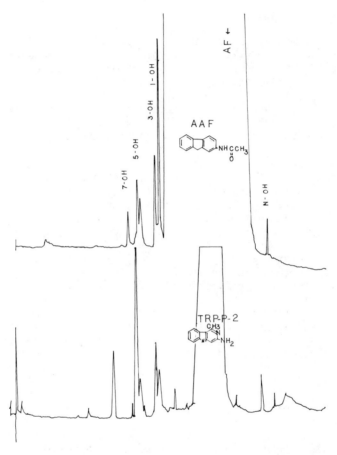

Figure 3. Microsomal metabolism of Trp–P–2 and AAF. HPLC profiles of organic solvent extracts of the metabolized mutagens. Rat livers (3-MC microsomes) were used. HPLC was performed with a stainless steel reverse phase C-18 column.

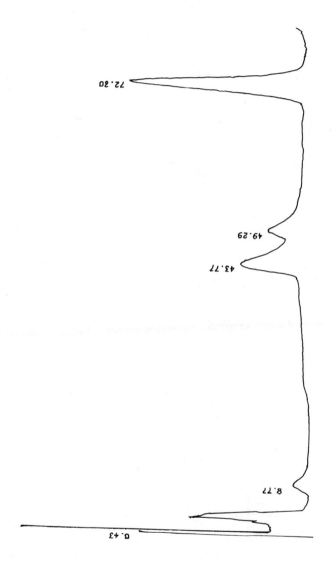

Figure 4. Microsomal metabolism of norharman. HPLC profile of ethyl acetate extract. A similar reaction was performed for control, in which microsomes were not added and there were no metabolites eluted. HPLC was performed with a C-18 radial compression module.

Comutagenic Action of Harman and Norharman: When the reconstituted MFO system, which contained 3-MC induced cytochrome P-448,
was used to study the effects of Norharman and Harman on the
hydroxylation of Benzo(a)pyrene, they both showed an enhancement
effect under the optimal enzymatic conditions. Norharman, however,
showed a larger activity increase in Benzo(a)pyrene hydroxylation
than Harman(Figure 5). It ascertains that the inhibitory effects
of these carbolines on mutagenicity are not dependent on cytochrome P-448 in the sense of simple substrate inhibition.
    One may argue that there could be some contribution of the
comutagenic activity played by the other multiple forms of cytochrome P-450 than that of cytochrome P-448 in the 3-MC microsomes.
It is true that there are two other major forms of cytochrome
P-450 have been purified from 3-MC induced rat-liver microsomes
(34) and four other major forms other than cytochrome P-448 have
been purified from β Naphthoflavone rat   microsomes(30). Although
the comutagenic actions of these compounds have not been studied
with these purified forms of cytochrome P-450, the availability
of the antibody IgG fraction to the purified cytochrome P-448
allowed us to study this mechanism on the microsomal level.
    The HPLC profiles in Figure 6 shows an overall decrease in
Benzo(a)pyrene metabolite formation upon the addition of IgG P-448
fraction. Interestingly the peak corresponding to the 3,6-dione
decreases in relative percentage of all the ethyl acetate extractable metabolites. When the reconstituted purified cytochrome
P-448 system was used, the presence of Norharman enhanced the
formation of 3,6-dione(Figure 7). The results shown here strongly
suggest that the comutagenic action of Norharman is cytochrome
P-448 dependent.

Conclusion

    There are several postulates that can be made based on the
data shown in this work and those published earlier .

Translocation of Mutagens and Comutagens across Cellular membranes
Is Enhanced by β Carboline Metabolites: γ-Carbolines(Trp-P-1 and
Trp-P-2) and β-carbolines(Harman and Norharman) are readily water
soluble and hence is insoluble, relatively, in hydrophobic
membranes. The β-carbolines after they are hydroxylated can
fluidize membranes therefore it renders the hydrophobic polycyclic such as Benzo(a)pyrene more accessible to the membrane
embedded MFO system. In mammalian cells, this can be a two step
mechanism: The MFO in the endoplasmic reticulum may first hydro-
xylate the comutagens and the hydroxylated comutagens then fluidize the nuclear membrane enabling the hydrophobic polycyclics to
be in contact with the MFO system which is embedded in the nuclear
envelope(37). The activation of mutagens by nuclear cytochrome
P-450 would cause the subsequent DNA binding which then triggers
the initiation of mutagenesis.

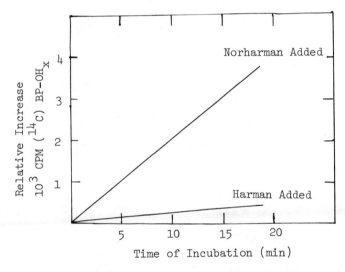

Figure 5. Metabolism of comutagens by cytochrome P-448. The purified enzymes used were the reconstituted cytochrome P-448 system. The relative increase was computed by substrating the ethyl acetate extractable radioactivity in counts per minute from that of a corresponding control experiment in which BP was metabolized in the absence of comutagens.

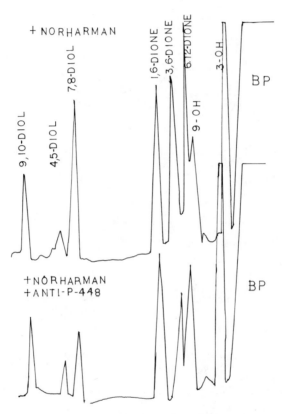

Figure 6. Microsomal metabolism of aryl hydrocarbon in the presence of co-mutagens. HPLC was performed with two connected stainless steel C-18 col-umns.

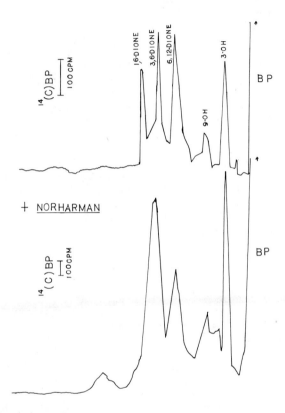

Figure 7. Metabolism of aryl hydrocarbon by the purified cytochrome P-448 in the presence of norharman. HPLC was performed as described in Figure 6.

The Enhancement or the Inhibitory Effect of the β-Carbolines Is
a Net Result of Substrate Inhibition and Membrane Fluidization:
We showed earlier(18) that the presence of Harman or Norharman
did not interfere the reversible noncovalent DNA binding for
Trp-P-2, but inhibited irreversible covalent DNA binding in vitro
upon the metabolic activation by the crude microsomal fraction
isolated from 3-MC pretreated rat livers.
    Drug intercalation stabilizes the DNA duplex. The unstable
A-T rich regions in a DNA duplex normally can have transiently
denatured structure in an otherwise fully duplex in aqueous solution of physicological conditions. Ethidium bromide, a classical
intercalator and a positively charged molecule of planar structure
can even renature fully denatured closed circular DNA(38). The
inhibitory effect of Ethidium bromide upon single stranded DNA
nuclease is another evidence for the stabiliztion of DNA duplex
by the intercalative drug(39). We must recognize that Norharman
and Trp-P-2 being positively charged intercalators also can
stabilize the DNA duplex. If Norharman destabilized the DNA duplex,
the comutagens would not have unwound the supercoiled DNA, In fact,
Norharman was shown to unwind supercoiled DNA(17). Therefore,
we cannot envision that the comutagen binding to DNA would in any
way facilitate the DNA binding of the mutagens either in the
covalent or noncovalent mode.
    The alternative explanation must involve the MFO system. The
possible mechanism for the inhibitory effect or enhancement effect
of Norharman upon covalent DNA binding and mutagenicity must be
the results of the net balancing of substrate inhibition and
membrane fluidization of the microsomal membrane or of the lipid
vesicles in the reconstituted MFO system. A schematic pathway
of the metabolism of these tryptophan pyrolysis products is
postulated as shown in Figure 8.

Plausible Mechanism for Adduct Formation of Trp-P-2 and DNA:
Hashimoto et al(40) have identified one of the major DNA adduct
[2] for Trp-P-2[1](Figure 9). The covalent binding site on the
guanine is at the C-8 position. The exocyclic amino group in
pyrido(4,3b)indoles is a prerequisite for expression of mutagen-
icity(19). Since the structurally related 2-aminofluorene(AF)[3]
exerts mutagenicity through the activated species N-hydroxy-AF[4],
it seems that the mutagenic pyrido(4,3-b)indoles may be activated
in the same fashion since the exocyclic amino group is required in
the expression of the mutagenicity for Trp-P-2. As we have shown
that a peak of similar retention as that of the N-OH AF was
observed in the Trp-P-2 profile and, the well known function of
N-demethylation by the hydroxylation of the cytochrome P-450 system,
we thus propose the following mechanism for the C-8 guanine adduct
formation:
    It is quite plausible that the metabolically activated Trp-P-2
is the corresponding hydroxylamine [5] or its esters [6]. The
electron-deficiency nature of imino group in guanine molecule may

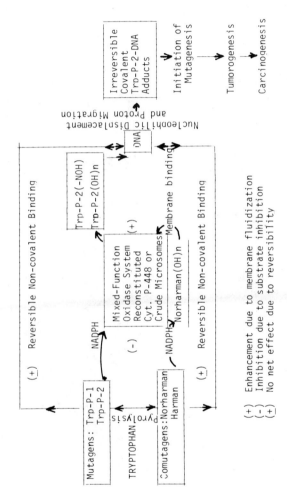

Figure 8. A schematic pathway for the chemical mutagenesis and comutagenesis of the tryptophan pyrolysis products.

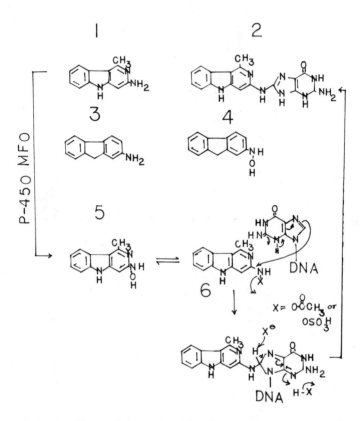

Figure 9. A plausible mechanism for adduct formation of Trp–P–2 and DNA.

create the nucleophilicity of the C-8 atom in that molecule through electron-proton shift. Nucleophilic displacement of good leaving groups such as, carboxylate or sulfate esters, in the activated Trp-P-2 by guanine at the C-8 position, followed by a proton migration, would give the identified adduct [2].

Literature Cited

1. Kosuge, T., Tsuji, K., Wakabayashi, K., Okamoto, T., Shudo,K., Titaka, Y., Itai, A., Sugimura, T., Kawachi, T., Nagao,M., Yahagi, T., and Seino, Y. Chem. Pharm. Bull. 1978, 26, 611-9.
2. Sugimura, T., Kosuge, T., Tsuji, K., Wakabayashi, K., Iitaka, Y., and Itai, A. Proc. Japan Acad. Sci.1977,53,58.
3. Sugimura, T., Sato, S., Nagao, M., Yahagi, T., Matsushuima,T., Seino, Y., Takeuchim T."Fundamentals in Cancer Prevention"; University of Tokyo Press, Tokyo, 1976;191-215.
4. Poindexter, E. H. and Carpenter, R.D.Phytochemistry,1962,1, 215-221.
5. Nagao, M., Honda, M.,Seino,Y., Yahagi,T. and Sugimura, T. Cancer Letters, 1977,2,221-226.
6. Matsumoto, T., Yoshida, D., Mizusaki, S. and Okamoto H. Mutat. Res. 1977,481,279-286.
7. Akimoto, H., Kawai, A., Nomura, H.,Nagao, M., Kawachi, T., and Sugimura, T. Chem. Lett. 1977, 1061-4.
8. Sugimura, T., Nagao,M., Kawachi, T., Honda, M., Yahagi, T., Seino, Y., Sato, S. and Matsukura, N. in "Origins of Human Cancer", Hiatt, H.H., Watson, J.D. and Winsten, J.A.(Cold Spring Harbor Laboratory, Cold Spring Harbor, NY), Eds., 1977,1561-1577.
9. Levitt, R.C., Legraverend, C., Nebert, D. W., and Pelkonen, O. Biochem. Biophys. Res. Comm. 1977, 79, 1167-75.
10. Chang, C., Castellazzi,M., Glover, T.W. and Trosko, J. E. Cancer Res. 1978, 38, 4527-33.
11. Ames, B.N. Sims, P. and Grover, P.L. Science, 1972,176,47-9.
12. Ames, B.N., Gurney, E. G., Miller, J. A. and Bartsch, H. Proc. Natl. Acad. Sci. USA 1972, 69, 3128-32.
13. Skopek, T. R., Liber, H. L., Krolewski, J. J. and Thilly, W. G. Proc. Natl. Acad. Sci. USA 1978, 75, 410-4.
15. Coon, M.J., Vermilion, J. L., Vatsis, K. P., French, J.S., Dean, W. L.,and Haugen, D. A."Concepts in Drug Metabolism" Ed., Jerina, D.M.ACS Series, Washington.D. C., 1977; p.46-71.
16. Coon, M.J., and Vatsis, K.P."Polycyclic Hydrocarbons and Cancer"Gelboin, H.V., and Tso, P.O.P., Eds; Academic Press: New York,1978,, Vol. I, p.335-360.
17. Hayashi, K., Nagao, M. and Sugimura, T. Nucl. Acid. Res.1977, 4, 3679-85.
18. Lau, P. P. and Luh, Y. Biochem. Biophy. Res. Comm. 1979,89(1), 188-194.
19. Pezzuto,J.M., Lau, P. P., Luh, Y., Moore,P.D;Wogan,G,N.and Hecht,S.Proc.Natl.Acad.Sci.USA.1980,77,1427-31.

20. Akimoto,H., Kawai, A. and Nomura, H. Chem. Lett. 1977,1061-4.
21. Matsumura, E., Ariza,M. and Ohifuji,T.Bull. Chem. Soc.Japan,
    1970,43,3210.
22. Ninomiya, K., Shioiri, T., and Yamada, S.Chem. Pharm. Bull.
    (Tokyo) 1974, 22, 1398.
23. Robinson, R.and Thornley, J. Chem. Soc. 1925, 125,2169.
24. Schindler, W. Helv. Chim. Acta.1957, 40, 2156.
25. Antony, W. C. J. Org. Chem. 1960, 25, 2409.
26. Takeda, K., Ohta, T., Shudo, K., Okamoto,T., Tsuji, K. and
    Kosuge, T. Chem. Pharm. Bull. Japan, 1977, 25(6), 2145-6.
27. Ikeda, M., Matsugashita, S. and Tamura, Y., J. Chem. Soc.
    Perkin Trans I, 1976,2587-90.
28. Umezewa, K., Shirai, A., Matsushima, T., and Sugimura, T.
    Proc. Natl. Acad. Sci. USA. 1978, 75, 928-30.
29. Caserio, M.C."Selective Organic Transformations" Thygarayan,
    Wiley,Eds; London, Vol I, p.272.
30. Lau, P. P. and Strobel, H. W. J. Biol. Chemistry,1982,257(9),
    5257-62.
31. Dignam, J. D., and Strobel, H.W. Biochemistry, 1977,16,1116-
    23.
32. Lu, A.Y.H., Strobel, H.,and Coon, M.J. Mol. Pharmacol.1970,
    6, 213-220.
33. Lau, P. P., Pickett, C.B., Lu, A.Y.H. and Strobel, H.W.
    Arch. Biochem. Biophys. 1982, 218(2), 472-7.
34. Ryan, D. E., Thomas, P. E., Korzeniowski, D. and Levin, W.
    J. Biol. Chem. 1979, 254, 1365-74.
35. Holder, G., Yagi, H., Dansette, P., Jerina, D. M., Levin, W.,
    Lu, A.Y.H. and Conney, A.H. Proc. Natl. Acad. Sci. USA 1974
    71(11), 4356-60.
36. Peura, P., Mackenzie, P., Koivusaari, U.and Lang, M. Mol.
    Pharm. 1982, 22, 721-24.
37. Bresnick, E., Vaught, J. B., Chuang, A.H.L., Stoming, T.A.
    Bockman, D. and Mukhtar, H. Arch. Biochem. Biophys. 1977,181,
    257-69.
38. Lau, P. P. and Gray, H. B. Nucl. Acid. Res. 1980, 8, 673-701.
39. Lau, P. P. and Gray, H. B. Nucl. Acid. Res. 1979, 6, 331-57.
40. Hashimoto, Y., Shudo, K., and Okamoto, T. Chem. Pharm. Bull.
    1979, 27(4), 1058-60.

RECEIVED June 3, 1983

Mutagen Formation in Processed Foods

C. A. KRONE and W. T. IWAOKA[1]

Institute for Food Science and Technology, University of Washington (WH-10),
Seattle, WA 98195

The role of cooking in the formation of mutagenic
substances in food is well established. Broiling,
grilling and frying of foods, especially those high
in protein, can produce substances which cause
mutation in bacterial and mammalian in vitro systems.
A large class of foods which also undergoes heat
treatment but which has been overlooked in mutagen
studies is commercially processed foods. This paper
describes a survey of mutagenicity in various
commercially heated foods, investigates the process
of mutagen formation in two canned products and
discusses the implications for the food industry and
regulatory agencies if the mutagens formed during
processing are eventually found to be carcinogenic.

Many carcinogens and mutagens have been detected in cooked foods.
These compounds may be present as a result of smoke condensation
on the product during heat treatment or of thermal degradation of
food components. The crust of charcoal-broiled beefsteak can
contain between 8 and 50 µg benzo(a)pyrene/kg (1). Wood smoked
meats and fish contain a variety of polycyclic aromatic hydrocarbons (2). Fish and beef grilled over a gas flame contain
substances which are mutagenic in the Ames Salmonella assay (3).
Some of these mutagens have been identified as pyrolysis products
of the amino acids tryptophan and glutamic acid (4,5). The
potent mutagens 2-amino-3 methylimidazo [4,5-f] quinoline (IQ),
2-amino-3,4 -dimethylimidazo [4,5-f] quinoline (MeIQ) and 2-amino-
3, 8-dimethylimidazo [4,5-f] quinoxaline (Me-IQ$_x$) were also
isolated from broiled fish and beef (6,7). The above heat treatments used temperatures >300°C; however, mutagenic substances can
also form when foods are cooked at the lower temperatures more
commonly employed in North America. Felton et al.(8) have shown

[1] Current address: Department of Biochemistry and Biophysics, University of Hawaii
at Manoa, Honolulu, HI 96822

that mutagens are formed in a wide variety of beef, pork, poultry, fish and egg products when they are broiled or fried at 200-300°C. Both the length of cooking time and temperature have been shown to be important factors in mutagen formation during cooking. Pariza et al. (9) found that ground beef fried at 143°C contained few mutagenic substances even after cooking for 20 min to a well done state. However, frying at 190°C for less than 10 min led to significant quantities of mutagens. Krone and Iwaoka (10) showed that the mutagenicity of fish fried at 190°C increased rapidly after a 6 min lag period. In general, longer cooking times and higher temperatures increase the extent of mutagen formation during cooking.

The Maillard browning reaction is also often implicated in the development of mutagens in heated foods. Dichloromethane extracts of browning reaction model systems (heated sugar plus amine mixtures) are mutagenic in the Ames test using S. typhimurium strains TA98 and TA100 with and without microsomal activation (11,12). Substances which induced chromosome aberrations in Chinese hamster ovary (CHO) cells and mitotic recombinations and mutation in Saccharomyces cerevisiae strain D5 are also found in these browning model systems (13). Caramelized sugars and commercial caramel powder (used as a colorant in beverages, beer, gravy mixes, soups, etc.) possess chromosome damaging activity in CHO cells (14). Mutagens were reported to be present in heated high starch content foods (potatoes, pancakes, biscuits, toasted bread) and were attributed to browning reactions (15). These mutagens may, however, have been artifacts, caused by the use of ammonium ions ($(NH_4)_2SO_4$ and NH_4OH) in the mutagen extraction procedure. It has been shown by Iwaoka et al (16) that when sodium analogs of the ammonium compounds (Na_2SO_4 vs. $(NH_4)_2SO_4$ and NaOH vs. NH_4OH) were used, no mutagens detected in a commercial biscuit product. Significant quantities of mutagens were produced when ammonium ions were present during the extraction of the same biscuit product. In a limited survey of foods which had undergone Maillard browning (cornflakes, rice cereal, crackers, coconut cookies, bread crumbs), Pariza et al (17) detected low levels of mutagenicity of most products.

Nearly all of the above studies involved heating processes which take place in the home, while foods heat processed at the commercial level have been substantially overlooked. Battered and breaded products (which are partially cooked before freezing and distribution) undergo Maillard browning which, as has been mentioned above, can produce mutagenic substances. Canning of food products involves relatively low temperatures compared to frying (~115°C vs. ~200°C) but requires extended processing times of greater than one and one half hours. Considering the influence of both time and temperature, the presence of mutagenically active substances in canned foods seemed probable. This paper reports on the mutagen content of a variety of commercially heated foods and investigates the process of mutagen formation in two canned products.

Materials and Methods

Food Samples. Commercially processed frozen and canned products were purchased at local markets. The frozen products were subjected to the aqueous extraction procedure described below, without further heating (directly from the package) or after being heated by the method recommended by the manufacturer. For the canned products, the entire contents of each can was extracted using the methanol procedure. In the studies on the process of mutagen formation during canning, two products were used, ground beef and pink salmon. These products were placed in 307 x 200.25 size cans, sealed with a vacuum sealer and retorted for 85 min at 117°C. Prior to canning some portions of ground beef were also dispersed in an equal weight of water, the mixture heated to 100°C for 10 min and the solids separated from the stock by filtering through glass wool. The filtered solids and stock were placed in separate cans, sealed and heat processed as above. Several precanning treatments were also performed on fresh pink salmon. The fish were cut into steaks (~2 cm thick) and one portion frozen overnight at -18°C. Fresh and thawed frozen steaks were wrapped in foil and steamed (100°C) for 1 hr. The fluid which left the fish tissue during steaming (stock) was drained from the flesh, and the stock and remaining flesh were packed in separate cans and processed.

Aqueous Extraction Procedure. The frozen products (mostly battered and breaded seafoods) were homogenized with four volumes (w/v) of distilled water, saturated with Na_2SO_4 and adjusted to pH 2.5 with HCl. When the proteins had precipitated the homogenate was filtered through glass wool and Whatman No. 1 filter paper, using slight suction. The filtrate was extracted three times with 20 ml glass distilled dichloromethane (CH_2Cl_2) per 100 ml aqueous to give the acidic organic extract. The aqueous phase was adjusted to pH 10 with 50% NaOH and again partitioned three times with CH_2Cl_2 (basic organic extract). The organic extracts were dried over Na_2SO_4 and evaporated to dryness in a rotary evaporator. The residues were dissolved in a known volume of dimethylsulfoxide (DMSO) and aliquots tested in the Ames assay.

Methanol Extraction Procedure. The canned foods were homogenized with three volumes (w/v) of methanol, the homogenate filtered through Whatman No. 1 filter paper overlaid with glass wool. The methanol was removed from the filtrate by rotary evaporation and the residue that remained was dissolved in a volume of distilled water (w/v) equal to four times the original weight of food product. This aqueous mixture was adjusted to pH 2.5 and partitioned three times with CH_2Cl_2 as in the above procedure. The aqueous phase was made basic (pH 10) and extracted three times.

The CH_2Cl_2 extracts were dried, evaporated and dissolved in DMSO as described previously.

Mutagenicity Testing. Aliquots of each extract equivalent to 80 g of original food product (80 g Eq) were tested for mutagenicity according to the procedure described by Ames et al (18) using Salmonella typhimurium strain 1538, TA98, and TA100. Extracts were tested with and without the addition of 80 μl Arochlor induced rat liver microsome preparation (S9) per plate. Results are reported either as mean revertants produced ± standard deviation (the mean number of spontaneous revertants have been subtracted from the total colonies on each plate) or as a mutagenic activity ratio (MAR) which equals the number of revertants on plates with food extracts divided by the number of spontaneous revertants.

Results and Discussion

In a typical commercial fish stick operation, fish sticks or portions are cut from frozen blocks of flesh, the pieces are breaded and battered, cooked in vegetable oil (~200°C), packaged and refrozen. The degree of browning that occurs during cooking varies with time of cooking, type of breading, etc. Small pieces of breading may be detached during the cooking process, darken rapidly, sometimes adhering to other pieces of product and possibly contributing to mutagen content. The mutagenic activity of the acidic and basic extracts of a variety of battered and breaded seafood products is shown in Table I.

Table I. Mutagenicity of Acidic and Basic Extracts of Seafood Products

	MAR* (80 g Eq)	
Product	Acidic Extract	Basic Extract
Breaded fish fillets	1.8	1.6
Breaded clams	1.3	1.2
Breaded shrimp	1.1	0.9
French fried fish sticks	1.8	2.2
Whitemeat fish in batter	0.4	0.7
Minced shrimp sticks	1.0	1.9

*Mutagenic Activity Ratio = $\dfrac{\text{No. of revertants on plates with extract}}{\text{No. of spontaneous revertants}}$

S. typhimurium strain 1538 with 80 μl S9
(mean spontaneous = 24 revertants)

Using the criterion that an MAR of 2.5 indicates a positive test, none of the products assayed appeared to contain mutagenic substances. In general, when these products were heated both according to manufacturers' instructions and to an overcooked state, mutagen content did not increase appreciably until heated twice the recommended times (Table II).

Table II. Effect of Additional Heating on Mutagenicity of
Processed Seafoods[a]

Product	Heating Method	Time (min)	MAR (80 g Eq)
Breaded fish fillets	--	0	1.6
	Bake (190°C)	20	2.7
	" "	30	2.8
	" "	40[b]	5.9
Breaded shrimp	--	0	0.9
	Deep fry (200°C)	2	0.9
	" " "	4[b]	2.8

[a]Basic extracts with S. typhimurium strain 1538 plus 80 μl S9.
[b]These times are twice the recommended heating times.

Only the most extensively overheated samples (which are nearly charred) began to show significant mutagenicity. The finding that in general these browned foods were nonmutagenic (even though browning model systems do produce mutagens) may indicate that the mutagens are bound to or associated with high molecular compounds and thus not extracted by the procedure used here.

Canned foods are another class of commercially processed foods which are widely consumed by the public. These products are subjected to extensive heat processing to achieve commercial sterility; thus mutagen formation seemed to be a distinct possibility. A variety of canned meat, poultry, seafoods and vegetable products were therefore surveyed for mutagenicity (Tables III and IV).

Extracts of raw products (beef, chicken, turkey, salmon and clams) exhibited no mutagenicity; neither did the extracts of the vegetable products tested (tomatoes, peas, green beans, beets and corn). Beef and beef-containing products generally possessed mutagenic activity while seafoods were more diverse in their mutagenic response; canned pink salmon displayed the highest levels of any of the canned foods tested, tuna packed in water and sardines were without mutagenicity. The chemical identity of the mutagens in these canned products is unknown at this time. They do, however, exhibit the same Salmonella strain specificity and extraction behavior as mutagens found in grilled fish and

Table III. Mutagenicity of Basic Extracts from Selected Canned
Meat and Poultry Products

Products	MAR (80 g Eq)[a]	Product	MAR (80 g Eq)[a]
Beef broth	13.0	Corned beef hash	3.0
Beef stew (retort pouch)	7.4	Spaghetti w/meatballs	2.6
Roast beef hash	6.0	Chunk turkey	2.2
Chili w/beef (brand #1)	4.9	Chunk chicken	1.3
Chili w/beef (brand #2)	4.4	Ham	1.0
Roast beef	4.6	Vienna sausage	0.8

[a] S. typhimurium strain TA98 with S9 mix.

Table IV. Mutagenicity of Basic Extracts from Canned Seafoods

Product	MAR (80 g Eq)[a]	Product	MAR (80 g Eq)[a]
Pink salmon (brand #1)	17.6	Tuna (oil pack)	3.8
Pink salmon (brand #2)	11.9	Minced clams	3.8
Red salmon (brand #1)	8.5	Tuna (water pack)	1.6
Red salmon (brand #2)	7.3	Sardines	1.3
Mackerel	7.2		

[a] S. typhimurium strain TA98 with S9 mix.

beef, several of which have recently been shown to produce hepa-
tomas when fed to rats and mice (19). If the mutagens in the
canned products are also isolated, identified and found to be
carcinogenic, they may pose a risk to humans because of the
significant quantities of canned foods consumed. In the U.S. in
1980 about 3 billion pounds of meat products and 1.4 billion
pounds of seafoods were processed by canning (20). Some of the
implications for the food industry and regulatory agencies if
the substances formed during canning do prove harmful will be
pointed out below.
      The National Research Council in its recent report on Diet,
Nutrition and Cancer (21) urged that efforts be made to reduce or
eliminate mutagens in foods. An understanding of the process of
mutagen formation is essential to the development of methods to
modify mutagen formation during canning. Two products, ground
beef and pink salmon, were subjected to several precanning treatments to investigate the effects on mutagen formation.
      Ground beef was mixed with an equal weight of distilled
water and boiled for 10 min. The solids were then separated from
the fluids (stock) by filtration and portions of each were

extracted immediately or placed in cans, sealed and processed for 85 min at 117°C. Table V shows the results of mutagenicity tests on the basic extracts from these samples.

Table V. Mutagenicity of Ground Beef and Beef Stock

Precanning Treatment	Sample	MAR (80 g Eq)[a]
None	Ground beef (canned)	3.7
Boil	Solids (not canned)	0.9
Boil	Solids (canned)	1.4
Boil	Stock (not canned)	3.2
Boil	Stock (canned)	9.3

[a] S. typhimurium strain 1538 with S9 mix.

Mutagens were formed when ground beef was canned. The mutagenicity decreased when the ground beef was washed with water prior to canning. The wash water (stock) apparently extracted precursors which could form mutagens upon heating; the canned stock produced an MAR more than twice that of the canned untreated meat.

Pink salmon was treated prior to canning by steaming, freezing or combined freezing then steaming. The stock which left the flesh during steaming (13% of the total weight) was collected and also canned. Table VI shows the effects of these precanning treatments on the mutagenicity of canned pink salmon.

Table VI. Variations in Mutagenicity of Salmon After Different Precanning Treatments

Pretreatment/samples	Revertants produced mean ± SD (n=4)	MAR (80 g Eq)[a]
None/flesh (canned)	98 ± 24	4.3
Steam/flesh (not canned)	10 ± 7	1.3
Steam/flesh (canned)	232 ± 37	8.7
Steam/stock (not canned)	11 ± 14	1.4
Steam/stock (canned)	1022 ± 89	35.0
Freeze/flesh (canned)	270 ± 32	10.0
Freeze, steam/flesh (canned)	237 ± 25	8.9
Freeze, steam/flesh (not canned)	18 ± 32	1.6
Freeze, steam/stock (canned)	1182 ± 240	40.4
Freeze, steam/stock (not canned)	36 ± 48	1.2

[a] S. typhimurium strain TA98 with S9 mix (mean spontaneous = 23-30).

The steaming and/or freezing pretreatments all appeared to
increase the mutagenicity of the canned product. These pretreatments would lead to disruption of cells within the tissue,
possibly allowing more intimate contact between the reactants
during the duration of heat processing. During heat processing
of the untreated fresh tissue, the cellular structure also is
disrupted as the heat penetrates the flesh, but this process
occurs rather slowly due to the resistance to heat transfer that
exists in a solid product of this type.

As was the case with the ground beef stock, the canned fish
stock exhibited higher mutagenicity than the flesh. However, the
steaming was not nearly as effective in removing the mutagen
precursors from the fish as washing of the ground beef had been.
This was undoubtedly due in part to the physical form of the
ground beef in which much cellular disruption had taken place due
merely to grinding. The large proportion of water used for
rinsing the beef was probably also an important factor in the
more efficient removal of mutagen precursors. This also, however,
resulted in dilution of the precursors, explaining the apparently
lower mutagenicity of the beef stock compared to the fish stock
(which was equal to only about 13% of the original weight of
fish).

The results of this study with canned foods bring up several
issues which have not been dealt with in the past. Up to the
present time, studies dealing with mutagens in heated foods have
been concerned with mutagens formed during the cooking process.
In that case, the consumer has some control over how he cooks his
food and has a choice of methods which can reduce or eliminate
mutagen production. For example, he can use low temperature
techniques such as microwaving or steaming rather than frying or
grilling. However, the consumer has no choice in the case of
canned foods where the only way to avoid these substances is to
not purchase the product.

If the compounds in canned foods are indeed carcinogenic,
some questions that need to be addressed are, "Should these
compounds be regulated or should the foods be regulated because
of a possible health hazard? If they are to be regulated, what
provisions of the current regulations apply?"

The first legislation that comes to mind is the Delaney
clause because it deals with carcinogens, but when the clause is
closely examined one finds that it deals only with food additives.
Thermal processing adds nothing to the product other than heat.
Heat processing could possibly be compared to food irradiation in
that both are different types of food processing techniques and
food irradiation is considered an "additive" by FDA and subject
to its regulations on additives.

However, heat or thermal processing is not considered an
additive, therefore, the mutagens could also not be dealt with
under Section 409 of the Food, Drug and Cosmetic Act which deals
with unsafe food additives, or Section 406 of the same Act which

deals with tolerances for added poisonous ingredients in foods. These mutagens (or carcinogens) also probably can't be considered a carcinogenic "constituent" as defined in the FDA's latest "constituents" policy where a carcinogenic impurity is allowed to be present with a non-carcinogenic additive.

The section where mutagens/carcinogens formed as a result of processing possibly could be regulated is in Section 402 of the Food, Drug and Cosmetic Act dealing with adulterated food. This section says that: "...A food shall be deemed to be adulterated if it bears or contains any poisonous or deleterious substances which may render it injurious to health ...".

One organization, the Council for Agricultural Science and Technology (CAST), in its report No. 89 (22), decided to categorize naturally occurring carcinogens and carcinogens formed during cooking under this Section 402. Apparently, however, if these carcinogens (naturally occurring or formed) are present in minute concentrations, CAST does not consider them to constitute a threat to public health which would justify action against them. The FDA has stated that in regulating natural potential hazardous constituents, it would consider the benefits of the food and the impact a prohibition would have on the available food supply. The FDA also stated that they would not remove from the food supply a deleterious substance that is a nutrient, widely used and entrenched in the food system unless it posed a significant health risk (23).

The meaning of the phrases, "injurious to health" in Section 402 of the Food, Drug and Cosmetic Act and "significant health risk" mentioned above are vague in reference to occurrences or formation of mutagens in foods and must be clarified before meaningful decisions can be made. For example, does a significant health risk" exist if these mutagens are determined to be mammalian carcinogens but found in low levels in canned foods?

It clearly appears that our current regulations have difficulty in consistently dealing with low and uncertain risks such as we find in canned foods and that we do need a change in the way we evaluate potential hazards in foods. The Food Safety Council's proposed food safety evaluation process (24), in which a systematic sequence is followed for evaluation of the safety of a food component, may be a major step in that direction.

Acknowledgments

This research was supported in part by the University of Washington Sea Grant Office, Institute for Food Science and Technology and the Egtvedt Food Research Fund.

Literature Cited

1. Lijinsky, W.; Shubik, P. Science 1964, 145, 53–55.
2. Howard, J.W.; Tesque, R.T.; White, R.H.; Fry, B.E. J. Am. Oil Chem. Soc. 1966, 49, 596–601.
3. Nagao, M.; Honda, M.; Seino, Y.; Yahagi, T.; Sugimura, T. Cancer Lett. 1977, 2, 221–26.
4. Sugimura, T. "Naturally Occurring Carcinogens–Mutagens and Modulators of Carcinogenesis"; Miller, E.C.; Miller, J.A.; Hirono, I.; Sugimura, T.; Takayama, S., Eds.; University Park Press: Baltimore, 1979, p. 241.
5. Yamamoto, T.; Tsuji, K.; Kosu, T.; Okamoto, T.; Shudo, K.; Takeda, K.; Iitaka, Y.; Yamaguchi, K.; Seino, Y.; Yahagi, T.; Nagao, M.; Sugimura, T. Proc. Jpn. Acad. 1978, 54B, 248–50.
6. Kasai, H.; Yamaizumi, Z.; Wakabayashi, K.; Nagao, M.; Sugimura, T.; Yokoyama, S.; Miyazawa, T.; Spingarn, N.E.; Weisburger, J.H.; Nishimura, S. Proc. Jpn. Acad. 1980, 54B, 278–83.
7. Kasai, H.; Yamaizumi, Z.; Shiomi, T.; Yokoyama, S.; Miyazawa, T.; Wakabayashi, K.; Nagao, M.; Sugimura, T.; Nishimura, S. Chem. Lett. 1981, 485–88.
8. Bjeldanes, L.F.; Morris, M.M.; Felton, J.S.; Healy, S.; Stuermer, D.; Berry, P.; Timourian, H.; Hatch, F.T. Fd. Chem. Toxicol. 1982, 20, 357–69.
9. Pariza, M.W.; Ashoor, S.H.; Chu, F.S.; Lund, D.B. Cancer Lett. 1979, 7, 63–69.
10. Krone, C.A.; Iwaoka, W.T. Cancer Lett. 1981, 14, 93–99.
11. Spingarn, N.E.; Garvie, C.T. J. Agric. Food Chem. 1979, 27(1), 1319–21.
12. Mihara, S.; Shibamoto, T. J. Agric. Food Chem. 1980, 28(1), 62–66.
13. Powrie, W.D.; Wa, C.H.; Rosin, M.P., Stich, H.F. J. Food Sci. 1981, 46, 1433–38.
14. Stich, H.F.; Stich, W.; Rosin, M.P.; Powrie, W.D. Mutation Res. 91, 129–136.
15. Spingarn, N.E.; Slocum, L.A.; Weisburger, J.H. Cancer Lett. 1980, 9, 7–12.
16. Iwaoka, W.T.; Krone, C.A.; Sullivan, J.J.; Meaker, E.H.; Johnson, C.A.; Miyasato, L.S. Cancer Lett. 1981, 11, 225–230.
17. Pariza, M.W.; Ashoor, S.H.; Chu, F.S. Food Cosmet. Toxicol. 1979, 17, 429–30.
18. Ames, B.N.; McCann, J.; Yamasaki, E. Mutation Res. 1975, 31, 347–364.
19. Sugimura, T. Cancer 1982, 49(10), 1970–84.
20. "The Almanac of the Canning, Freezing and Preserving Industries," Edward E. Judge and Sons: Westminster, Maryland, 1981.
21. "Diet, Nutrition and Cancer", National Research Council, National Academy Press: Washington, D.C. 1982.

22. Council for Agricultural Science and Technology. Report No. 89. "Regulations of Potential Carcinogens in the Food Supply"; Ames, Iowa, June 1981.

23. "Regulations of Cancer Causing Food Additives - Time for a Change", Report to Congress of the U.S., Comptroller General, December 1981.

24. Food Safety Council. "A Proposed Food Safety Evaluation Process"; Nutrition Foundation, Inc.: Washington, D.C. 1982, p. 7-8.

RECEIVED June 28, 1983

Biological Properties of Heated Dietary Fats

J. C. ALEXANDER

Department of Nutrition, College of Biological Science, University of Guelph,
Guelph, Ontario, Canada N1G 2W1

Thermal oxidation of dietary fats, with the formation of potentially toxic derivatives during heating and processing, is related to the conditions
used in the home and the food service industry.
During deep-fat frying many volatile and non-
volatile compounds are formed, some of which can be
toxic depending on the level of intake. Many chemical and biological studies have been carried out,
and experimental findings indicate that possible
dietary hazard should be greater as the severity of
the treatment of the fat is increased. Observations with animals fed these fats have shown adverse effects ranging from depression in growth,
diminished feed efficiency, increased liver size,
fatty necrosis of the liver and numerous other organ lesions. Specific effects on biological tissues can be verified by selected techniques including histopathological evaluations, biochemical
parameters, and tissue culture in monolayers.
Fractionation of heated fat samples serves to concentrate a number of the unnatural components, and
incorporation of these materials into rat diets
has enabled experimenters to observe distinct reactions by the animals. Practical processing and
frying operations usually produce low levels of
nutritionally undesirable products, but it is
worthwhile to recognize their possible adverse biological effects.

The biological properties of thermally oxidized fats have
been studied for many years. Evaluation of laboratory-heated and
commercially-used fats in diets for animals have included feed
consumption, weight gain, and feed efficiency (1-4), pathology
(5-9), organ weights (4, 10), enzyme assays (11), and total lipid

content and tissue fatty acid composition (12-15). A variety of thermally oxidized fats was included and results ranged from mild responses to substantial adverse effects on the animals. Questions remain regarding the potential toxicity of laboratory-heated or commercially used frying fats.

Evidence indicates that secondary oxidation products such as monomeric, dimeric and polymeric compounds accumulate in the heated fats and may subsequently be ingested with the fried foods. Johnson et al. (16) observed that thermally oxidized oil is not so rapidly hydrolyzed as the corresponding unheated oil. Nolen (5) found when feeding male dogs diets containing a 15% level of fresh or heated partially hydrogenated soybean oil that the heated fat reduced the absorption, growth rate and feed efficiency. These products rather than peroxides are the principal factors in adverse effects seen with thermally oxidized fats. Paik et al. (17) studied mice dosed with methyl linoleate hydroperoxides or autoxidized methyl linoleate containing secondary oxidation products. Mortality was 50% and 100% respectively. Congestion in tissues, fatty degeneration and necrosis were observed, and the amount of impairment correlated with the type of material fed. The conclusions were confirmed by histopathological observations, and volatile low molecular weight compounds containing carbonyl groups were suspected of being involved. The reactivity of fatty acids increases with the degree of unsaturation, but the distribution and geometry of double bonds also influence the extent of oxidation (18). Double bonds become conjugated or lost as they are involved in reactions forming various secondary products, some of which have been identified as cyclic compounds, scission products, dimers and larger molecules (19-23). The severity of conditions (aeration, temperature and heating time) plays an important role in the degree of deterioration of frying fats (1). Perkins and Kummerow (24) confirmed the earlier observations of Crampton et al. (25) that the non-urea-adductable portion of heated fats was most toxic to animals. These concentrates, containing monomeric and dimeric derivatives, are more toxic than the larger polymers due to better absorption (2, 10, 26). Urea filtrate of heated fat, fed to rats, resulted in a 30% reduction in the oxidation of palmitic acid to CO_2 (27). Animals given low levels of vitamins and thermally oxidized fats in their diet at a fixed protein concentration responded poorly compared to those which received fresh fats and the same amount of vitamins (3). A real positive response was obtained in the presence of the heated fat when the protein level was increased. Tappel (28) suggested that chemical deteriorative effects due to free radicals produced in heated fats (hydroxyl and hydroperoxyl) might be slowed by increased amounts of dietary antioxidants. Fukuzawa and Sato (29) selected 12-keto-oleic acid as a degradation product of lipid peroxidation and compared its effects on rat tissues with those of a vitamin E deficiency. Both increased fluorescent production in the liver, as well as hemolysis and plasma alkaline phosphatase level in the blood.

Because of the severity of some problems reported when experimental animals are fed compounds from thermally oxidized food fats there is justified concern about effects some of these derivatives could have on consumers. Early work which showed adverse effects on animals was complicated by improper protection of the diet leading to vitamin deficiencies. However, in studies with used frying fats, Alexander (30) found that frequent diet preparation and feeding, and the use of antioxidants and refrigeration could avoid these difficulties. In recent years, a number of well conducted studies have produced considerable evidence that oxidized and abused frying fats contain potentially toxic constituents.

Experimental

To evaluate the biological effects of thermally oxidized fats, isolated concentrates of fatty acid derivatives were prepared. Fats used were corn oil (CO) olive oil (OO) low erucic acid rapeseed oil (LE) and lard (LA). The heating conditions were those of Gabriel et al. (7). Each fat was heated in a stainless steel beaker for 72 hr at a controlled temperature of 180°C. Each day it was stirred continuously with a mechanical stirrer for 12 hr and by hand every hr for 12 hr to ensure aeration and mixing. Distillation and urea treatment concentrated the cyclic and branched chain degradation products. Intubation experiments with rats were used as short-term studies to determine the toxicity of the distillable non-urea-adductable (DNUA) fractions obtained from ethyl esters produced from thermally oxidized fats (31,32). A urea adduction method modified from that of Eisenhauer and Beal (33) was used to produce the DNUA concentrates. All rats were intubated daily with 0.5 ml of either DNUA materials from thermally oxidized fats or the respective fresh fats, using a rubber stomach tube (no. 8 catheter) on a syringe. Body weights were recorded daily, and the animals were examined on a regular basis to detect early symptoms of toxicity. After approximately three days, due to morbidity, the animals were killed. Histopathological examination of the heart, liver and kidneys of the rats was carried out to quantitate tissue damage, and lesions in the organs were graded as described by Gabriel et al. (7). Organ weights were recorded and portions were frozen in liquid nitrogen for lipid analysis (34). Fatty acid methyl esters were prepared from the neutral and polar lipid fractions of the organs (35,36) and analyzed for component fatty acids by GLC. Types of lesions found in the tissue sections were graded as to incidence and severity on a scale from zero for normal, to three for necrotic tissue, in the following anatomical structures:

Heart: Myocardial nuclei
                Nuclei of vascular media and endothelium
                Interstitial tissue and myofibers

Liver: Hepatocellular nuclei
                Hepatocellular cytoplasm
                Kupffer and endothelial cells
Kidney: Glomeruli
                Tubules
                Vessels and interstitial tissues
        Animal tissue cells grown in culture medium in the form of a
monolayer are a useful biological living model to observe physiological, morphological or metabolic changes in the presence of
compounds added to the medium. Bird and Alexander (15, 37) reported on effects of thermally oxidized corn oil and olive oil
on in vitro heart cells. The DNUA from fat thermally oxidized as
described earlier (7) was isolated. Free fatty acids from the
fresh fat controls or from the DNUA of the heated fats were prepared (38).
        Primary cultures of neonatal heart cells were prepared from
2-5 day old rats by the method of Rogers (39) as monolayered
coverslip cultures. The hearts were excised aseptically and
transferred to a petri dish containing phosphate-buffered saline.
The tissue was chopped finely and separated into single cells by
trypsinization using 0.25% trypsin solution (15). Leighton tubes
containing a culture medium supplied with 5% fetal calf serum were
seeded with 2 x 10^5 cells/ml of medium. Four day old cultures
were exposed to fresh and heated fatty acid fractions (60 or 100
μg/ml) in the form of an emulsion with bovine serum albumin dissolved in phosphate-buffered saline (PBS). The required concentration of each free fatty acid fraction, dissolved in hexane,
was transferred to a 100 ml sterilized bottle, and the solvent
was evaporated completely. The solution of bovine serum albumin
(40 mg/ml of PBS) was added to the lipid fractions. A ratio of
free fatty acid fraction to bovine serum albumin of 1:60 (w/w)
was maintained. The bottle was screw-capped and incubated at 40°
with occasional shaking for two hr. This incubation was sufficient to obtain an emulsion of free fatty acids ready for administration into the culture medium (15).
        Cellular lipid was extracted by means of the procedure of
Folch et al. (40) and fractionated by thin layer chromatography
(TLC). Glass plates coated with Silica Gel G of 0.5 ml thickness
and a solvent system containing heptane/isopropyl ether/acetic
acid (60:40:3) were used (41). Cultures of heart cells were observed periodically with a Nikon inverted microscrope with phase
contrast optics. For detailed morphology, replicate cultures
also were stained with May-Grunwald-Giemsa stain (42). Intracellular lipid accumulation was assessed subjectively with the
phase contrast microscope, and a numerical scale ranging from zero
to four was used. The zero value was given to cells showing no
lipid droplets, as in those grown in the medium containing 5%
fetal bovine serum without additional lipid. A value of four was
given to a field consisting of cells exhibiting abundant fat
droplets where most of the extranuclear space appeared to be
occupied with lipid (38).

Stained cover slip cultures from each treatment group were observed under the x40 objective to estimate the effect of various treatments on growth pattern and cell morphology. Twenty random fields were selected, and the number of cells in each field, the number of cells in various stages of mitosis, and the number of pyknotic nuclei were recorded. The mitotic index and percent pyknotic cells were calculated as percentages based on the total number of cells observed in 20 random fields and were not average values of replications. The cellular protein was quantitated by the method of Lowry et al. (43) as modified by Oyama and Eagle (44).

Results

Intubation of the rats with three of the heated fat DNUA samples, heated olive oil (HOO), heated lard (HLA) and heated low erucic acid rapeseed oil (HLE) resulted in early signs of physiological stress. Within 10 hr the animals became disoriented and nervous and feed and water consumption were reduced. A loss of body weight was observed. Rats given DNUA from heated corn oil (HCO) were indistinguishable from those given the fresh fats (Table I). Average weight of the animals at the start of the experiment was 59 g.

Table I. Body Weights of Rats Intubated with Different Dietary Fats

Dietary Fat	Body Weight[1] (g)
CO	75[a]
HCO	70[a]
OO	70[a]
HOO	49[b]
LE	62[a]
HLE	48[b]
LA	71[a]
HLA	49[b]

[1]Numbers with the same superscripts are not significantly different ($P < 0.05$).

Gross pathology of animals in the HOO, HLA and HLE groups showed distended stomachs, gastric ulceration, and little ingesta

in the intestines. Interstitial edema was observed in the lungs,
heart and kidneys, as well as multiple focal hemorrhaging of the
liver. All lesions were without scarring, indicative of short
duration. Figures 1 and 2 show the average histological scores
for heart, liver, and kidneys. Although the HCO animals gained
weight and appeared normal their hearts and livers exhibited some
tissue damage. The extreme morbidity observed in the other three
heated fat groups was reflected in the substantial histological
grades for their organs.

The myocardial nuclei were activated and increased in size
with extensive chromatin condensation, but most of the damage to
the heart was confined to interstitial tissues and blood vessel
walls, indicated by disruption of the vascular endothelium
(Figure 3). In the liver there was hepatocellular dissociation
with nuclear activation such as pyknosis, and cytoplasmic vacuolation due to accumulation of fatty material (Figure 4). Numerous mitotic hepatocytes were observed in the kidney. Various
stages of tubulonecrosis were found in the uriniferous tubules
(Figure 5). Cellular and granular debris blocked some of the
tubules.

Tables II and III show relative organ weights expressed as
percent body weight for six rats, and percent organ lipids.

Table II. Relative Organ Weights and Total Organ
Lipids (CORN OIL and OLIVE OIL)[1]

Dietary	Heart		Liver		Kidney	
Fat	Wt. (%)	Lipid (%)	Wt. (%)	Lipid (%)	Wt. (%)	Lipid (%)
CO	0.42^a	5.4^b	3.7^c	7.4^b	1.0^c	5.9^{bc}
HCO	0.44^a	6.1^{ab}	5.4^{bc}	6.3^b	1.3^{ab}	8.4^a
OO	0.43^a	5.1^b	4.3^{bc}	6.6^b	1.2^{bc}	5.5^c
HOO	0.45^a	7.3^a	8.3^a	6.7^b	1.5^a	7.8^{ab}

[1]Numbers with the same superscripts are not significantly different (P<0.05).

No changes in total heart lipids and weights were observed
in the HCO group but the other three fats produced a substantial
increase in amount of lipid. Both livers and kidneys in the test
groups showed weight increases, some of which were highly significant. In certain cases lipid accumulation contributed to these
increases.

Although there were a number of changes in the tissue fatty
acids of the test rats compared to the controls, the most notable

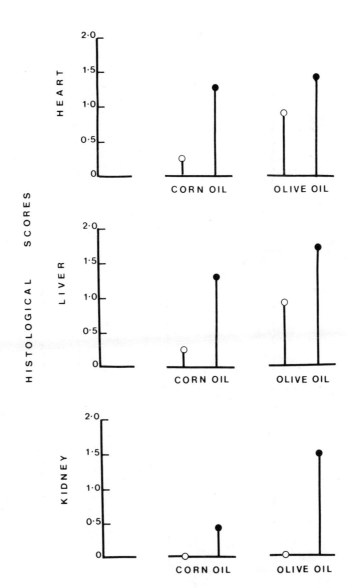

Figure 1. Histological scores for organs of rats intubated with fresh fats (○) or DNUA of heated fats (●). (Reproduced with permission from Ref. 31. Copyright 1979, Geron-X Inc.)

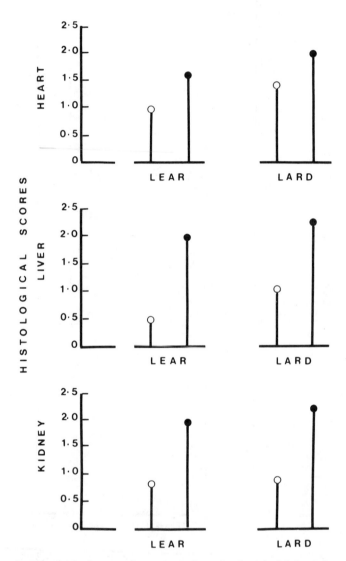

Figure 2. Histological scores for organs of rats intubated with fresh fats (○) or DNUA of heated fats (●). (Reproduced with permission from Ref. 32. Copyright 1979, Geron-X Inc.)

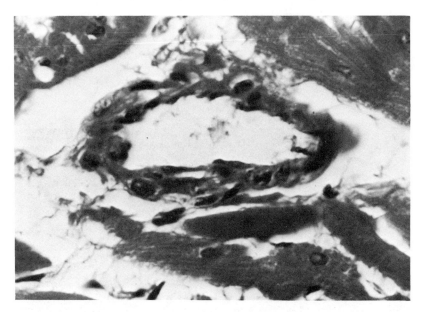

Figure 3. Heart of rat intubated with DNUA–HLA. Blood vessel wall has lost its integrity, and endomysium is very prominent. Hematoxylin and eosin, ×750. (Reproduced with permission from Ref. 32. Copyright 1979, Geron-X Inc.)

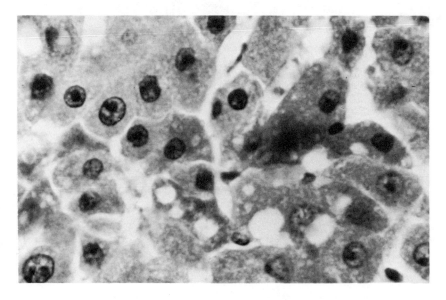

Figure 4. Liver of rat intubated with DNUA–HLA. Pyknosis and fragmentation of necrotic hepatocytes. Hematoxylin and eosin, ×500. (Reproduced with permission from Ref. 32. Copyright 1979, Geron-X Inc.)

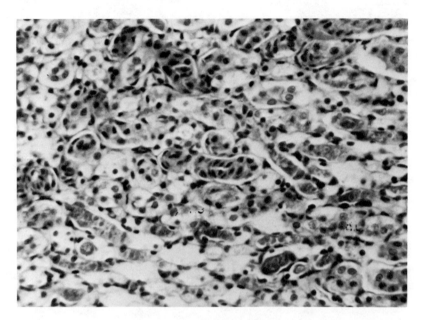

Figure 5. Kidney of rat intubated with DNUA–HLE. Cellular and granular casts fill lumina of uriniferous tubules. Hematoxylin and eosin, ×344. (Reproduced with permission from Ref. 32. Copyright 1979, Geron-X Inc.)

Table III.   Relative Organ Weights and Total Organ
Lipids (LEAR and LARD)[1]

Dietary Fat	Heart Wt. (%)	Heart Lipid (%)	Liver Wt. (%)	Liver Lipid (%)	Kidney Wt. (%)	Kidney Lipid (%)
LE	0.47^a	5.2^b	4.4^b	7.9^a	1.2^{ab}	7.4^a
HLE	0.44^a	9.3^a	7.0^a	7.8^a	1.4^a	5.9^a
LA	0.41^a	4.7^b	4.4^b	5.9^b	1.0^b	6.9^a
HLA	0.42^a	7.7^a	8.8^a	9.5^a	1.6^a	6.7^a

[1]Numbers with the same superscripts are not significantly different (P<0.05).

changes were decreases in neutral heart and kidney lipid oleic acid with concomitant increases in linoleic acid for groups given HOO, HLA and HLE (Tables IV, V and VI). These effects were not observed for the group given HCO.

Table IV.   Fatty Acid Composition of Neutral Heart Lipids

Dietary Fat	Oleic Acid (%)	Linoleic Acid (%)
CO	19.5	36.2
HCO	20.1	35.0
OO	36.4	25.8
HOO	19.1	46.5
LE	34.8	26.4
HLE	19.4	48.2
LA	44.7	18.1
HLA	15.2	51.8

Treatment of cultured rat heart cells with HCO or HOO (15) resulted in lower concentrations of oleic, linoleic and arachidonic acids in the phospholipids (PL). However, there were marked increases in arachidonic acid and decreases in oleic acid in the triacylglycerols (TG), and linoleic acid also declined substan-

Table V.   Fatty Acid Composition of Neutral Liver Lipids

Dietary Fat	Oleic Acid (%)	Linoleic Acid (%)
CO	19.5	32.9
HCO	15.2	29.1
OO	29.6	16.1
HOO	24.7	22.6
LE	30.1	23.1
HLE	26.8	25.2
LA	29.6	22.4
HLA	28.2	24.1

Table VI.   Fatty Acid Composition of Neutral Kidney Lipids

Dietary Fat	Oleic Acid (%)	Linoleic Acid (%)
CO	23.3	36.0
HCO	21.1	30.5
OO	42.1	20.0
HOO	22.3	31.1
LE	37.5	21.1
HLE	30.5	30.4
LA	37.7	22.4
HLA	24.8	32.3

tially due to HCO (Table VII. Pooled samples from four cell cultures were used.

Rat heart cells in culture, exposed to thermally oxidized fat components, (37) took up and incorporated more exogenous 1-^{14}C-palmitic acid into the cell TG fraction that when the cells were treated with fresh fats (Table VIII). Particularly with the HCO compared to CO, much less of the radioactivity from labeled palmitic acid was deposited in the PL fraction. Also with the

Table VII. Fatty Acids of Phospholipid and Triacylglycerol
Fractions of Heart Cells

Treatment	Phospholipid			Triacylglycerol		
	18:1 (%)	18:2 (%)	20:4 (%)	18:1 (%)	18:2 (%)	20:4 (%)
CO	33.4	13.3	4.9	23.2	24.2	10.0
HCO	27.8	6.3	1.7	12.7	2.9	43.4
OO	38.9	5.2	3.5	51.3	7.7	11.7
HOO	22.8	2.3	2.6	13.4	16.9	28.0

Table VIII. Incorporation of ^{14}C-Radioactivity into
Phospholipids and Triacylglycerols of Heart Cells

Treatment	Phospholipid[1]			Triacylglycerol[1]		
	12 (h)	24 (h)	48 (h)	12 (h)	24 (h)	48 (h)
CO	80.4	73.1	65.1	4.2	6.7	8.9
HCO	38.6	43.8	48.4	40.2	28.8	23.4
OO	46.2	46.0	48.8	31.7	31.4	27.3
HOO	38.6	38.4	38.0	42.7	42.8	44.3

[1]Incubation times and average values for five samples.

HCO, when the incubation period was extended beyond 12 hr, there
was a decline in the radioactivity retained in the TG fraction of
the heart cells. When the two fresh fats were compared for ^{14}C
incorporation into the lipid classes, the OO resulted in at least
three times as much activity in the TG fraction.

The most consistent change in cultures exposed to heated fats
was associated with intracellular lipid accumulation, which occurred rapidly (Figure 6). Prolonged exposure produced abnormal
spherical cells filled with lipid droplets. They contained con-
stricted, centrally located nuclei. Karyorrhexis and karyolysis
were observed, and vacuolation and a network appearance were pronounced due to oxidized fat (Figure 7). The pyknotic nuclei as a
percentage of the total number of cells in 20 random fields were
increased due to heated fat fractions (Table IX), and accompanied
the cytoplasmic changes seen earlier. Lipid droplet accumulation
was estimated as shown in Table X, and the free fatty acids from
the fresh fats induced less lipid accumulation. Nevertheless,
the values for OO were as high as those for HCO.

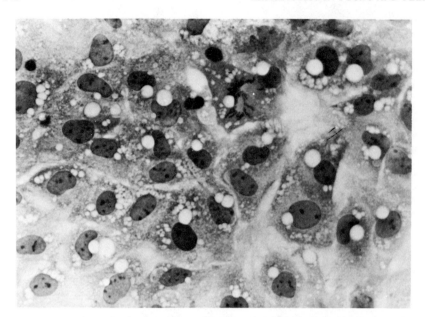

Figure 6. Cell culture from rat heart treated with DNUA–HOO free fatty acids (60 μg/mL) for 48 h. A dividing cell with a broken chromosome can be seen (May-Grunwald-Giemsa, ×400). (Reproduced with permission from Ref. 38. Copyright 1981, Tissue Culture Association Inc.)

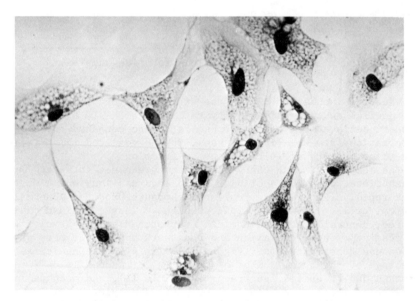

Figure 7. Cell culture from rat heart treated with DNUA–HOO free fatty acids (100 μg/mL) for 96 h. Condensed nuclei and extensively vacuolated cytoplasm can be seen (May-Grunwald-Giemsa, ×400). (Reproduced with permission from Ref. 38. Copyright 1981, Tissue Culture Association Inc.)

Table IX. Percent Pyknotic Cells in Heart Cell Cultures

Treatment	Concentration in Medium	
	60 µg/ml	100 µg/ml
CO	0.28	0.21
HCO	0.54	2.90
OO	0.50	3.50
HOO	0.86	5.90

Table X. Lipid Droplet Accumulation in Heart Cells

Treatment	Concentration in Medium (µg/ml)	Lipid Accumulation Score[1]
CO	60	1.2
HCO		2.6
CO	100	1.4
HCO		3.4
OO	60	2.4
HOO		3.0
OO	100	3.4
HOO		4.0

[1]Obtained by a visual estimation of lipid droplets
in five microscopic fields of heart cells in culture
under an inverted phase contrast microscrope (10 x
40). Range 0 to 4.

Mitotic indices as a percentage of total number of cells in
20 random fields are shown in Table XI. Heated fat suppressed
the rate of mitosis with the greater effect shown by HOO. In
Figure 8, some tripolar spindles were observed among the dividing
cells in the presence of HOO.

Discussion

Toxic properties of thermally oxidized fats are concentrated
in the non-urea adductable monomers and dimers (45, 46). Usual

Table XI. Mitotic Index of Heart Cell Cultures

Treatment	Concentration in Medium (µg/ml)	Percentage of Dividing Cells
CO	60	0.41
HCO		0.31
CO	100	0.35
HCO		0.20
OO	60	0.44
HOO		0.31
OO	100	0.22
HOO		0.14

frying procedures may produce only small quantities of toxic
materials, but such substances may be selectively absorbed in
fried foods (47). With acute animal experiments involving intubation, adverse effects were seen even after the first treatment
indicating rapid absorption. Reduction of feed intake would result in protein-energy deficiency with ensuing weight loss. Components of the DNUA or their metabolites may have depressed feed
intake centers in the brain. Ohfuji and Kandea (48) have documented a feed intake depressing effect of oxidized fats. Increases in relative liver and kidney weights without corresponding
increases in lipid contents may be attributed to some edema of
the organs as well as deposition of protein normally used for
synthesis of new tissue in the hepatocytes. Miller and Landes
(6) found a significant increase in hepatic protein in rats fed
heated soybean oil.

Histological evaluation showed cardiac lesions including
disruption of the endothelial sheath and chromatin condensation
(32) which could lead to impaired oxygen and nutrient transport
into the myocardium. Livers had accumulated lipid in large vacu-
oles in the cytoplasm, and along with necrotic foci there was
invasion by cellular and fibrous elements. In the kidney there
was intense proteinuria, and the lumina of the uriniferous tubules were filled with cellular debris. Tubulonecrosis leads to
impaired filtration and detoxification of the blood.

Alteration of tissue fatty acid concentration by oxidized
fats may indicate the impairment of transport and enzyme systems
by effects on lipoprotein synthesis and function (31). Clark et
al. (49) showed that lipoproteins are susceptible to alterations
of both structure and function by reaction with agents that pro-

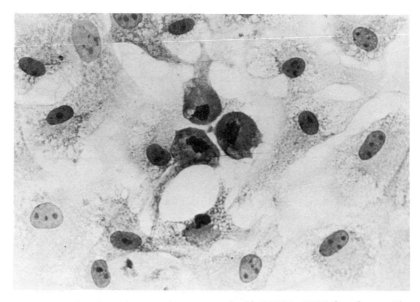

Figure 8. Cell culture from rat heart treated with DNUA–HOO free fatty acids (60 μg/mL) for 48 h. Pyknotic nuclei and tripolar spindle can be seen (May-Grunwald-Giemsa, ×400). (Reproduced with permission from Ref. 38. Copyright 1981, Tissue Culture Association Inc.)

mote lipid peroxidation. The sites of the lesions in major organs could indicate that toxic fatty materials cause an impairment in active transport across membranes and inhibit metabolic activity.

Cultured heart cells responded rapidly to fatty acids administered to the medium. Heated fat produced lower levels of unsaturated fatty acids in the PL fractions, and a greatly increased level of arachidonic acid in the TG fractions (15). In the livers of rats fed heated fats, Rao et al. (50) showed a rapid rate of elongation and desaturation of fatty acid chains.

Palmitic acid is preferentially taken up by the myocardium and used for synthetic reactions or as an energy source (51), and it has been shown to be important in the beating activity of heart cells in culture (52). Treatment of cells with heated fats resulted in a substantially reduced incorporation of labeled palmitic into the PL fraction, and an increased incorporation into the TG fraction (37). This would indicate that PL synthesis was inhibited due to heated fat treatment, and there was an impaired mobilization of TG fatty acids. Oleic acid is known to promote fat accumulation in tissue culture cells (53). The HOO treatment which provided most oleic acid gave the highest TG values.

The cytotoxicity studies associated with oxidized fats indicate that they interfered with cellular metabolism and differ-

entiation, and caused necrotic changes (38). Cytoplasmic vacuolation observed in stained cultures represented intracellular
lipid accumulation. This excess on exposure to heated fats could
reflect an accelerated uptake from the medium by the cells, or
an inhibition of their intracellular mobilization for cellular
functions. Landes (14) showed that heated fats were oxidized
slowly by the myocardium of animals fed thermally oxidized peanut
oil in their diet. Since heated fat exposure increased the number
of pyknotic cells and decreased the mitotic index, these aberrations suggest detrimental effects of oxidized fat components
either through their physical presence, or through interference
with biochemical activity.

During deep-fat frying, depending on conditions used, many
volatile and non-volatile compounds may be formed. Possible
dietary hazard depends on severity of treatment, and level of
intake. Animal studies have shown adverse effects including decreased growth and feed efficiency, increased liver size, fatty
necrosis of organs, and numerous other lesions. Practical processing and frying usually produce low levels of undesirable
products, but it is worthwhile to recognize their possible adverse
biological effects.

Acknowledgments

The author is grateful to the following persons for assistance in obtaining the data: Dr. V.E. Valli, Dr. R.P. Bird,
Dr. P.K. Basrur, and Mr. H.G. Gabriel. Financial support was
provided by the Natural Sciences and Engineering Research Council,
and the Ontario Ministry of Agriculture and Food.

Legend of Symbols

DNUA (distillable non-urea adductable fraction)
CO (corn oil); HCO (heated corn oil)
OO (olive oil); HOO (heated olive oil)
LE (low erucic acid rapeseed oil); HLE (heated low erucic acid
rapeseed oil)
LA (lard); HLA (heated lard)

Literature Cited

1.   Poling, C.E.; Warner, W.D.; Mone, P.E.; Rice, E.E. J. Am.
     Oil Chem. Soc. 1962, 39, 315.
2.   Nolen, G.A.; Alexander, J.C.; Artman, N.R. J. Nutr. 1967,
     93, 337.
3.   Hemans, C.; Kummerow, F.A.; Perkins, E.G. J. Nutr. 1973,
     103, 1665.
4.   Alexander, J.C. J. Am. Oil Chem. Soc. 1978, 55, 711.
5.   Nolen, G.A. J. Nutr. 1973, 103, 1248.
6.   Miller, J.; Landes, D.R. J. Food Sci. 1975, 40, 545.

7. Gabriel, H.G.; Alexander, J.C.; Valli, V.E. Can. J. Comp. Med. 1977, 41, 98.
8. Gabriel, H.G.; Alexander, J.C.; Valli, V.E. Lipids 1978, 13, 49.
9. Alexander, J.C. J. Toxicol. Environ. Health 1981, 7, 125.
10. Poling, C.E.; Eagle, E.; Rice, E.E.; Durand, A.M.; Fisher, M. Lipids 1970, 5, 128.
11. Andia, G.A.; Street, J.C. Agric. Food Chem. 1975, 23, 173.
12. Kaunitz, H.; Johnson, R.E.; Pegus, L. J. Am. Oil Chem. Soc. 1965, 42, 770.
13. Yoshida, H.; Shibahara, A.; Kajimoto, G. Yukagaku 1975, 24, 575.
14. Landes, D.R. Nutr. Rep. Internat. 1975, 12, 19.
15. Bird, R.P.; Alexander, J.C. Lipids 1979, 14, 836.
16. Johnson, O.C.; Perkins, E.G.; Sugai, M.; Kummerow, F.A. J. Am. Oil Chem. Soc. 1957, 34, 594.
17. Paik, T.H.; Hochino, T.; Kaneda, T. Eiyo to Syokuryo (Food and Nutrition) 1976, 29, 85.
18. Barrett, C.B.; Henry, C.M. Proc. Nutr. Soc. 1966, 25, 4.
19. Endres, J.G.; Bhalerao, V.R.; Kummerow, F.A. J. Am. Oil Chem. Soc. 1962, 39, 118.
20. Endres, J.G.; Bhalerao, V.R.; Kummerow, F.A. J. Am. Oil Chem. Soc. 1962, 39, 159.
21. Artman, N.R.; Alexander, J.C. J. Am. Oil Chem. Soc. 1968, 45, 643.
22. Perkins, E.G.; Anfinsen, J.R. J. Am. Oil Chem. Soc. 1971, 48, 556.
23. Paulose, M.M.; Chang, S.S. J. Am. Oil Chem. Soc. 1973, 50, 147.
24. Perkins, E.G.; Kummerow, F.A. J. Am. Oil Chem. Soc. 1959, 36, 371.
25. Crampton, E.W.; Common, R.H.; Farmer, F.A.; Wells, A.F.; Crawford, D. J. Nutr. 1953, 49, 333.
26. Michael, W.R.; Alexander, J.C.; Artman, N.R. Lipids 1966, 1, 353.
27. Shue, G.M.; Douglass, C.D.; Firestone, D.; Friedman, L.; Friedman, L.; Sage, J.S. J. Nutr. 1968, 94, 171.
28. Tappel, A.L. Fed. Proc. 1973, 32, 1870.
29. Fukuzawa, K.; Sato, M. J. Nutr. Sci. Vitaminol. 1975, 21, 79.
30. Alexander, J.C. Lipids 1966, 1, 254.
31. Gabriel, H.G.; Alexander, J.C.; Valli, V.E. Nutr. Rep. Internat. 1979, 19, 515.
32. Gabriel, H.G.; Alexander, J.C.; Valli, V.E. Nutr. Rep. Internat. 1979, 20, 411.
33. Eisenhauer, R.A.; Beal, R.E. J. Am. Oil Chem. Soc. 1968, 45, 619.
34. Entenman, C. J. Am. Oil Chem. Soc. 1961, 38, 534.
35. Morrison, W.R.; Smith, L.M. J. Lipid Res. 1964, 5, 600.

36. Johnston, P.V. "Basic Lipid Methodology"; Special Publi-
     cation 19, College of Agriculture, University of Illinois:
     Urbana, 1971; p. 49.
37. Bird, R.P.; Alexander, J.C. Lipids 1978, 13, 809.
38. Bird, R.P.; Basrur, P.K.; Alexander, J.C. In Vitro 1981,
     17, 397.
39. Rogers, C.G. Lipids 1974, 9, 541.
40. Folch, J.; Lees, M.; Stanley, G.H. J. Biol. Chem. 1957,
     226, 497.
41. Andersen, D.B.; Holub, B.J. J. Nutr. 1976, 106, 529.
42. Paul, J. "Cell and Tissue Culture"; 4th Edition; Williams
     and Wilkins: Baltimore, 1970; p. 129.
43. Lowry, O.H.; Rosenbrough, N.J.; Farr, A.L.; Randall, R.H.
     J. Biol. Chem. 1951, 193, 265.
44. Oyama, V.I.; Eagle, H. Proc. Soc. Exp. Biol. Med. 1956,
     91, 305.
45. Firestone, D.W.; Horwitz, W.; Friedman, L.; Shue, G.M.
     J. Nutr. 1961, 73, 85.
46. Hutchison, R.B.; Alexander, J.C. J. Org. Chem. 1963, 28,
     2522.
47. Watt, B.K.; Merrill, A.L. "Composition of Foods"; U.S.
     Department of Agriculture Handbook No. 8. 1975.
48. Ohfuji, T.; Kaneda, T. Lipids 1973, 8, 353.
49. Clark, D.A.; Foulds, E.L.; Wilson, F.H. Lipids 1969, 4, 1.
50. Rao, M.K.G.; Hemans, C.; Perkins, E.G. Lipids 1973, 8, 341.
51. Opie, L.H. Am. Heart J. 1968, 76, 685.
52. Gerschenson, L.E.; Harary, I.; Mead, J.F. Biochim. Biophys.
     Acta 1967, 131, 50.
53. Moskowitz, M.S. in "Lipid Metabolism in Tissue Culture
     Cells", Rothblat, G.H.; Kritchevsky, D. Ed.; Wistar
     Symposium Monograph No. 6, Wistar Institute Press:
     Philadelphia, PA, 1967; p. 49.

RECEIVED June 6, 1983

Mutagens in Cooked Food

L. F. BJELDANES

Department of Nutritional Sciences, University of California, Berkeley, CA 94720

J. S. FELTON and F. T. HATCH

Biomedical and Environmental Research Program, Lawrence Livermore Laboratory, University of California, Livermore, CA 94550

With the development of simple and rapid methods for detecting agents which modify genetic material of cells (i.e., Ames bacterial assay) has come the realization that mutagens are widespread in our environment (1). The attention of several research groups has turned toward examining mutagenic activity of foods. As a result of this extensive research effort the occurrence of mutagenic substances in certain heated foods and food components is now well documented. Proteins and several amino acids yield highly mutagenic substances when pyrolyzed at temperatures above 300°C (2-4). Similar temperatures were reported to be necessary to generate appreciable mutagenicity in pyrolyzed food samples (5). Under pyrolytic conditions, carbohydrate and lipid components and foods rich in them tend to exhibit less mutagenic activity than samples rich in proteins or amino acids. Evidence compiled by several research groups indicates that mutagenic activity is also induced in certain foods cooked under conditions less severe than required for pyrolysis (6-9). In these studies mutagenic activity is detected in fried and broiled protein-rich food (beef), and at a higher level than in cooked carbohydrate-rich food (10). Broiled fish samples also contain mutagens (11). In addition, extended boiling of beef stock results in mutagen formation (6,8).

Reviewed herein are the results of our work to determine the effects of food type and cooking conditions on mutagenicity of cooked protein-rich foods. Results of our efforts to isolate and identify mutagens from fried beef are also described.

Mutagenicity of cooked protein-rich foods

Published information on dietary practices in the U.S. was examined in order to establish priorities for mutagenicity testing of cooked foods. Analysis of diet surveys conducted by the U.S.D.A. (1964-66) and U.S. Department of H.E.W. (1971-75) provided a listing of the major sources of dietary protein in the U.S. (Table 1) based on per capita consumption (12). Milk was clearly the most significant dietary source of protein and beef was the most significant meat source.

All of the foods tested were submitted to various heat treatments (13,14). The initial survey included two sets of cooking times and temperatures for each food. One set approximated common practice in the United States, and the other utilized more severe conditions that generally resulted in a very well done, though not burned, sample. In some cases, when significant mutagenic activity was detected in the initial screening, a more detailed investigation of the dependence of mutagenicity on cooking time and temperature was carried out. Except in cases in which mixtures of food were examined, no seasonings or other additives were used. When normal procedures required cooking oil, corn oil was used. For the initial surveys most samples were cooked in stainless steel pans. Broiled samples were prepared in ceramic cooking dishes. The more detailed investigations of frying conditions were conducted on an electrically heated stainless steel griddle. Temperatures given in the tables were measured in each experiment with the empty utensil, on top of a household electric range or electric griddle, at the heat control setting that was used in cooking the food sample.

Special heating conditions were used for certain foods. Eggs were fried in the form of patties in addition to the more conventional forms. Egg patties were prepared by heating egg mixture or egg fraction for 1 hour at 95°C in a petri plate, a procedure that by itself causes no mutagen to form. Milk samples were heated to vigorous reflux for periods up to 240 min. or were reduced in volume by 50% and 25% by vigorous boiling.

Cooked samples were deboned if necessary and when an obviously browned outer portion or crust was present on the cooked food, this material was separated from the inner portion and extracted for bioassay. Results of bioassays of the inner portions of foods were uniformly negative except for small amounts of mutagenic activity that appeared when samples were fried at the highest temperatures.

Cooked foods were homogenized and extracted with acetone as previously described (9). The organic base fraction, which contained all of the detectable mutagens, was dissolved in DMSO and assayed with Salmonella tester strains TA 1538 or TA 98 (15). Aroclor-induced rat liver S-9 fraction was used for metabolic activation of mutagens. The number of revertants induced per 100 gram wet weight equivalents (100 gE), i.e., per 100 grams of uncooked food, was extrapolated from the linear portions of dose-response curves.

In this initial survey, mutagenicity in cooked protein-rich foods was found to be dependent on the type of food and the

Table 1.   Ten highest ranking food items from the two data sets

	per capita mean daily protein intake (g) from food item	
	HANES	USDA
Whole milk	8.9	11.7
Ground beef	4.2	4.5
Beef steak	4.0	4.5
White bread	3.3	4.1
Eggs	3.1	3.7
Pork chops	1.6	*1.7
Fried chicken	1.4	2.5
Beef, braised or pot roasted	1.3	*0.7
Ham	1.0	2.5
Roast beef	0.9	1.8

* Rank order for USDA and HANES data are identical except for these 2 food items.

degree of heating.   Whereas all of the foods tested developed
mutagenic activity under some cooking conditions, only the most
severe conditions consistently produced activity in milk, cheese,
tofu,beans, and organ meats (Table 2).   Extensive discoloration
or charring was generally obvious in the mutagenic milk, cheese
and tofu samples.   Nonmutagenic samples of these later foods were
not markedly discolored.

Data presented in Tables 2-4 show results of more severe
heat treatments.   Mutagenic activity was generally reduced in
samples treated under milder conditions than indicated in the
tables.   None of the bean samples was burned or considered
inedible.   Several samples were weakly mutagenic and one sample
(baked pinto beans) contained moderate mutagenic activity (3,650
revertants/100 gE).   Many of the organ meat samples showed weak
activity, with sauteed kidney and brain samples being the most
active   (900   revertants/100   gE).   None   of   the   organ   meat
preparations was charred.

The griddle-fried and the oven-broiled samples of rock cod
showed moderate mutagenic activity (1,300-2,000 revertants/100
gE) (Table 3).   The more extensively fried trout, salmon, and red
snapper yielded 2,500-3,100 revertants/100 gE, while halibut
yielded about 1,100 revertants/100 gE.   The remainder of the rock
cod samples, and the sole, shrimp, and batter-fried seafood from
a   commercial galley exhibited negligible or small amounts of
mutagenic activity.   These results are comparable to results of
Krone and Iwaoka (16).

Preparation of chicken under several relatively moderate
conditions produced low or moderate levels of mutagenic activity
(Figure   1).   Moderate   mutagenic   activity   (1,000-4,000
revertants/100 gE) was detected in very well done to partially
charred   chicken   samples.   Undetectable   or   weak   (<500
revertants/100 gE) activity was present in chicken samples which
were not overcooked.   High activity (16,500 revertants/100 gE)
was detected in one sample of broiled breast meat.   In general,
white chicken meat samples tended to be more mutagenic than dark
meat cooked under similar conditions.

Cooked egg products showed variable levels of mutagenic
activity depending on the type of product and the conditions of
cooking.   As indicated in Table 4, very little mutagenic activity
was formed in eggs and egg products unless severe cooking
conditions were used.   The mutagenic samples, eggs fried sunny-
side up at $310^{\circ}C$ for 6 min. and pancakes cooked at high
temperatures, did not approach the levels of mutagenic activity
found in meats cooked at lower temperatures for shorter periods.
Baked meringues and custards and pancakes fried at $350^{\circ}C$ were
non-mutagenic.   Egg patties fried at pan temperatures above
$225^{\circ}C$ showed levels of mutagenicity that depended on the time
and temperature of frying (Table 4).   Degree of browning appeared
to correspond to levels of mutagenic activity of the egg patties.
The highest levels of activity (>10,000 revertants/100gE) were

Table 2. Mutagenic activity in food samples under different cooking conditions

Sample	Cooking method	Time (min)	Temperature (°C)	TA1538 revertants per 100gE*
Whole milk	Boiling	60	100	NS†
Whole milk	25% boildown	65	100	440
Sharp cheddar cheese	Baked	30	232	63
Sharp cheddar cheese	Fried	5	375	NS
American cheese	Baked	20	232	360
American cheese	Fried	5	375	94
Pinto bean	Boiling	78	100	75
Kidney bean	Boiling	90	100	140
Pinto bean	Boiling then frying (no oil)	4	450	NS
Kidney bean	Boiling then frying (no oil)	10	450	380
Pinto bean	Boiling then baking	60	176	3650
Pinto bean	Boiling then baking	120	176	460

Continued on next page

Table 2. Continued

Kidney bean	Boiling then baking	60	176	140
Kidney bean	Boiling then baking	120	176	140
Pinto bean	Boiling then frying w/oil	8	450	NS
Kidney bean	Boiling then frying w/oil	8	450	150
Tofu	Deep-fried brown	15	162	400
Liver (beef)	Pan-fried	4.5/side	310	210
Heart (beef)	Baked	165	163	81
Heart (beef)	Braised	2.5 then	450 then	
Kidney (beef)	Baked	135	275	230
Kidney (beef)	Sauteed	60	149	310
Brains (beef)	Sauteed	7	450	830
		2 then	450 then	
Brains (beef)	Broiled	15	100	920
		12/side	260	85

*gE = gram net weight equivalents of uncooked food.

†Not significantly different from the spontaneous reversion rate, based on failure to meet two separate criteria: first, that the highest dose point be more than two standard deviations above the historical spontaneous rate for our laboratory ($22 + 6.2$ s.d.); second, that the linear regression fit to the data show a significant slope at the 95% confidence level for the doses included.

Table 3. Mutagenic activity in seafood samples under different cooking conditions

Type of fish	Cooking method	Time (min)	Temperature (°C)	TA1538 revertants per 100 gE
Rock cod	Griddle-fried	6/side	200	1330
Rock cod	Baked	45	204	NS*
Rock cod	Broiled	12/10/side‡	300	1990
Sole	Pan-fried	2/side	280	170
Halibut	Pan-fried	5.5/side	280	1080
Trout	Pan-fried	6.5/side	280	3100
Salmon	Pan-fried	6/side	280	2800
Red snapper	Pan-fried	5.5/side	280	2500
Shrimp	Deep-fat fried	15	190	NS
Seafood galley	Batter-fried	§	§	180

*See footnote to Table 2.

‡Twelve minutes on the first side and ten minutes on second side.

§Commercially cooked.

Table 4. Mutagen formation in eggs and egg products.

Sample	Cooking method	Temperature (°C)	Time (min)	TA1538 revertants per 100 gE
Eggs	Fried--up	310	6	290
Eggs	Fried--over	310	6	NS*
Eggs	Hard-boiled	100	50	NS
Eggs	Baked/shirred	190	60	NS
Meringue	Baked	177	90	NS
Custard	Baked	204	75	NS
Pancakes	Fried	475	3	190
Patties	Fried	250	6	1000
Patties	Fried	300	6	40000

*See footnote to Table 2.

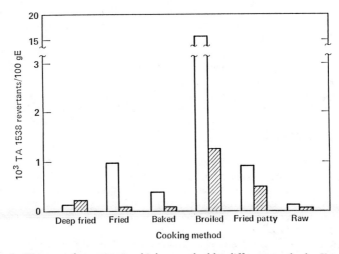

Figure 1. Mutagen formation in chicken cooked by different methods. Key: open bars, white meat; and shaded bars, dark meat. Conditions: deep fried, 12 min at 101 °C; fried, 15 min first side and 10 min second side at 103 °C; baked, 50 min at 190 °C; broiled, 17 min per side at 274 °C; fried patty, 6 min per side at 200 °C; and raw, uncooked.

detected in samples which began to show some charring (i.e., samples fried at >300°C for >4 min/side).

The most consistently elevated mutagenic activity was detected in meat products of beef and pork muscle. Information presented in Figure 2 compares mutagenic activity of various meat products fried for 6 min/side at pan temperatures from 150°C–300°C. Samples cooked at 200°C were considered well done but not charred. Mutagenic activity in these samples ranged from approximately 2,000 revertants/100 gE for bacon to about 9,000 revertants/100 gE for pork sausage. Samples fried in the 275–280°C range or above for 6 min/side showed generally higher activity and were partially charred. For comparison, lamb chops fried at 210°C pan temperature for 5 min/side (well done, not charred) showed mutagenic activity of 14,100 revertants/100 gE.

From the results of this initial survey it became obvious that mutagenicity of protein-rich food was related to the type of food and degree of cooking. In order to study the effect of cooking in more detail and to determine the contribution of major meat constituents to mutagenicity of heated samples, ground beef patties or reconstituted samples were fried for various times at one or a series of temperatures on stainless steel or other cooking surfaces (17).

Cooking Surface. The mutagenic activities of the basic fraction from hamburger cooked on the different surfaces are shown in Table 5. Meat cooked on aluminum, cast iron, stainless steel and Teflon surfaces contained the highest activity of the samples tested. Meat cooked on the ceramic and enamel surfaces contained less mutagenic activity.

A more detailed investigation of the effects of cooking surface on mutagen production was conducted by measuring mutagenic activity of meat cooked at 200°C for various times on Teflon, ceramic and stainless steel surfaces (Figure 3). Mutagen production on the stainless steel and ceramic surfaces was reproducible with lower activity observed in samples cooked on the ceramic surface. Mutagen production on the Teflon surface was somewhat variable between experiments. However, the overall trend of mutagenicity in samples fried for various times on Teflon was similar to the trend for samples fried on stainless steel.

Evidence from these cooking–surface experiments suggests that there is not likely to be a specific role of surface metal in catalysis of mutagen production. The general indications from data presented in Table 5 are that all the metal surfaces and the Teflon surface produce similar levels of activity in fried samples. The consistently lower activity produced on the ceramic and enamel surfaces can be ascribed to reduced cooking rate for these samples. Thus, weight loss during cooking, moisture content, red reflectance (data not shown) as well as general

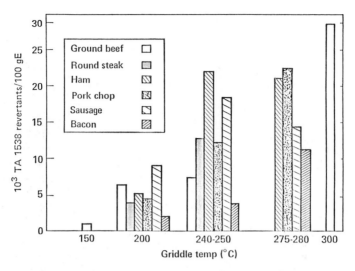

Figure 2. Comparative mutagenesis of fried red meats. All meats were fried for 6 min per side on a stainless steel griddle.

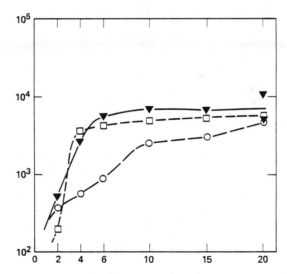

Figure 3. Effect of cooking surface on mutagenicity of fried beef. All cooking surfaces were equilibrated to 200 °C before cooking. Key: ▼, steel; □, Teflon; and ○, ceramic.

Table 5. Mutagenicity of organic base fractions from ground beef fried on different surfaces at 200°C for 6/min/side

	Number of experiments	Revertants[a]
Stainless steel (control	5	6270 ± 1200[b]
Stainless steel on aluminum	1	7160
Aluminum	1	4300 ± 2370
Teflon	4	4250
Cast iron	1	3550
Enamel	1	1425
Ceramic	2	900 ± 85

[a]Mutation frequencies per 100 gE in Salmonella strain TA1538 were determined by regression analysis from the linear portions of dose-response curves.

[b]Standard deviation of estimates from n experiments.

appearance of samples fried for 10 min on the ceramic surface are similar to those of samples fried for 6 min on the stainless steel at the same temperature setting. Mutagenicity of the samples fried for 10 min on the ceramic surface is also in the range of activity of the samples fried for 6 min on stainless steel. A possible advantage of the ceramic surface in minimizing mutagen production during frying is that, at a given temperature setting, rates of cooking and mutagen production are lower on the ceramic surface compared to the metal surfaces and therefore can be more easily controlled.

The effects of variation in meat composition on mutagenicity of cooked product were examined in reconstituted beef patties. Patties of variable water and fat content were prepared from freeze-dried meat. Appropriate amounts of distilled water were added back to the meat for the variable-water-content experiment. Defatted meat was prepared by petroleum ether extraction of freeze-dried material in a Soxhlet apparatus. Petroleum ether was removed <u>in</u> <u>vacuo</u> and the remaining oil was used to reconstitute the meat samples, which were also reconstituted to their original water content. Reconstituted meat samples had the compositions indicated in Figures 4 and 5.

Mutagen production is strongly dependent on the amount of moisture initially present in the meat above approximately 40%. Below this level mutagen production is low and appears to be independent of moisture level.

The relative fat content of meat appears to have little effect on mutagenicity of cooked samples. Maximum mutagenicity was detected in defatted samples with a slight decrease in activity with increasing fat content.

These results suggest that adequate water is required for mutagen production perhaps as a heat-transfer agent or as a reaction medium for water-soluble intermediates. The observed independence of mutagen production and content of fat, an excellent heat-transfer agent, suggests that water may be serving the latter purpose. Whereas the requirement of water as a reactant in mutagen formation cannot be ruled out based on the present results, fat is clearly not required as a reactant. The results provide evidence that increased fat levels may even lead to a slight decrease in mutagenicity in fried meat possibly due to loss of mutagens into the cooking juices.

The present results appear to be inconsistent with the results of others who have reported low mutagenicity of low-fat meat (18). However, the present study was carried out with reconstituted samples from totally dehydrated and defatted meat. The consistency of the reconstituted samples was similar to, but certainly different from, the consistency of ground beef. These physical effects of total dehydration and defatting may contribute to the differences in the observed results using reconstituted and normal low-fat ground beef.

An analysis was conducted of the influences of time and

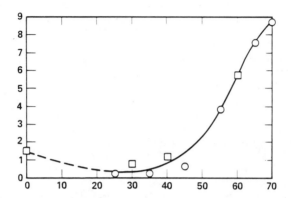

Figure 4. Effects of variation of initial water content on mutagenicity of ground beef. Samples are fried at 200 °C for 6 min per side and the basic fraction is tested for activity in the Salmonella *mutagenesis assay. (The □ and ○ are data from two separate experiments.) The original fat-to-protein ratio of approximately 0.8 in the ground beef was maintained in these samples.*

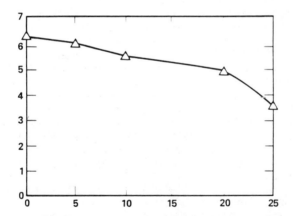

Figure 5. Effects of variation of initial fat content on mutagenicity of ground beef. Samples are fried at 200 °C for 6 min per side and the basic fraction is tested for activity in the Salmonella *mutagenesis assay. An amount of water equal to that removed in freeze-drying was added to each sample. Graded amounts of the extracted fat were added to the reconstituted samples before cooking.*

temperature of frying on mutagenicity of ground beef. Ground beef patties were fried for 2-20 min/side with pan surface temperatures ranging from 150-300°C. The levels of mutagenic activity in patties fried under these conditions are indicated in Figure 6. At all temperatures studied, induced mutagenicity increases rapidly until about 10 min/side of cooking, followed by only a moderate increase (300°C samples) or no further increase in mutagenicity at longer times. An increase in frying temperature from 150°C to 200°C had a marked effect on mutagenic activity. This temperature change caused as much as a 20-fold increase in activity of patties fried for 6 min/side. In contrast, the temperature increase from 200°C to 250°C was associated with no significant increase in activity of the 6 min-samples. Interestingly, the increase in frying temperature from 250°C to 300°C was again associated with a marked increase (approximately 6-fold) in activity of the fried meat. This renewed increase in activity at the higher temperatures may be due to the formation of mutagens different from those formed at the lower temperatures.

These results do not provide evidence for a general lag period of cooking before mutagen production becomes readily detectable. A lag period of approximately 4-5 min. has been reported for mutagen production in meat patties fried by a process which involved turning patties at 1-2 min. intervals ([19]) or when timing was initiated when heating of the frying surface was begun ([18]). Our frying procedure involved application of meat to a preheated surface and incorporated a single turn of the patty during heating, a technique which appears more closely to approximate the conventional cooking process. This technique, by allowing a more continuous heating of one side of the patty than the multiple turn method, results in more rapid cooking on one side and yields higher levels of mutagenicity early in the cooking process.

<u>Isolation of mutagens from fried ground beef.</u> Prior to proceeding with a large scale extraction and fractionation of mutagens from fried beef, an effort was made to maximize mutagen yield from the initial extraction procedure ([20]). Total mutagenic activity in ground beef fried under standard conditions (6 min/side, 200°C) was estimated to be in the range of 300-400 revertants/gE based on corrected measurements of activity in an initial aqueous acid extract. By contrast, methods employing $(NH_4)_2SO_4$ to precipitate proteins from an acid extract or an initial extraction with acetone provided mutagenicity yields of only about 25 revertants/gE and 60 revertants/gE, respectively. Use of a mixed solvent $(CH_3OH:CH_2Cl_2:H_2O, 45:45:10, v:v:v)$ improved the mutagenicity yield to approximately 100 revertants/gE. Our best recovery of mutagenicity was obtained with the use of an XAD-2 resin to absorb active substances from an initial aqueous acid extract.

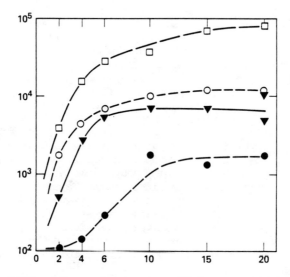

Figure 6. Effects of time and temperature of frying on mutagenicity of ground beef. Standard sized patties were fried on a stainless steel griddle and the basic extract was assayed for mutagenicity. Key: □, 300 °C; ○, 250 °C; ▼, 200 °C; and ●, 150 °C.

By this method, recoveries in the range of 200–250 revertants/gE were obtained. An outline of this fractionation scheme is presented in Figure 7.

The procedure which included the XAD–2 resin to remove active substances from an initial aqueous acid extract was scaled up to process a 40 kg batch of ground beef.

The active eluent from the XAD–2 column was stripped of volatile solvents and the remaining aqueous mixture was made basic with a few drops of concentrated NaOH. This mixture was extracted with petroleum ether and the combined organic phases were back-extracted with acetonitrile which was added to the aqueous phase. The aqueous phase was then extracted with acetonitrile. The combined acetonitrile phases were dried with a single partition against saturated NaCl (aq.) and reduced in volume.

Samples were then chromatographed on a preparative C–8 bonded phase column at low pressure under the conditions specified in Figure 8. Results of the <u>Salmonella</u> assay of collected fractions are also given in Figure 8. The results shown in the figure indicate two major bands of mutagenic activity which are resolved under these preparative conditions. These bands are designated CE (for earlier, more polar) and CL (for later, less polar).

All material eluting in the E-band region was pooled to give a combined early (<u>CE</u>) fraction. The principal mutagenic material of this fraction was obtained as a single subfraction following two chromatographic sequences using a C–8 semi-preparative column with methanol/water containing 100 ppm triethylamine as the eluting solvent. The composition of this subfraction ($\alpha 3$) was then investigated in comparison with the known mutagens IQ(3-methyl-1,3,6,9-tetraazacyclopenta[a]naphthalen-2-amine) and MeIQx(3,8-dimethyl-1,3,6,9-tetraazacyclopenta[a]naphthalen-2-amine.

Co-injection of <u>MeIQx</u> with $\alpha 3$ gave a chromatogram showing an enhancement in the latest UV peak of $\alpha 3$ and thus suggesting the presence of this compound. Results of further fractionation of the CE-derived fraction on a normal phase HPLC system indicated the presence of two distinct areas of mutagenic activity. The major active substance coeluted with MeIQx. Ultraviolet (λ_{max} 274) and mass spectral (m/e; 213,197,185,144) properties of this substance are consistent with the MeIQx assignment. The minor active component did not coelute with any of the standard mutagens isolated from food or pyrolysis experiments and is unidentified.

The active fractions corresponding to the later band of activity (CL) from the original low pressure chromatography were combined. This material was rechromatographed on the C–8 semi-preparative column with methanol/water as the eluting solvent. The three major bands of mutagenic activity were combined into fractions designated <u>CL–I</u>, <u>CL–II</u> and <u>CL–III</u>.

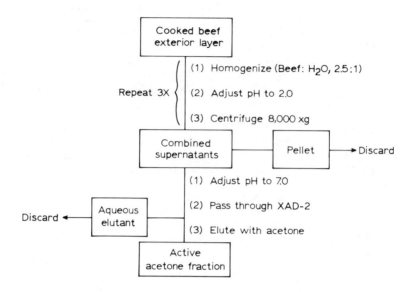

Figure 7. Acid–XAD–2 extraction scheme.

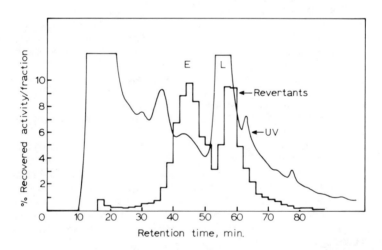

Figure 8. UV absorbance chromatograms (262 nm) and Salmonella *assay results on fractions collected in the low-pressure preparative separation of fried beef extracts.*

Chromatographic specifications: Solvent—25% A in A + B for 30 min to 80% A over 40 min and held (A = acetonitrile + 100 ppm triethylamine, B = water + 100 ppm triethylamine). Flow rate— 5.05 mL/min. Column—EM Lobar RP-8, 2.5 × 31 cm, 40–63 μm packing. Amount injected—1.5 kgE.

Two consecutive chromatographic runs of CL-II resulted in the isolation of a single mutagenic substance. Spectral characterization of the active material (CL-II-B) is in progress.

It should be noted that IQ, MeIQ (the 4-methyl derivative of IQ) and MeIQx elute earlier than CL-II-B (around 30 min) and Trp-P-1 (9H-1,4-dimethyl-3,9-diazafluoren-2-amine) and the product of soybean pyrolysate (9H-1,9-diazafluoren-2-amine both elute much later (greater than 90 min). Only Glu-P-1 (8-methyl-1,4b,9-triazafluoren-2-amine) elutes near the active compound (around 47 min).

Band CL-III was also submitted to rechromatography by reversed phase HPLC. The mutagenic profile of the corresponding fractions indicates that this fraction contains many substances at least several of which appear to be mutagenic.

At this stage of our studies it is possible to estimate the contribution of the major mutagenic fractions to the total activity of the fried meat. The toal activity is nearly equally divided between the CE and CL fractions. Of the mutagenic activity in the CE fraction perhaps 80-90% is due to MeIQx with 10-20% due to a less polar, unidentified substance. Approximately 70% of the activity of the CL fraction is due to a single unidentified substance. The remaining 30% of the mutagenic activity of this later eluting fraction appears to arise from several unidentified components.

Literature Cited

1. Nagao, M., Sugimura, T. & Matsushima, T., Ann. Rev. Genet. 1978, 12, 117.
2. Matsumoto, T., Yoshida, D., Mizusaki, S. & Okamoto, H., Mutation Res. 1977, 48, 279.
3. Matsumoto, T., Yoshida, D., Mizusaki, S. & Okamoto, H., Mutation Rns. 1978, 5, 281.
4. Nagao, M., Honda, M., Seino, Y., Yahagi, T., Kawachi, T. & Sugimura, T., Cancer Lett. 1977, 2, 335.
5. Uyeta, M., Kanada, T., Mazaki, M. & Taue, S., J. Food Hyg. Soc. Japan (Shokuhin Eiselgaka Zasshi) 1978, 19, 216.
6. Commoner, B., Vithayathil, A.J., Dolara, P., Nair, S., Madyastha, P. & Cuca, G.C., Science 1978, 201, 913.
7. Pariza, M.W., Ashoor, S.H., Chu, F.S. & Lund, D.B., Cancer Lett. 1979, 7, 63.
8. Spingarn, N.E. & Weisburger, J.H., Cancer Lett. 1979, 7, 259.
9. Felton, J., Healy, S., Stuermer, D., Berry, C., Timourian, H., Hatch, F.T., Morris, M. & Bjeldanes, L.F., Mutation Res. 1981, 88, 33.
10. Spingarn, N.E., Slocum, L.A. & Weisburger, J.H., Cancer Lett. 1980, 9, 7.

11. Kasai, H., Nishimura, S., Nagao, M., Takahashi, Y. & Sugimura, T., Cancer Lett. 1979, 7, 343.
12. Plumlee, C., Bjeldanes, L.F. & Hatch, F., J. Amer. Diet. Assoc. 1981, 79, 446-9.
13. Bjeldanes, L.F., Morris, M.M., Felton, J.S., Healy, S., Stuermer, D., Berry, P., Timourian, H., & Hatch, F.T., Food Chem. Toxicol. 1982, 20, 365.
14. Bjeldanes, L.F., Morris, M.M., Felton, J.S., Healy, S., Stuermer, D., Berry, P., Timourian, H. & Hatch, F.T., Food Chem. Toxicol. 1982, 20, 365.
15. Ames, B.N., McCann, J. & Yamasaki, E., Mutation Res. 1975, 31, 347.
16. Krone, C.A., & Iwaoka, W.T., Cancer Lett. 1981, 14, 93.
17. Bjeldanes, L.F., Morris, M.M., Timourian, H., & Hatch, F.T., J. Agric. Food Chem. 1982, in press.
18. Spingarn, N.E., Garvie-Gould, C., Vuolo, L.L., & Weisburger, J.H., Cancer Lett. 1981, 12, 93.
19. Pariza, M.W., Ashoor, S.H., Chu, F.S., & Lund, D.B., Cancer Lett. 1979, 7, 63.
20. Bjeldanes, L.F., Grose, K.R., Davis, P.H., Stuermer, D.H., Healy, S.K. & Felton, J.S., Mut. Res. Lett. 1982, 105, 43.

RECEIVED July 8, 1983

D-Amino Acids in Processed Proteins: Their Nutritional Consequences

L. RAÚL TOVAR

Departamento de Alimentos, DEPg, Facultad de Química, Universidad de México, México 04510, D. F.

DANIEL E. SCHWASS

Western Regional Research Center, U.S. Department of Agriculture, ARS, Berkeley, CA 94710

Racemization of amino acyl residues in food proteins is a reaction that can take place during processing and cooking. This review deals with the occurrence and detection of alkali- and heat-induced racemization in proteins. Differences between calcium hydroxide- and sodium hydroxide-induced racemization and the effects of treatment with these alkalis on protein bioavailability is discussed.

Amino acids in animal and plant proteins appear to occur solely as L-isomers. However, D-amino acids are observed widely in nature as constituents of bacterial cell walls and of several antibiotics (1-3). In addition, the heat and alkali treatments used in food processing can produce racemization of amino acids (4-6).

Food proteins are often treated with alkali to improve their functional properties. For example, soy protein is treated with alkali and heat during extrusion to produce textured fibers for use as meat analogues and extenders which are widely marketed for human consumption (7). Several studies have shown that soy protein treated with alkali contains significant amounts of racemized amino acids (8-10).

Another example of a protein-containing material that is processed with alkali is corn, which traditionally has been treated with aqueous lime, ashes or caustic soda (11,12). Tortillas, a primary source of protein for a large portion of the Mexican population, are prepared by simmering corn in a 1% lime solution. The pH reached during this process is about 12.4, and 175°C temperature is used during the final stage of cooking. Limited racemization of protein in tortillas has been reported (13).

0097–6156/83/0234–0169$06.00/0

Harsh treatments used during food processing can have deleterious effects on the nutritional quality of the processed protein. Decreases in digestibility (enzymatic hydrolysis) (8,10,
14-18) and availability (absorption by the gut) (14,16,17,19) of
heat and alkali treated proteins have been observed. There is
evidence that racemization may play an important role in the
decreased nutritional quality of some treated proteins (8,14,16),
and for this reason, this review will focus on the methods used
to detect racemization, the effects of alkali on racemization,
and the nutritional effects of protein racemization.

Analytical Procedures for Determination of D-Amino Acids

Historically, optical isomers have been difficult to separate
and measure. Table I lists several methods for isomer analysis
arranged in order of their development. Because optical isomers
differ in configuration but not reactivity, melting point or
other physical properties, it was necessary for earlier investigators to measure changes in the optical rotation of polarized
light (15,20-22).
In 1935, Krebs published a technique for isomer analysis
that employs D-amino acid oxidase, an enzyme which selectively
deaminates D-isomers. This method allowed measurement of D-amino
acids via the resultant keto acids that were formed or by recovery
of intact L-amino acids (28). Other enzymatic methods based on
L-amino acid decarboxylases (25,43), L-amino acid acylases and
amidases (44) also have been used. Other biologically-based
techniques employing selective utilization of L-amino acids by
microorganisms appeared as early as 1949 (29,30), but due to
their complexity, have not been used widely.
A major difficulty in isomer analysis was the isolation of
individual amino acids from a mixture. This problem was solved
in the mid-1950's with the advent of ion exchange chromatography
(45). With this technology, amino acids could be separated
quickly and subsequently analyzed for their isomer composition.
Under certain conditions, ion exchange chromatography also can be
used to separate optical isomers. Amino acids with more than one
asymmetric center (diastereomers), such as isoleucine and threonine, are separable into isomers (about the α-carbon) directly
using ion exchange amino acid analyzers because the "allo" forms
of these compounds have physical properties different from their
non-allo counterparts (31). Most protein amino acids have only
one asymmetric carbon (the α-carbon) however, and must be coupled
to another optically active molecule such as N-carboxy-L-leucine
(using the carboxy anhydride) before they can be separated by ion
exchange (32,33). This technique is fairly cumbersome however.
A preliminary separation of the amino acid mixture is necessary
before derivatization with the anhydride, due to the inability of

TABLE I.   Main Analytical Tools Utilized to Determine D-Amino
Acids in Several Materials[a]

Method	D-Amino acid detected	Remarks	Reference
Polarimetry	Total amino acids in proteins or hydrolysates, or pure amino acids	Cumbersome separation of each amino acid from protein hydrolysates	15-19 20-23
Enzymatic	Most amino acids	One assay for each amino acid	24-28,
Microbio- logical	Most amino acids	One assay for each amino acid	23,24 29,30
IEC[b]	Most amino acids	Excellent for Alloile-Ile separation but difficult for L-L and L-D dipeptides	31-33
GC&GC-MS[b]	Most amino acids	Met and Trp partially damaged during hydrolysis. D/L Ratios of amino acids are determined in a single step	34-39
HPLC[b]	Most amino acids	No derivatiza- tion required	40-43

[a]These include processed proteins and foods, animal tissue,
geological and extraterrestial materials.

[b]IEC = Ion exchange chromatography; GC = Gas chromatography;
MS = Mass spectrometry; HPLC = High pressure liquid chromatography; aa = amino acid.

an ion exchange amino acid analyzer to resolve a complete mixture of derivatized isomers.

The most widely used technique for the estimation of amino acid isomers is gas-liquid chromatography. Two basic strategies have been used to separate isomers by this technique. Both approaches appeared in the mid-1960's, and both involve derivatization of the amino acids to suitably volatile acyl-esters (46,47). One method is similar in concept to the separation of disastereomers by ion exchange chromatography discussed above. In one step of the two step derivatization, the amino acids are esterified with an optically active agent. This procedure creates molecules with two centers of asymmetry which can be separated on a non-optically active liquid (stationary) phase (46). This method allows any laboratory equipped with a gas chromatograph to perform isomer analyses.

The second gas chromatographic method employs an optically active liquid phase (47). The amino acids are derivatized to acyl-esters to improve volatility; however, in this case, both the acylation and esterification agents are optically inactive. Because the L-amino acid derivatives interact preferentially with the optically active stationary phase, the isomers can be separated. However, use of this technique was limited because the optically active liquid phases were not stable to sufficiently high temperatures to separate all the derivatized amino acids. In 1977, Bayer and coworkers reported covalent coupling of an optically active moiety (L-valine) to a silicone liquid phase (48). This phase has high thermal stability and allows analysis in approximately one hour.

The principal advantages of gas chromatographic methods over ion exchange methods are that isomers of most amino acids may be determined in a single chromatographic step and the analysis time is much shorter. Furthermore, it is possible to couple an optically active column in the gas chromatograph to a mass spectrometer which allows analysis of incompletely separated peaks and correction of the results for racemization that may occur during acid hydrolysis of the protein sample when deuterium chloride is used for hydrolysis instead of hydrochloric acid (39).

There are three basic approaches for using high performance liquid chromatography (HPLC) for the separation of amino acid isomers, and each of these is based on technology which emerged during the course of development of traditional liquid chromatography (for a review, see 49). Takaya, et al. (50) have reported a method using non-optically active, reverse-phase HPLC for separation of derivatized amino acid diastereomers. This is essentially the approach of Manning and Moore (33), using L-phenylalanine-N-carboxy anhydride or L-leucine-N-carboxy anhydride as a derivatization agent to provide a second center of asymmetry. While analysis times are short (40 min. or less) for most isomers, the conditions (pH, temperature, solvent polarity) necessary for separation vary substantially over the amino acids. This drawback prohibits analysis in a single run.

A second approach to isomer separation by HPLC is to use a non-optically active stationary phase and an optically active solvent. If the amino acids can interact with both the stationary and mobile phases, but one of the isomers interacts more strongly with the mobile, optically active phase, separation of the isomers is possible (49). In 1979, several laboratories reported methods involving the use of chiral mobile-phases containing zinc(II) or copper (II) complexed to an L-amino acid (51-53). A distinct advantage of these methods is that they do not require derivatization of the sample prior to analysis. However, separation of a complete mixture of amino acids (such as that obtained from a protein hydrolysate) has not been reported.

The third approach to isomer separation by HPLC is based on the use of chiral stationary phases. The phase may be inherently optically active (e.g., powdered d-quartz or starch) or may be a non-optically active material coated with or reacted with an optically active moiety. As early as 1938, enantiomers of a camphor compound were separated on a lactose column (54), and twenty years later, alumina coated with α-tartaric acid was used to separate isomers of mandelic acid and phenylglycine-methyl ester (55). In 1960, a patent was granted for the separation of D,L-proline on a lactose column (56). Davankov's laboratory was the first to report separation of amino acid isomers on polymeric resins derivatized with optically active amino acids (57). However, separation of amino acid enantiomers by these techniques has been hampered by long separation times (ca. 10 hr) and the difficulty in synthesizing supports of sufficient quality for modern HPLC (spherical particles, small size, uniform chemical modification). Separation of amino acid isomers on a column consisting of silica bonded with L-amino acids and complexed with copper (II) has been reported by Gubitz and Jellenz (42). Short analysis times for separation of mixtures of single D,L-amino acids were reported (ca. 30 min), but complex mixtures have not been separated.

With further development it is likely that a HPLC method will be able to separate complex mixtures of amino acid isomers. The high speed and efficiency of HPLC, coupled with the ability to run samples without prior derivatization would be an ideal situation. The likelihood that such a method could be scaled up for commercial preparation of pure isomers is also a strong impetus for its successful development.

Factors Causing Racemization in Food Systems

The first observations of racemization of amino acids in proteins were made near the beginning of the century (4-6). In these experiments, proteins were exposed to moderate temperatures and strongly alkaline conditions. Several reactions including partial hydrolysis of the proteins, some destruction of amino acyl residues, formation of inter- and intra-chain crosslinks and racemization of amino acyl residues occurred. These studies showed that several proteins suffered rapid declines in optical activity when treated with alkali.

Dakin (15) and later Dakin and Dudley (19) determined the optical properties of some amino acids obtained by hydrolyzing the products resulting from the action of caustic soda on gelatin and casein. Some amino acids like leucine, glutamic acid, aspartic acid, arginine, lysine and phenylalanine showed loss of optical activity indicating a racemic mixture and implying that racemization was complete. These workers were also among the first to report that racemized proteins were particularly resistant to the action of proteolytic enzymes.

Treatment of proteins with alkali can alter their conformation, with the extent of alteration depending on concentration of the base, duration of treatment and the temperature. Hydroxide ions can denature the protein and induce hydrolysis of amide groups of glutamine and asparagine, causing the protein to be more water soluble.

A mechanism for the base-catalyzed racemization reaction has been proposed (58). The reaction occurs via removal of the

$$\underset{\text{L-Amino Acid}}{\overset{\displaystyle \overset{O}{\underset{\|}{}}}{\underset{\substack{\overset{}{\underset{\text{HN}}{}}\overset{}{\underset{/}{}}\text{R} \\ \text{P}_1 \\ \text{OH}^{\ominus}}}{\overset{\text{C-NH-P}_2}{\underset{|}{\overset{|}{\text{C}}}}}} \quad \underset{-H^+}{\overset{+H^+}{\rightleftarrows}} \quad \underset{I}{\overset{\displaystyle \overset{O}{\underset{\|}{}}}{\underset{\substack{\text{P}_1\text{-HN-C-R} \\ \overset{..}{\ominus}}}{\overset{\text{C-NH-P}_2}{\underset{|}{|}}}}} \quad \underset{-H^+}{\overset{+H^+}{\rightleftarrows}} \quad \underset{\text{D-Amino Acid}}{\overset{\displaystyle \overset{O}{\underset{\|}{}}}{\underset{\substack{\text{R} \; \text{NH} \\ \text{H} \\ \text{P}_1}}{\overset{\text{C-NH-P}_2}{\underset{|}{\overset{|}{\text{C}}}}}}}$$

P_1 = Portion of protein chain containing the amino terminus group

P_2 = Portion of protein chain containing the carboxyl terminus

α-methine hydrogen, giving rise to a carbanion intermediate (I). This is followed by the rapid readdition of a proton with equal probability of forming either the D- or L-amino acyl residue, assuming there are no conformational, structural or other effects external to the residue which may bias the reprotonation. This general mechanism appears to be operative within the pH range 1 to 13, although the rate of racemization is proportional to the hydroxide concentration only above pH 8 (59). Below this pH, the racemization rate depends on the electron-withdrawing ability of the amino acid sidechain, and below pH 1, acid-catalyzed enolization at the α-carbon and α-carboxy group may occur (59). Acid-catalyzed racemization of amino acids is well known (60), and that caused during acid hydrolysis of protein samples may be determined most directly using mass spectrometry if deuterium chloride is used for hydrolysis instead of hydrochloric acid (39).

In addition to high pH, increases in the length of treatment and increases in temperature are factors which promote increased racemization. Friedman, et al. (61) have shown that for casein, half of the amount of aspartic acid that will racemize within 24 hours (at 65°C in 0.1N NaOH) will do so within the first hour. Others have shown similar results for proteins such as soy isolate and lactalbumin, with 60% to 80% racemization occurring with the first hour at 100°C (0.1N NaOH)(62).

Heat alone can induce racemization in proteins. Bovine plasma albumin and cod fillets, after heating at 145°C, were partially racemized: isoleucine racemization (measured as D-alloisoleucine by ion exchange analysis) was observed in both test materials (63). Hayase et al. (64,65) roasted several proteins and poly-L-amino acids at 180°-300°C (see Table II for results with casein). Aspartic and glutamic acid were the most racemized amino acids of those detected in the heat-treated proteins. Interestingly, lysine was almost completely racemized in the roasted poly-L-lysine. These workers suggested that the ε-amino group promotes the dissociation of the α-hydrogen atom. D-Alloisoleucine was formed in the roasted proteins: neither L-alloisoleucine nor D-isoleucine were detected, indicating that racemization mainly occurs at the α-carbon of the amino acyl residues.

Early work supports the conclusion that free amino acids and dipeptides are more resistant to racemization upon exposure to alkali than proteins (15,22). These observations have been re-examined recently by Whitaker (68) who hypothesized that amino acid residues in proteins undergo more racemization than do free amino acids due to the electron densities of the amino and carboxylate groups of the free amino acids which interfere in the abstraction of the α-proton by the hydroxide ion.

Recent studies have shown that in addition to the structure of the amino acyl residue, the position of the residue in the peptide (or protein) can have a major effect on racemization (69). Therefore, at the end of an exposure to alkali, and depending on the severity of the treatment, a mixture of the original protein and several D-amino acyl residue-containing proteins is likely to result. The latter are not necessarily identical, i.e., the D-amino acyl residues may be located at different positions along the primary structure of the protein, thereby giving rise to a heterogenous mixture of racemized proteins.

TABLE II. Percent D-Amino Acid Content $\left(\frac{D}{D+L}\right)$ x 100 of Several Proteins

Amino acid	Heat Casein[a]		Proteins Casein[b]	
	230°C	250°C	(8)	(67)
Alanine	10.3	31.5	8.1	11.1
Valine	4.4	14.0	1.2	4.0
Threonine[e]	nd	nd	44.0	nd
Isoleucine[e]	3.8	18.0	nd	nd
Leucine	5.1	14.1	2.4	4.7
Proline	1.0	7.5	nd	nd
Serine	nd	nd	33.0	nd
Methionine	nd	nd	20.7	nd
Aspartic acid	27.9	46.9	20.4	28.0
Phenylalanine	0	19.0	23.8	19.4
Glutamic acid	18.0	36.0	11.1	15.6
Lysine	nd	nd	4.4	nd

[a]Casein was roasted either at 230° or 250° under air for 20 min (65)
[b]Aqueous solutions of casein in 0.1N NaOH at 65° for 3 hr (8,66)
[c]3.8% aqueous solution of fish protein concentrate (FPC) in 0.1N
solution of either NaOH or Ca(OH)$_2$ at 85° for 4 hr

Each value was an average of duplicate samples (14)

upon Exposure to Different Processing Conditions

Alkali		
FPC[c]		Collagen[d]
NaOH	Ca(OH)$_2$	
10.3	10.0	5.0
4.0	3.0	nd
nd	nd	nd
nd	nd	nd
4.0	3.0	6.6
3.0	3.0	6.6
39.0	28.0	36.3
nd	nd	nd
25.0	32.0	18.4
21.0	14.0	12.5
18.0	16.0	10.0
9.0	9.0	8.8

[d]Collagen was maintained 113 hr at room temperature in a 3% aqueous lime solution (67)

[e]%D-threonine and %D-isoleucine expressed as ([D-allo-amino acid]/ ([L-amino acid]+[D-allo-amino acid])) x 100

While several laboratories have shown that severe racemization of proteins can occur during treatment with sodium hydroxide (6,18,22-24,61,62), the effects of other alkalis used in food processing are documented less well. Jenkins, et al. (70) have observed substantial differences in the degree of racemization caused by lime or caustic soda treatment of zein. Lime causes only 50% to 90% of the racemization observed for several amino acyl residues compared to when caustic soda is used. Because a substantial amount of calcium ion remained bound to the protein (approx. 10,000 ppm) compared to 1/20th that amount of sodium ion for the caustic soda-treated zein, it is possible that divalent calcium may stabilize the protein making it less susceptible to racemization. Tovar (14) observed increases of 40% to 50% in serine and phenylalanine racemization and a decrease of 30% aspartate racemization for caustic soda-treated fish protein concentrate compared to lime-treated protein (see Table II). These studies indicate that different alkalis have different effects on racemization of proteins; specifically, lime may cause less racemization than caustic soda at a similar pH.

Nutritional Effects of Racemized Protein

Several studies have compared _in vitro_ enzyme digestibilities between alkali-treated and untreated proteins, and decreases are routinely observed for the treated samples (8,16,18,17,24,61, 71). For instance, as early as 1908, Dakin showed that alkali-treated casein was much more resistant to hydrolysis by enzymes than the untreated protein (71). However, in addition to racemization, crosslinking reactions between amino acids also may occur when proteins are exposed to alkali (72). Of the products formed during alkali-induced crosslinking (73-75), lysinoalanine has been credited with causing a histologically unique lesion in the kidneys of rats fed soy protein treated with caustic soda (76-78). Since that time, most of the _in vivo_ studies which fed alkali-treated protein have investigated the effects of lysino-alanine, using several animal species (79). Because the phenomena of racemization and crosslinking occur under the same conditions, and crosslinked amino acids are measured more readily than racemization, few _in vivo_ studies have been performed specifically on the effects of racemization.

Tovar (14) performed an experiment designed to evaluate the _in vivo_ effect of D-amino acids in alkali-treated protein without the presence of lysinoalanine. In addition, either lime or caustic soda were used to investigate whether these alkalis had different effects _in vivo_. Zein was exposed to 0.1N alkali for 4 hours at 85°C. Because lysine is absent from zein, no lysinoalanine formation was observed. Diets were prepared using untreated or alkali-treated zein and were supplemented with casein and free amino acids to meet the nutritional requirements of the rat. Supplements were adjusted to offset minor losses of amino acids suffered during alkali treatment, and levels of alkali-treated protein were adjusted to provide levels of D-serine (measured by gas chromatography) which have been shown to cause kidney lesions in the rat (80). When these diets were fed to weanling rats, animals on the lime-treated zein diets showed significantly less weight gain (3.96g/rat/day) than animals on the untreated zein diet (4.49g/rat/day). Animals fed caustic soda-treated zein diets suffered alopecia and diarrhea, and depressed weight gain (0.29g/rat/day).

From these results, it can be concluded that caustic soda treatment is much more deleterious to zein than is lime treatment. Racemization of 9 of 11 amino acids in the caustic soda-treated zein was equal of or higher than that observed for the lime-treated protein (70). However, the mechanism by which nutritional quality is reduced is not clear. In a related study, Schwass, et al. investigated lime and caustic soda effects on pronase digests of treated zein, and observed similarly reduced levels of uptake of both treated materials by perfused rat jejunum (16). Therefore, the reduced nutritional quality of caustic soda-treated zein observed by Tovar (14) may be due to impaired metabolic utilization at a step subsequent to intestinal absorption.

Species Variation of Amino Acid Availiability

The potential of an ingested D-amino acid to be used for protein synthesis appears to depend on whether or not there is a mechanism for its conversion to the L-enantiomer. Evidence gathered in several studies showed that most of the essential amino acids in the D-form are not used by human adults. Berg reviewed the utilization of D-amino acids in humans and rats (81). An updated version of Berg's data, including results from more recent studies on availability of D-amino in the chick (82, 83), showed that some essential amino acids in the D-form are better utilized by the chick and the rat than by humans (Table III).

Extensive amino-aciduria was observed in both normal infants and infants with kwashiorkor when fed a diet that contained D-amino acids (114). It appeared that the D-isomers present were incompletely utilized and this accounted for most of the excretion.

Although it had been stated that D-methionine was utilized by man (91), D-methioninuria as well as fecal methionine sulfoxide were consistently observed when a soy formula containing D,L-methionine was fed to infants (93,94). As a result of these findings, use of D,L-methionine was forbidden in infant formulas based on soy (115). Recently, in a metabolic study (95) using nitrogen balance as a criterion for utilization, D-methionine was

Table III. Utilization of D-Amino Acids for Nitrogen Equilibrium
in the Adult Human and for Growth in the Weanling Rat
and Chick[a,b]

Amino Acid	Human		Rat		Chick (82,83)
Leucine	NU	(84)	U	(85)	U
Isoleucine	NU	(84)	NU[c]	(86,87)	PU
Valine	NU	(88)	NU	(89,90)	PU
Threonine	NU	(91)	NU[c]	(92)	NU
Methionine	NU	(93-95)	U	(96)	U
Phenylalanine	PU	(97)	U	(98)	U
Tyrosine	nd		U	(99)	U
Histidine	nd		PU	(100)	PU
Lysine	NU	(101)	NU	(102)	NU
Tryptophan	NU		U	(108-110)	PU[d]
Cystine	nd	(103-107)	NU[c]	(111-112)	U

[a]U = utilized; NU = not utilized; PU = partially utilized; nd =
not determined
[b]The number in parenthesis identifies the references
[c]Only L-isoleucine and L-threonine of the four possible isomers
of each of these amino acids support growth in the young rat.
Mesocystine supports growth only half as well as L-cystine
[d]As well as Ref. 110 and 113

not used as well as the L-enantiomer. It appears that D-methionine may have contributed mainly sulfur to the sulfate pool rather
than being converted to L-methionine.
     Evidence (104,116) suggests that D-tryptophan is not fully
utilized by human subjects and may have harmful effects. Further
studies showed that D-tryptophan did not maintain nitrogen balance
in normal young men (106), and in another study (117), urine from
normal human subjects, after ingestion of D-tryptophan, contained
a considerable portion of this compound as well as D-kynurenine.
In contrast, the rat utilizes D-tryptophan completely; however,
food intake is significantly less in D-tryptophan-fed rats than
in rats fed a diet containing L-tryptophan (110). The metabolic
conversion of the D- to the L-enantiomer takes place in the rat
liver and kidney: D-amino acid oxidase plays a key role in this
conversion (109). Indole pyruvic acid can be converted to L-tryptophan by a stereospecific transaminase apparently absent in
humans. The chick, on the other hand, utilizes only 7-40% of the
D-tryptophan (82,83,110, 113). This wide range of values is probably due to different experimental conditions. D-tryptophan and

other D-amino acids can be absorbed in these species by a diffusion system and these isomers inhibit the absorption of the L-enantiomers (118).

In summary, while HPLC techniques hold the greatest promise of short analysis times and the convenience of no derivatization of samples, these techniques are not yet available. At this time, gas chromatography using covalently bonded chiral stationary phases is the method of choice. This method is sufficiently accessible that measurement of racemization in protein materials can be done on a routine basis. The current state-of-the-art in isomer analysis is this gas chromatographic technique coupled with mass spectrometry.

It has been well established that the three major factors involved in racemization are pH, temperature and time of treatment, with isomerization increasing with increasing pH (above 8), increasing temperature and increasing time. While exposure to extremes of pH and temperature may be short for most processed materials, it is clear that racemization of the most labile residues (e.g. serine, aspartate) occurs fairly rapidly. Because alkali-induced racemization can cause decreased nutritional quality, treated protein materials should be assayed for racemization. Decreases in nutritional quality due to processing should be avoided, especially in situations where protein intake may be at marginal levels. Furthermore, the choice of alkali for a particular treatment may affect the level of racemization observed in a protein material. Studies of the effects of different alkalis should be extended to other proteins which are important in the food industry.

The evidence reviewed here also shows that while crosslinking reactions occur under the same conditions as racemization, and crosslinking can contribute to decreased bioavailability, racemization alone can have a dramatic effect. Part of this effect is likely to be due to the observation that, except for D-phenylalanine, D-amino acids are not utilized by humans.

Acknowledgments

The authors wish to thank Dr. John W. Finley for helpful discussions and Beverly E. Powell and Sonia Semoloni for typing the manuscript.

Reference to a company and/or product named by the Department is only for purposes of information and does not imply approval or recommendation of the product to the exclusion of others which may also be suitable.

Literature Cited

1. Corrigan, J.J. Science, 1969, 164, 142.
2. Beatty, I.M.; Magrath, D.I.; Ennor, A.H. Nature, 1959, 183, 591.
3. Auclair, J.; Patton, R. Rev. Can. Biol., 1950, 9, 3.
4. Kossel, A.; Weiss, F. Z. Physiol. Chem., 1909, 59, 492.
5. Kossel, A.; Weiss, F. Z. Physiol. Chem., 1909, 60, 311.
6. Kossel, A.; Weiss, F. Z. Physiol. Chem., 1910, 68, 165.
7. Rosenfield, D., Hartman, W.E. J. Am. Oil Chem. Soc., 1974, 51, 91A.
8. Bunjampamai, S.; Mahoney, R.R.; Fagerson, I.S. J. Food Sci., 1982, 47, 1229.
9. Hayashi, R.; Kameda, I. Agr. Biol. Chem., 1980, 44, 891.
10. Friedman, M.; Zahnley, J.C.; Masters, P.M. J. Food Sci., 1981, 46, 127.
11. Katz, S.H.; Hediger, M.L.; Valleroy, L.A. Science 1974, 184, 765.
12. DelPaso y Troncoso, F. Papeles dela Nueva España, Succ. de Rivadeneyra, Madrid, 1906, 4, 1.
13. Tovar, L.R.; Carpenter, K.J. Arch. Latinoam. Nutr., 1982, 32.
14. Tovar, L.R. Ph.D. Thesis, Univ. Calif., Berkeley, 1981.
15. Dakin, H.D. J. Biol. Chem., 1912, 13, 357.
16. Schwass, D.E.; Tovar, L.R.; Finley, J.W. This publication.
17. deGroot, A.P.; Slump, P. J. Nutr., 1969, 98, 45.
18. Hayashi, R., Kameda, I., J. Food Sci., 1980, 45, 1430.
19. Dakin, H.D.; Dudley, H.W. J. Biol. Chem., 1913, 15, 263.
20. Allers, A.R. Biochem. Zeitschr., 1907, 6, 272.
21. Kossel, A., Weiss, F. Z. Physiol. Chem., 1909, 59, 492.
22. Levene, P.A.; Bass, L.W. J. Biol. Chem., 1929, 82, 171.
23. Tannenbaum, S.R.; Ahren, M.; Bates, R.P. Food Tech., 1970, 24, 604.
24. Provansal, M.M.P., Cuq, J.L.A.; Cheftel, J.C. J. Agric. Food Chem., 1975, 23, 938.
25. Najarr, V.A. Methods Enzymol., 1957, 3, 462.
26. Cutierrez, J.L.; Soriano, J.; Tovar, L.R. Unpublished data, 1982.
27. Hoeprich, P.D. J. Biol. Chem., 1965, 240, 1654.
28. Krebs, H. A. Biochem. J., 1935, 29, 1620.
29. Prescott, J.M.; Schweigert, B.S.; Lyman, C.M.; Kuiken, K.A. J. Biol. Chem., 1949, 178, 727.
30. Snell, E.E. Methods Enzymol., 1957, 3, 477.
31. Hamilton, P.B. Anal. Chem., 1963, 35, 2055.
32. Hirschman, R.; Strachen, R.G.; Schwan, H.; Schoenewaldt, E.F.; Joshua, H.; Barkemeyer, B.; Veber, D.F.; Paleveda, W.J. Jr.; Jacob, T.A.; Beesley, T.E.; Denkewalter, R.G. J. Org. Chem., 1967, 32, 3415.
33. Manning, J.M.; Moore, S. J. Biol. Chem., 1968, 243, 5591.
34. Pollock, G.E.; Frommhagen, L.H. Anal Biochem', 1968, 24, 18.

35. Nakaparskin, S.; Birret, P.; Gil-Av, E.; Oro, J. J. Chromatogr. Sci., 1970, 8, 177.
36. Mackenzie, S.L.; Tenaschuck, D. J. Chromatogr., 1979, 171, 195.
37. Mackenzie, S.L.; Tenaschuck, D. J. Chromatogr., 1979, 173, 53.
38. Frank, H.; Nicholson, G.J.; Bayer, E. J. Chromatogr. Sci., 1977, 15, 174.
39. Liardon, R.; Lederman, S.; Ott, U. J. Chromatogr., 1981, 203, 385.
40. Davankov, V.A.; Zolotarev, Yu. A.; Kurganov, A.A. J. Liq. Chromatogr., 1979, 2, 1191.
41. Nimura, N.; Suzuki, T.; Kasahara, Y.; Kinoshita, T. Anal. Chem., 1981, 53, 1380.
42. Gübitz, G.; Jellenz, W. J. Liq. Chromatogr., 1981, 4, 701.
43. Gale, E.F. in "Methods of Biochemical Analysis", Glick, D., Ed.; Interscience Publishers: New York, 1954, Vol IV, p. 285.
44. Greenstein, J.P. Methods Enzymol., 1957, 3, 554.
45. Moore, S., Spackman, D.H., Stein, W.H. Anal. Chem., 1958, 30, 1185.
46. Pollock, G.E., Oyama, V.I., Johnson, R.D. Gas Chromatog., 1965, 3, 174.
47. Gil-Av, E., Feibush, B. Charles-Sigler, R. Tetrahed. Lett., 1966, 10, 1009.
48. Frank, H., Nicholson, G.J., Bayer, E. J. Chromatog. Sci., 1977, 15, 174.
49. Buss, D.R., Vermeulen, T. Ind. Eng. Chem., 1968, 60(8), 15.
50. Takaya, T., Kashida, Y., Sakakibara, S. J. Chromatog., 1981, 215, 279.
51. LePage, J.N., Lindner, W., Davies, G., Seitz, D.E., Karger, B.L. Anal Chem., 1979, 51, 433.
52. Hare, P.E., Gil-Av, E. Science, 1979, 204, 1226.
53. Gilon, C., Leshem, R., Tapuhi, Y., Grushka, E. J. Am. Chem. Soc., 1979, 101, 7612.
54. Henderson, G.M. Rule, H.G. Nature, 1938, 141, 917.
55. Karagounis, G., Charbonnier, E., Floss, E. J. Chromatog., 1959, 2, 84.
56. Garmaise, D. L., Colucci, J. U.S. Patent 2, 957, 886, 1960.
57. Davankov, V.A., Rogozhin, S.V. J. Chromatog., 1971, 60, 280.
58. Neuberger, A. Adv. Protein Chem., 1948, 4, 297.
59. Bada, J.L. J. Amer. Chem. Soc., 1972, 94, 1371.
60. Manning, J.M. J. Amer. Chem. Soc., 1970, 92, 7449.
61. Friedman, M., Zahnley, J.C., Masters, P.M. J. Food Sci., 1981, 46, 127.
62. Schwass, D.E., Finley, J.W. Manuscript in preparation.
63. Bjarnason, J.; Carpenter, K.J. Br. J. Nutr., 1970, 24, 313.

64. Hayase, F.; Kato, H.; Fujimaki, M. Agr. Biol. Chem., 1973,
     37, 191.
65. Hayase, F.; Hiromachi, K.; Fujimaki, M. J. Agric. Food Chem.,
     1975, 23, 491.
66. Masters P.M.; Friedman, M. J. Agric. Food Chem., 1979, 27,
     507.
67. Neiss, H.G. Leder 1981, 32, 113.
68. Whitaker, J.R. in "Chemical Deterioration of Proteins",
     Whitaker, J.R.; Fujimaki, M., Eds.; ACS Symposium Series 123,
     American Chemical Society, Washington, D.C., 1980, p. 145.
69. Smith, G.G.; de Sol, B.S. Science, 1980, 207, 765.
70. Jenkins, W.L., Tovar, L.R., Carpenter, K.J., Schwass, D.E.,
     Liardon, R. Manuscript in preparation.
71. Dakin, H.D. J. Biol. Chem., 1908, 4, 437.
72. Whitaker, J.R., Feeney, R.E. in "Protein Crosslinking-Nutri-
     tional and Medical Consequences"; Friedman, M., Ed.; Plenum
     Press: New York, 1977, p. 155.
73. Ziegler, K. J. Biol. Chem., 1964, 239, 2713.
74. Ziegler, K., Melchert, I., Lurken, C. Nature, 1967, 214,
     404.
75. Asquith, R.S., Garcia-Dominguez, J.J. J. Soc. Dyers Colour,
     1968, 84, 155.
76. Woodard, J.C.; Alvarez, M.R. Archs. Path., 1967, 84, 153.
77. Woodard, J.C. Lab. Invest., 1969, 20, 9.
78. Woodard, J.C.; Short, D.D. J. Nutr., 1973, 103, 569.
79. Finley, J.W. This publication.
80. Kaltenbach, J.P., Ganote, C.E., Carone, F.A. Exp. Molec.
     Pathol., 1979, 30, 209.
81. Berg, C.P. in "Protein and Amino Acid Nutrition", Albanese,
     A.A., Ed.; Academic Press: New York, 1959 p. 57.
82. Sugihara, M.; Morimoto, T.; Kobayashi, T.; Ariyoshi, S. Agr.
     Biol. Chem. 1967, 31, 77.
83. Sunde, M.L. Poultry Sci., 1972, 51, 44.
84. Rose, W.C.; Eades, C.H., Jr.; Coon, M.J. J. Biol. Chem.,
     1955, 216, 225.
85. Rechcigl, M.; Loosli, J.K.; Williams, H.H. J. Biol. Chem.,
     1958, 231, 829.
86. Greenstein, J.P.; Levintow, L.; Baker, C.G.; White, J. J.
     Biol. Chem., 1951, 188, 647.
87. Albanese, A.A. J. Biol. Chem., 1945, 157, 613.
88. Rose, W.C.; Wixom, R.L.; Lockhart, H.D.; Lambert, G.F. J.
     Biol. Chem., 1955, 217, 987.
89. Wretlind, K.A.J. Acta Physiol. Scand., 1956, 36, 119.
90. Womack, M.; Snyder, B.B.; Rose, W.C. J. Biol. Chem., 1957,
     224, 793.
91. Rose, W.C.; Coon, M.J.; Lockhart, H.B.; Lambert, G.F. J.
     Biol Chem., 1955, 215, 101.
92. West, H.D.; Carter, H.E. J. Biol. Chem., 1938, 122, 611.

93.   Efron, M.L.; McPherson, T.C.; Shi, V.E.; Welsh, C.F.;
      McCready, R.A. Am. J. Dis. Child, 1969, 117, 104.
94.   Stegink, L.D.; Schmitt, J.L.; Meyer, P.D.; Kain, P.H. J.
      Pediatr., 1971, 79, 648.
95.   Zezulka, A.Y.; Calloway, D.H. J. Nutr., 1976, 106, 1286.
96.   Wretlind, K.A.J.; Rose, W.C. J. Biol. Chem., 1950, 187, 697.
97.   Rose, W.C.; Leach, B.E.; Coon, M.J.; Lambert, G.F. J. Biol.
      Chem., 1955, 213, 913.
98.   Rose, W.C.; Womack, M. J. Biol. Chem., 1946, 166, 103.
99.   Bubl, E.C.; Butts, J.S. J. Biol. Chem. 1948, 174, 637.
100. Cox, G.J.; Berg, C.P. J. Biol. Chem., 1934, 107, 497.
101. Rose, W.C.; Borman, A.; Coon, M.J.; Lambert, G.F. J. Biol.
      Chem., 1955, 214, 579.
102. Berg, C.P. J. Nutr. 1936, 12, 671.
103. Albanese, A.A.; Davis, V.I.; Lein, M. J. Biol. Chem., 1948,
      172, 39.
104. Albanese, A.A.; Snyderman, S.E.; Lein, M.; Smetak, E.M.;
      Vestal, B. J. Nutr., 1949, 38, 215.
105. Baldwin, H.R.; Berg, C.P. J. Nutr. 1949, 29, 203.
106. Rose, W.C.; Lambert, G.F.; Coon, M.J. J. Biol. Chem., 1954,
      211, 815.
107. Clayton, B.E.; Heeley, A.F.; Heeley, M. Br. J. Nutr., 1970,
      24, 573.
108. du Vigneaud, V.; Doffman, R.; Loring, H.S. J. Biol. Chem.,
      1932, 98, 577.
109. Ohara, I. Nutr. Rep. Int., 1979, 20, 833.
110. Ohara, I.; Otsuka, S.; Yugari, Y.; Ariyoshi, S. J. Nutr.,
      1980, 110, 634.
111. du Vigneaud, V.; Sealock, R.R.; Van Etten, C. J. Biol Chem.,
      1932, 98, 565.
112. Loring, H.S.; Dorfman, R.; du Vigneaud, V. J. Biol. Chem.,
      1933, 103, 399.
113. Wilkening, M.C.; Schweigert, B.S. J. Biol. Chem., 1947, 171,
      209.
114. Schendel, H.E.; Antoins, A.; Hansen, J.D.L. Pediatrics.,
      1959, 23, 662.
115. U.S. Food and Drug Administration (1973) Federal Register
      38 No. 143 Part II: 20037.
116. Berg, C.P.; Rohse, W.G. J. Biol. Chem., 1947, 170, 725.
117. Langner, R.R.; Berg, C.P. J. Biol. Chem., 1955, 214, 699.
118. Shorrock, C.; Ford, J.E. Br. J. Nutr., 1978, 40, 185.

RECEIVED July 8, 1983

Absorption of Altered Amino Acids from the Intestine

DANIEL E. SCHWASS—Western Regional Research Center, U.S. Department of Agriculture, ARS, Berkeley, CA 94710

L. RAÚL TOVAR—Departamento de Alimentos, DEPg, Facultad de Química, Universidad de México, México 04510, D. F.

JOHN W. FINLEY[1]—Nutritional Biochemistry, Ralston Purina, Checkerboard Square, St. Louis, MO 63188

Heat or alkaline treatment of protein-containing materials may cause racemization of a portion of the amino acids as well as crosslinking between amino acids. Very little is understood about how these altered amino acids interact with transport systems for normal amino acids and peptides in the gut. This study was designed to examine the effects of racemization on *in vitro* digestibility of alkali-treated protein and on *in vivo* uptake of digested, treated protein, in the absence of crosslinking. We report that significant decreases in *in vitro* digestibility and *in vivo* availability can be attributed to racemization effects.

Two major chemical modifications of proteins that occur during alkaline treatment are crosslinking and racemization. Lysine, ornithine (via arginine), cystine and O-substituted serine can participate in base-catalyzed reactions forming the crosslinked amino acids lysinoalanine, ornithinoalanine and lanthionine (1-4). Under the same conditions, inversion can occur when the α-hydrogen of an amino acid residue is abstracted by the base, resulting in a planar, optically inactive carbanion (7), as illustrated in Figure 1. The carbanion may be reprotonated from either face of the plane, which causes inversion when this occurs from the opposite face.

The formation of lysinoalanine (LAL) in treated proteins has been the subject of several investigations (for reviews, see 6,7) since it was discovered that alkali-treated soy protein could cause a kidney lesion in rats and LAL appeared to be responsible (8). Human toxicity has not been established and no lesions were observed in rhesus monkeys, mice, hamsters, dogs and Japanese quail fed diets including free LAL or protein containing LAL (8, and see 7).

[1] Current address: Department of Pediatrics, University Hospitals and Clinics, University of Iowa, Iowa City, IA 52242

In addition to LAL, D-serine has been shown to be nephrotoxic in rats, with lesions similar to those observed after LAL administration (9). When included in the diet, D-serine causes necrosis of the proximal tubule of the kidney which can be fatal (10). Although rats are sensitive to D-serine, several other species such as dogs, hamsters, rabbits and mice do not develop lesions (8,11). Toxicity has not been established for humans.

Over and above the toxic effects of D-serine, which are likely to be negligible in a realistic diet, several studies have provided evidence that racemization of amino acyl residues in alkali-treated and heat-treated proteins decreases digestibility. Dakin, in 1908, was the first to examine the effects of alkali treatment on *in vitro* digestibility (12). He showed that treated casein was highly-resistant to pepsin, trypsin and erepsin hydrolysis. Dakin and Dudley followed up the *in vitro* studies with an experiment in which dogs were fed alkali-treated casein, and found that the protein was largely unabsorbed and was recoverable in the feces (13).

In 1969, deGroot and Slump also demonstrated decreases for *in vitro* digestibility of alkali-treated soy protein isolate and decreases in absorption of some amino acids by everted intestinal sacs (14). These workers also observed decreases in net protein utilization for treated soybean meal, treated soy protein isolate and treated casein. These decreases in net protein utilization were correlated with increases in LAL formation. In these experiments, therefore, it was possible that protein utilization was hindered by the presence of LAL.

Provansal and co-workers (15) treated sunflower protein isolate with sodium hydroxide and observed formation of LAL, racemization of isoleucine and lysine (only these two were analyzed for racemization), and decreased *in vitro* digestibility by pronase. While these workers suggested that the decreased pronase hydrolysis may have been due to crosslinking reactions, they also pointed out that it was likely that other amino acids were also racemized which could compromise the nutritional quality of the protein.

More recently, Hayashi and Kameda (16) investigated the effects of alkali treatment on casein and soybean protein by looking at *in vitro* pepsin digestibility, racemization and LAL formation. These authors observed that pepsin released fewer amino acids from treated protein than control samples. They suggested that decreases in *in vitro* digestibility were due to racemization (which was measured indirectly by tritium exchange) and not crosslinking because they felt LAL formation occurred too slowly. However, it appears that LAL formation was high enough in these experiments to question this conclusion.

In 1981, Friedman, Zahnley and Masters measured the *in vitro* digestibility of alkali-treated casein by trypsin and chymotrypsin as a function of temperature, time and pH of the treatment (17). They also measured LAL formation and the racemization of aspartate and phenylalanine and observed that the decrease in digestibility occurred as both crosslinking and racemization increased. However, it was not possible from their results to determine whether crosslinking reactions or racemization had the greater effect on digestibility.

Because crosslinking and racemization both occur during alkaline treatment of proteins and an effect of both of these phenomena is to decrease nutritional quality (18), it is of interest to know if either process has a greater effect on protein digestibility and uptake. While there is no way known to prevent racemization during alkaline treatment, it is possible to prevent LAL formation by the addition of thiols during processing (19) or by acylation of the protein prior to processing (20).

The work of Bunjapamai, Mahoney and Fagerson (21) was the first successful attempt to separate the effects of racemization from crosslinking as measured by *in vitro* digestion. Alkali-treatment of citraconylated (lysine-blocked) or non-blocked casein resulted in racemized only (blocked) or racemized and LAL cross-linked (non-blocked) casein. *In vitro* multienzyme digestion of these preparations as well as untreated casein revealed similarly decreased digestibilities for the treated proteins whether crosslinked or not, indicating that the primary cause for reduction of casein digestibility was racemization.

It is important to know the separate effects of racemization and crosslinking for several proteins, especially those important in food systems. Therefore, the purpose of this study was to isolate racemization from crosslinking, examine the effects of racemization on *in vitro* digestibility of alkali-treated zein and *in vivo* accumulation of alkali-trated protein by isolated rat jejunum.

Zein, which is the major protein in corn, was chosen because it contains no lysine. This precluded the formation of LAL during alkali treatment. Therefore, any changes in digestibility or uptake could be attributed to racemization effects alone. Additionally, we were interested in comparing the effects of sodium hydroxide treatment with the effects of calcium hydroxide treatment because lime is used in the preparation of corn meal for use in tortillas. If the traditional lime treatment of corn meal is unnecessarily harsh, it could have important nutritional consequences because a large segment of the Mexican population obtains much of their dietary protein in the form of tortillas (22).

Materials and Methods

The basic outline of our experiment (Figure 2) was to treat zein with sodium hydroxide or calcium hydroxide causing racemization. The treated or untreated zein was then enzymatically hydrolyzed and values for digestibility determined. Samples of the

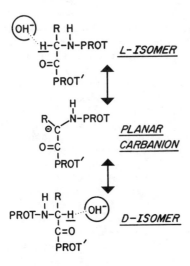

Figure 1. Mechanism of base-catalyzed inversion of an amino acyl residue in a protein.

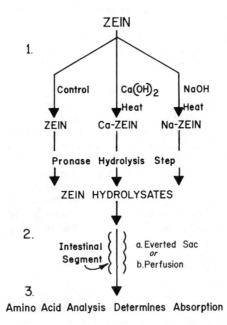

Figure 2. Outline of in vitro digestibility and in vitro (everted sac) or in vivo (intestinal perfusion) uptake experiments. Amino acid analysis of everted sac contents or of original and final intestinal perfusate allows uptake determination.

enzymatic hydrolysates were then presented to segments of rat intestine to determine uptake of the pre-digested treated or untreated material.

Alkali Treatment. Zein (ICN Nutritional Biochemicals, Cleveland, OH) was suspended in 0.1N sodium hydroxide or 0.1N calcium hydroxide, held at 85°C for 4 hours, neutralized with 2 N hydrochloric acid, cooled to 4°C (3 hours) and dialyzed against 25 volumes of 0.1N acetate buffer, pH 4.5 for 24 hours with one change at eight hours. Untreated zein was suspended in deionized water and taken through the dialysis procedure. After dialysis, the zeins were lyophilized. At this point, samples were taken for amino acid analysis (Durrum D-500, Dionex Corp., Sunnyvale, CA; or Beckman 121 MB, Palo Alto, CA) and isomer analysis.

Hydrolysis by Pronase. *In vitro* pronase (Calbiochem-Behring Corp LaJolla, CA) hydrolyses were performed according to the method of Rayner and Fox (23). Mixtures of zein, pronase and 40 mM borate buffer (pH 8.0) in the ratio 1 gm zein to 150 mg pronase to 100 ml buffer were placed in screw-cap flasks and the pH readjusted to 8.0 if necessary. A sample without zein was also prepared as a control. The suspensions were incubated at 40°C for 48 hours with shaking. After the incubation, a 3 ml aliquot was taken for amino acid analysis and the remainder was frozen at -20°C. The 3 ml of hydrolysate was mixed with 6 ml 1% aqueous picric acid and centrifuged for 30 minutes at 3000 rpm at 4°C to remove residual protein and peptides. Five ml of the supernatant was placed on a 1.2 cm by 9 cm AG-50W-X8(H+), 100-200 mesh cation exchange column (Bio-Rad Laboratories, Richmond, CA). Picric acid was washed from the column with deionized water and the bound hydrolysate was eluted with 3M ammonium hydroxide. The eluates were rotary evaporated at 60°C and washed twice with deionized water, before being dissolved in 0.2N citrate buffer (pH 2.2) for amino acid analysis.

Everted Sac Experiments. Hydrolysate solutions for use in the everted sac experiments were prepared by mixing 15 ml of the thawed pronase hydrolysates with 5 ml of a solution containing 4.50 g/l NaCl, 0.74 g/l KCl and 2.10 g/l NaHCO₃. The solutions were equilibrated with 95%:5% oxygen:carbon dioxide at 37°C (pH 8.0) and osmolality (Wescor, Inc., Logan, UT) was observed to be within 10% of 302 mOsm.

Everted intestinal sacs were prepared following the method developed by Wilson and Wiseman (25). Rats (mean weight of 210g, Simonsen Laboratories, Gilroy, CA) which were fed a chow diet (Ralston Purina, Inc., St. Louis, MO), were killed by a blow to the head after a 13 hour fast. The small intestine was sectioned at a distance of 10% of the total length of the intestine from pylorus to the ileo-caecal junction. Any residual, undigested food was washed out with chilled 0.9% NaCl before the intestine was turned inside out (everted). Two sacs from the duodenum end, of approximately 6 cm each, were made from each rat. The sacs were tied off from the ileal end and filled with 2 ml Krebs-Henseleit Ringer isotonic buffer, pH 7.4. The sacs were then transferred into Erlenmeyer flasks containing 20 ml of the sample solution. Incubation was carried out at 37° for 1 hour with constant stirring. At the end of the incubation period, the volume of the serosal fluid was measured and an aliquot taken for amino acid analysis.

Intestinal Perfusion Experiments. Hydrolysate solutions for use in the perfused intestine experiments were prepared by concentrating the pronase hydrolysates approximately two-fold in a rotary evaporator at 60°C (to inactivate pronase, 24) and mixing the equivalent of 157.5 mg (untreated zein), 289.2 mg (Ca(OH)$_2$-treated zein) or 150.0 mg (NaOH-treated zein) with 0.05M HEPES (Calbiochem-Behring Corp., LaJolla, CA) buffer (pH 8.0). The final solutions had a pH of 8.10 ± 0.05.

Intestinal perfusion experiments were performed using an adaptation of the technique of Smithson and Gray (26). Rats (mean weight of 220 gm fasted 13 hr.) were anesthetized with sodium pentobarbital (Abbot Laboratories, N. Chicago, IL) and a midline incision made in the abdomen which allowed access to the small intestine. A length of jejunum adjacent to the duodenum was isolated by inserting a tube catheter at both ends of the segment and the sample was perfused for 40 minutes. Even though the intestinal loop was outside the animal, it continued to receive blood from the intact circulatory system and remained quite viable over the course of the experiment.

Fifteen ml of the pronase hydrolysate solutions were circulated through the intestinal segments over a 40 minute interval at a rate of 0.39 ml/min at 37°C, using a peristaltic pump (Buchler "Polystaltic", Fort Lee, NJ). At the end of the perfusion interval, the perfusates were flushed from the system using 0.9% saline at 37°C and stored at -20°C for later analysis. The perfused segments of jejumum were excised and weighed. The frozen perfusates were thawed, adjusted to pH 6.5 with 0.1N hydrochloric acid, heated 10 minutes in a boiling water bath (to precipitate any protein sloughed from the mucosal cells), centrifuged 10 minutes and the supernatant collected. The deproteinized supernatants were made up to 25 ml with deionized water and an aliquot taken for hydrolysis in 6 N hydrochloric acid. Aliquots of the pronase hydrolysate solutions (which were not perfused) were also adjusted to pH 6.5, boiled, centrifuged and hydrolyzed as above. Amino acid analyses of the hydrolyzed samples were then performed.

Isomer Analysis. Isomer analyses were performed using an optically active Chirasil-Val 25m column (Applied Science, State College, PA) in a Hewlett-Packard 5840 gas chromatograph (Avon-

dale, PA) fitted with an inlet stream splitter and flame ionization detector. Hydrolysates were derivatized (27) using 3N hydrochloric acid in dry isopropyl alcohol for esterification and pen-
tafluoropropionic anhydride (Pierce Chemical Co., Rockford, IL)
for acylation.

Results and Discussion

The amino acid compositions of the untreated and treated
zeins are given in Table I, and are in reasonable agreement with
those of Boundy, et al. (28). As expected, no LAL was observed
in these materials.

Table II lists the amino acid compositions of the pronase
hydrolysates after picric acid precipitation (i.e. amino acids
released by pronase). For each amino acid but glycine, which was
present only in small quantities, decreases in released amino
acids were observed for the lime- and caustic soda-treated zeins.
These results are shown in Figure 3 where release is expressed as
a percent of that seen for untreated zein. The 32% decrease for
the Ca(OH)$_2$-treated zein and 41% decrease for NaOH-treated zein
indicates that the *in vitro* digestibility has been significantly
reduced by both of the alkali treatments.

Hayashi and Kameda have reported 40% to 70% decreases in pep-
sin-catalyzed hydrolysis of lysozyme, soybean protein, casein and
ribonuclease A due to alkali-treatment under slightly milder conditions than ours (16, 29). Friedman, Zahnley and Masters reported an 80% decrease in digestibility of sodium hydroxide-treated
casein measured as hydrolysis by trypsin (17). However, trypsin
is specific for lysyl residues and lysine levels decreased to
about half control values during the alkali-treatment, with a concomitant increase in LAL formation. The somewhat lower digestibilities reported by these laboratories compared to our observations may be due to LAL formation in the proteins other than zein.

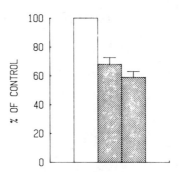

*Figure 3. In vitro pronase digestibilities of untreated zein (open bar), Ca (OH)$_2$-
treated zein (center, shaded bar) and NaOH-treated zein (right, shaded bar).
Results expressed as percent free amino acids released relative to control. Standard error bars are shown.*

TABLE I. Amino acid composition of the non-treated and alkali-treated
          zein obtained by acid hydrolysis, compared with published data[1]

Amino Acid[2]	g/16 g nitrogen					
	non-treated		Ca(OH)$_2$-treated		NaOH-treated	
				%		%
Cysteic acid	nd	[1.5]	nd	[1.3]	nd	
Methionine	nd	[2.0]	nd	[1.4]	nd	
Aspartic acid	6.6	[5.6]	6.6	[6.1] (100)	6.2	(94)
Threonine	3.5	[3.2]	2.6	[3.2] (74)	2.5	(71)
Serine	6.8	[6.9]	5.1	[6.3] (75)	4.8	(90)
Glutamic acid	27.7	[25.9]	25.5	[26.7] (92)	24.8	(90)
Proline	12.6	[11.0]	11.6	[9.6] (92)	10.8	(86)
Glycine	1.5	[1.4]	1.5	[1.2] (100)	1.4	(93)
Alanine	12.2	[10.6]	12.0	[11.2] (98)	11.4	(93)
Valine	4.4	[3.2]	4.4	[4.0] (100)	3.9	(89)
Isoleucine	5.2	[3.1]	4.8	[4.4] (92)	4.5	(87)
Leucine	25.8	[20.4]	27.6	[22.4] (107)	24.9	(97)
Tyrosine	6.8	nd	6.2	nd (91)	5.7	(84)
Phenylalanine	9.4	[7.4]	8.9	[7.8] (95)	8.2	(87)
Histidine	1.7	nd	1.6	nd (94)	1.5	(88)
Arginine	2.1	[1.6]	1.4	[1.5] (67)	1.8	(86)
Totals	126.3	[103.8]	119.8	[107.1]	112.4	

[1]Values in brackets are data gathered by Boundy et al. (28). Their
Ca(OH)$_2$ treatment was carried out at 75° for 15 minutes (concentration
of the alkali not indicated). Values in parentheses are percentages of
amino acid observed relative to the non-treated zein acid hydrolyzate;
nd = not determined.

[2]Lysinoalanine was not detected in any of the samples.

Table II. Amino acids released by the *in vitro* pronase hydrolysis in non-treated and alkali-treated zein[1]

Amino Acid	g amino acid/16 g of original nitrogen Zein					
	non-treated		Ca(OH)$_2$		NaOH	
Aspartic acid	0.4[2]		0.5[2]		0.0	[0]
Threonine[3]	–		–		–	
Serine[3]	–		–		–	
Glutamic acid[3]	–		–		–	
Proline	0.0	[0]	0.0	[0.0]	0.0	
Glycine	0.2	[13]	0.5	[33.3]	0.0	
Alanine	16.9[4]		11.7	[98]	8.8	[77]
Valine	3.4	[77]	2.6	[59]	2.3	[59]
Methionine	0.9		0.4		0.5	
Isoleucine	4.0	[77]	2.7	[56]	2.4	[53]
Leucine	27.7	[107]	22.9	[83]	19.4	[78]
Tyrosine	3.0	[44]	2.5	[40]	2.1	[37]
Phenylalanine	7.5	[80]	5.0	[56]	5.1	[62]
Histidine	0.5	[29]	0.4	[25]	0.3	[20]
Lysine	0	0	0.16		0.21	
Arginine	1.5	[71]	0.6	[38]	0.4	[22]
Cysteine	0.0		0.0		0.0	
TOTAL[5]	64.1		48.9		41.5	

[1] Corrections have been made for the reagent blanks in each test materials. Values in brackets refer to the percentage of the amino acid that has been released by pronase relative to its content in the zein acid hydrolyzates. These values represent one determination.

Continued on next page

Table II.--Continued

[2]No percentage can be given relative to the values in the acid
hydrolyzates because of a lack of data of actual content of
asparagine in non-treated and treated zein.

[3]Since asparagine and glutamine peaks overlapped with the threonine,
for serine and glutamic acid peaks in the zein hydrolyzates, values
for these amino acids are not included.

[4]An interfering peak overlapped with the alanine peak: this value
is higher than that obtained in acid hydrolyzates.

[5]Neither ammonia nor tryptophan is included.

Accumulation of the measured amino acids from the pronase
digests into everted sacs is shown in Figure 4. The results are
expressed as percent accumulation relative to control which was
directly measured in the contents of the everted sac by amino
acid analysis. Although accumulation in the calcium hydroxide-
treated cases is not greatly decreased compared to the control,
the sodium hydroxide-treated zein hydrolysate shows markedly decreased accumulation. However, serine shows significantly reduced uptake in both the lime- and soda-treated zeins. The reason for this observation is not clear.

The results from the everted sac experiments were that both
calcium hydroxide and sodium hydroxide treatment significantly
decrease *in vitro* digestibility, but that only sodium hydroxide
treatment affects uptake of the zein hydrolysates. Because of
the minimal effects of calcium hydroxide treatment on accumulation, we decided to reexamine the uptake phenomenon using an

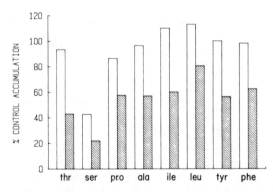

*Figure 4. Accumulation of free amino acids by everted gut sacs. Key: open bars,
pronase digests of Ca(OH)$_2$-treated zein; and shaded bars, pronase digests of
NaOH-treated zein. Results are expressed as percent relative to accumulation
for pronase digests of untreated (control) zein and represent duplicate determinations.*

in vivo technique that more closely approximated the physiological gut, as the everted sac technique has been criticized for lack
of proper oxygenation of the tissue (26).

Figure 5 shows the results for the uptake of several amino
acids from the pronase hydrolysate of untreated zein. One disadvantage of using this technique is that it is necessary to measure
both the original concentration of substrate as well as the concentration of substrate remaining after the uptake interval. The
accumulation must be determined by difference and has been expressed here as the percent of amino acid in the original hydrolysate taken up. These results show that the gut is able to remove
10 to 15% of the amino acids presented to it over a 40 minute
interval.

Figure 6 shows the results for the calcium hydroxide-treated
zein digest in the hatched bars, while the open bars are the control values, for ease of comparison. A generally similar pattern
of uptake was observed except most values were reduced about 5%,
(to about 60% control), indicating a decrease in amino acid uptake. This is in contrast to the results obtained using the
everted sac technique, where little difference was observed between control and calcium hydroxide-treated zein. Numbers below
the bars indicate the degree of racemization for the treated
zein, which will be discussed below.

The results for the sodium hydroxide treated zein are shown
in Figure 7. Again, the control values are given as open bars for
comparison. As in the calcium hydroxide-treated case, uptake is
reduced to the 5 to 10% level (about 50% control) with a generally
similar pattern of uptake over the amino acids. As in Figure 6,
numbers below the bars indicate the percent D-isomer present in
the treated zein. It is apparent that there is not a linear
correlation between the degree of racemization and the degree of
uptake inhibition in either the soda or lime-treated cases since
the accumulation of phenylalanine, for example, in the soda-
treated case is similar to the accumulation of alanine in the
soda-treated sample even though there is only one half as much
racemization of alanine.

This phenomenon may be explained if one considers that a
great deal of the amino acids are taken up in the form of peptides rather than by a process of essentially complete hydrolysis to free amino acids in the gut lumen. Evidence from many
laboratories including those of Matthews (30) and Adibi (31) has
shown that perhaps more than 50% of amino acid uptake can be
accounted for by transport of intact peptides. There appears
to be specificity for some portion of the peptide, but at this
time it is not clear how large the recognition sequence must be
(32). Although there has been no evidence excluding all peptides
containing more than three residues, several tetrapeptides have
been tested in mammalian systems and do not appear to be transported intact, while tripeptides are good substrates for uptake
(33).

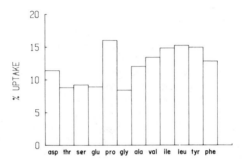

Figure 5. Uptake of amino acids from pronase hydrolysate of untreated zein by perfused jejunal segments. Results represent the portion of total amino acids taken up and are expressed as the percent of the difference between the original and final amino acid concentrations in acid hydrolysates of the perfusate (AA_o − AA_f) divided by the original concentration (AA_o):[(AA_o − AA_f)/(AA_o)] × 100. Duplicate determinations were run.

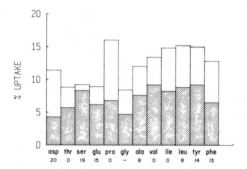

Figure 6. Uptake of amino acids from pronase hydrolysate of Ca(OH)$_2$-treated zein by perfused jejunal segments. Shaded bars show uptake for Ca(OH)$_2$-treated zein and open bars are control (see Figure 5) for ease of comparison. Results expressed as in Figure 5. Numbers below the bars indicate percent D-isomer in the treated hydrolysates.

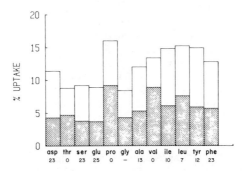

Figure 7.   Uptake of amino acids from pronase hydrolysate of NaOH-treated zein by perfused jejunal segments. Shaded areas show uptake for NaOH-treated zein and open bars are control (see Figure 5) for ease of comparison. Results are expressed as in Figure 5. Numbers below the bars indicate percent D-isomer in the treated hydrolysates.

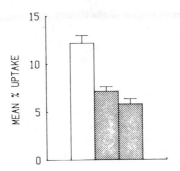

Figure 8.   Mean uptake of amino acids from pronase hydrolysates of untreated zein (open bar), Ca(OH)₂-treated zein (center, shaded bar) and NaOH-treated zein (right, shaded bar). Averages were taken over the 12 amino acids measured in Figures 5–7. Uptake is expressed as in Figure 5. Standard error bars are shown.

We are led by our results to speculate that if an amino acid residue is present in the peptide as the D-isomer, it may render that peptide unavailable for transport regardless of whether the inverted residue is an alanine, phenylalanine or any other amino acid. And each of the other L-residues in the peptide will be denied entry regardless of their identity or degree of racemization. So phenylalanine uptake might be decreased as much as alanine uptake because both of these amino acids finds themselves in D-isomer-containing peptides at about the same frequency.

A summary of the results from the perfused intestine experiment is shown in Figure 8. The results are expressed as the mean uptake of all the measured amino acids for the three zein hydrolysates. The results from this series clearly show that uptake has been reduced by both soda- and lime-treatments of zein, which is also consistent with the results of the pronase study which show that both calcium hydroxide and sodium hydroxide treatments decrease digestibility. However, it is not clear why the results for $Ca(OH)_2$-treated zein are different for the everted sac and perfusion experiments, but this may be related to the better viability of the *in vivo* perfusion technique.

In conclusion, racemization alone reduces *in vitro* digestibility as well as *in vivo* uptake of enzymatically digested protein. This supports in part the results of Bunjapamai, et al., (21) who concluded that racemization plays a greater role than crosslinking in reducing digestibility of treated protein.

These results suggest that racemization of certain non-essential residues such as aspartate may have indirect, negative effects on the availability of other, relatively non-racemized but essential residues. Therefore, conditions which cause racemization should be minimized during processing.

Acknowledgments

The authors wish to thank Dr. Gary M. Gray and his laboratory for demonstrating the intestinal perfusion techniques, Amy Noma for many amino acid analyses and B. E. Powell and Lillie Davis for typing the manuscript.

Literature Cited

1. Whitaker, J.R., Feeney, R.E. in "Protein Crosslinking - Nutritional and Medical Consequences"; Friedman, M., Ed.; Plenum Press: New York, 1977, p. 155.
2. Ziegler, K., J. Biol. Chem., 1964, 239, 2713.
3. Ziegler, K., Melchert, I., Lurken, C. Nature, 1967, 214, 404.
4. Asquith, R.S., Garcia-Dominguez, J.J., J. Soc. Dyers Colour, 1968, 84, 155.
5. Neuberger, A. Adv. Prot. Chem. 1948, 4, 297.

6. Gould, D.H., MacGregor, J.T. in "Protein Crosslinking-Nutritional and Medical Consequences"; Friedman, M., Ed.; Plenum Press: New York, 1977, p.29.
7. Finley, J.W. This publication.
8. deGroot, A.P., Slump, P., Feron, V.J., Van Beek, L., J. Nutr. 1976, 106. 1527.
9. Artom, C., Fishman, W.H., Morehead, R.P. Proc. Soc. Exptl. Biol. Med., 1945, 60, 284.
10. Morehead, R.P., Fishman, W.H., Artom, C. Am. J. Path. 1945, 21, 803.
11. Kaltenbach, J.P., Ganote, C.E., Carone, F.A. Exp. Mol. Pathol., 1979, 30, 209.
12. Dakin, H.D., J. Biol. Chem., 1908, 4, 437.
13. Dakin, H.D., Dudley, H.W., J. Biol. Chem., 1913, 15, 271.
14. deGroot, A.P., Slump, P., J. Nutr. 1969, 98, 45.
16. Hayashi, R., Kameda, I., J. Food Sci., 1980, 45, 1430.
17. Friedman, M., Zahnley, J.C., Masters, P.M., J. Food Sci. 1981, 46, 127.
18. deGroot, A.P., Slump, P., van Beek, L., Feron, V.J. in "Evaluation of Protein for Humans"; Bodwell, C.E., Ed.; AVI: Westport, Connecticut, 1977, p. 270.
19. Finley, J.W., Snow, J.T., Johnston, P.H., Friedman, M. in "Protein Crosslinking-Nutritional and Medical Consequences"; Friedman, M., Ed.; Plenum Press: New York, 1977, p. 85.
20. Friedman, M. in "Nutritional Improvement of Food and Feed Proteins"; Friedman, M., Ed.; Plenum Press: New York, 1978, p. 613.
21. Bunjapamai, S., Mahoney, R.R., Fagerson, I.S. J. Food Sci. 1982, 47, 1229.
22. Del Valle, F., Perez, J., J. Food Sci., 1974, 39, 244.
23. Rayner, C.J., Fox, M., J. Food Sci. Agric., 1976, 27, 643.
24. Ouchi, T. Agric. Biol. Chem., 1962, 26, 734.
25. Wilson, T.H., Wiseman, G. J. Physiol., 1954, 123, 116.
26. Smithson, K.W., Gray, G.M., J. Clin. Invest., 1977, 60, 665.
27. Schwass, D.E., Finley, J.W. Manuscript in preparation.
28. Boundy, J.A., Turner, J.E., Wall, J.S., Dimler, R.J. Cereal Chem., 1967, 44, 281.
29. Hayashi, R., Kameda, I., Agric. Biol. Chem., 1980, 44, 891.
30. Matthews, D.M., Craft, I.L., Geddes, D.M., Wise, I.J., Hyde, C.W., Clin. Sci., 1968, 35, 415.
31. Adibi, S.A., Phillips, E., Clin. Res., 1968, 16, 446.
32. Addison, J.M., Burston, D., Dalrymple, J.A., Matthews, D.M., Payne, J.W., Sleisenger, M.H., Wilkinson, S., Clin. Sci. Mol. Med., 1975, 49, 313.
33. Adibi, S.A., Kim, Y.S. in "Physiology of the Gastrointestinal Tract"; Johnson, L.R., Ed.; Raven Press: New York, 1981, p. 1073.

RECEIVED August 4, 1983

Lysinoalanine Formation in Severely Treated Proteins

JOHN W. FINLEY

Department of Pediatrics, The University of Iowa, Iowa City, IA 52242

Heat or alkaline treatment of foods, feeds or pure proteins can result in desirable changes in the food system but treatments can also lead to the formation of a series of xenobiotics, one of which is lysinoalanine. Alkaline treatment of proteins can be intended to improve flavor or texture (1-3), to destroy toxins or enzyme inhibitors and to promote solubilization of the protein for the purpose of isolation (4, 5). Heat treatment can be used for sterilization or to alter the physical characteristics of the protein or constituents of the food system.

An undesirable aspect of heat and alkaline treatment is that crosslinking compounds such as lysinoalanine are formed and can lead to severely impaired digestibility and reduced bioavailability of the protein. Such changes cannot be completely separated from the isopeptide formations (6), the Maillard reactions (7) and the racemization reactions (8) discussed elsewhere in this volume. In this chapter the chemistry, the analysis, the toxicology and the occurrence of lysinoalanine will be reviewed.

Chemistry of Lysinoalanine Formation

In 1964, Patchornik and Sokolovsky (9) observed the formation of an unusual amino acid when they treated S-dinitrophenylated ribonuclease with alkali. They concluded that the new amino acid was the result of an addition reaction between the ε-amino group of lysine and dehydroalanine. Later the same year, Bohak (10) reported the isolation of a new amino acid (N-ε-)D,L-2-amino-2-carboxyethyl)-L-lysine, from the acid hydrolyzte of alkaline treated proteins. The trivial name lysinoalanine (LAL) was assigned to the new amino acid. Patchornik and Sokolovsky (11) reported the importance of cystine in the formation of dehydroalanine in proteins. The observation was important in that dehydroalanine is an immediate precurser of LAL. Ziegler reported that alkaline treatment of wool also resulted in the formation of LAL and later found ornithinoalanine as well as LAL in alkaline-treated silk protein (12). Bohak (10) reported that LAL was

0097–6156/83/0234–0203$06.00/0

formed in a variety of alkaline treated proteins including lysozyme, papain, chymotrypsin, phosphovitin and bovine serum albumin.
The generally accepted route of formation of LAL is through
the formation of dehydroalanine from cysteine, cystine, serine or
phosphoserine through β-elimination reaction followed by Michael
addition between the dehydroalanine and the ε-amino group of
lysine. The formation of LAL from the oxidized derivatives of
cystine has been reported by Finley et al. (13). It was suggested
that oxidation of cystine to cystine monoxide may accelerate dehydroalanine formation and subsequent LAL formation. It was also
observed that very little LAL was formed through the β-elimination of cysteine. Mellet (14) proposed that the elimination reaction in serine residues was responsible for the formation of dehydroalanine in peptides. Whitaker and Feeney (15) have reviewed
the alkaline decomposition of phosphoserine and glycosylated
serine or threonine residues in proteins.

When cartilage is treated with alkali, there is complete or
nearly complete loss of cystine and glycosylated serine along with
the formation of substantial amounts of LAL in the protein. Lee
et al. (16) investigated the effects of alkali on antifreeze
glycoprotein. The protein was chosen because it contained no
sulfhydryls, disulfides or phosphates. Therefore, because it contained a substantial number of glycosylated threonine residues,
the β-elimination of the glycosylthreonine could be investigated
without interference from other dehydro-amino acid-forming residues in the protein. It was observed that the initial rate of
the β-elimination was dependent on the hydroxyl concentration but
not on protein concentration.

In a similar study, Sen et al. (17) investigated the β-
elimination in phosphoproteins. Phosphovitin was chosen for this
investigation because it contains 119 phosphoserine residues and
1 phosphothreonine residue. The rates of β-elimination were measured by change in absorbance of the protein at 241 nm after treatment with alkali. As with the glycoproteins, at low concentration
the initial rate of β-elimination was dependent on the hydroxyl
ion concentration. The rate of β-elimination was increased with
increased ionic strength and the addition of 1.12 x 10^{-3}M calcium
chloride increased the initial rate twenty times. The calcium
ion effect may be of great significance in that casein, which can
contain substantial amounts of calcium ion, is extremely susceptible to LAL formation. The primary source for dehydroalanine in
casein is phosphoserine. Other multivalent cations also influence
the rate of dehydroalanine formation in phosphoproteins. The addition of 0.0125 M magnesium chloride during alkaline treatment
resulted in the formation of 1320 ppm LAL in casein. Addition of
the same level of aluminum chloride resulted in casein containing
8060 ppm LAL. Addition of higher levels of potassium (0.225 M)
produced effects similar to those obtained with the lower levels
of di- and tri- valent metal ions.

Although lysine was not considered, products similar to LAL

and lanthionine were observed by Eiger and Greenstein (18) in an
early study of the addition reaction products of sulfydryls or
amines with dehydroalanine. The importance of lysine in these
addition reactions became apparent when the lysinoalanine crosslink was reported by Bohak (10).

The kinetics of the Michael addition reaction with acetonitrile on reduced protein studied by Cavins and Friedman (19)
served as an excellent model for later studies with N-acetyldehydroalanine methyl ester (20) where the formation of a variety
of dehydroalanine adducts of amino acids were reported. It is
necessary to use the dehydroalanine methyl ester in these studies
because the reaction kinetics are much faster than with the free
N-acetyldehydroalanine (21). The free amino compounds decom-
poses to ammonia and pyruvic acid when synthesis is attempted.
The reactivity of the methyl ester also more closely emulates
the reactivity of dehydroalanine residues in peptides. Gross et
al. (22) observed that dehydroalanine was present in the antibiotics cinnamycin and duramycin. Careful measurement of dehydroalanine in alkaline treated proteins was conducted by Sen et
al. (17) and Walsh et al. (23) by change in absorbance as described by Carter and Greenstein (24). The measurements were difficult in pure proteins and would not seem to lend themselves to
measurement of dehydroalanine in complex food protein systems.
We are aware of no reports finding dehydroalanine in food proteins. During acid hydrolysis the dehydroalanine is broken down
to ammonia and pyruvic acid; therefore, only the ammonia would
be detected in routine amino acid analysis. In summarizing the
many reactions of dehydroalanine in proteins, Friedman (25) reported that 14 crosslinked amino acids can be formed in proteins.
If one considers the isomeric forms that could exist, the number
expands to at least 53 derivatives.

Figure 1 summarizes the potential pathways involved in the
formation of dehydroalanine. It appears that dehydroalanine can
be formed in a variety of amino acids protein, suggesting that
any or all of the routes in Figure 1 could be involved in dehydroalanine formation. Table 1 contains results of partial
amino acid analysis of several alkaline treated proteins. The
results support the suggestion that both serine and cystine or
their derivatives can be sources of dehydroalanine and subsequently the lysinoalanine measured in the proteins. In casein
there is substantial LAL formation with a measurable loss in
serine. In isolated soy protein and lactalbumin it can be seen
that cystine shows the most significant losses. It should be
noted that a significant portion of the serine in casein is
present as phosphoserine. The relatively rapid β-elimination of
phosphoserine (15) accounts for the formation of considerable
quantities of dehydroalanine and subsequently the substantial
levels of LAL found in casein. In addition, as mentioned above,
the presence of calcium would accelerate dehydroalanine formation
from the phosphoserine present in the casein. The variability of

Table 1. Selected Amino Acid Analysis

Protein	Treatment Conditions	Units[a]	Lysine Untreated	Lysine Treated
Isolated Soy Protein	pH 12.2/40°C/1 hr.	1	5.7	5.6
	pH 12.2/40°C/2 hr.	1		5.2
	pH 12.2/40°C/4 hr.	1		5.4
	pH 12.2/40°C/8 hr.	1		5.1
	pH 12.2/80°C/4 hr.	1		4.7
Sun Flower Protein	0.1 N NaOH/55°C/1 hr.	2	11	10
	0.2 N NaOH/55°C/1 hr.	2		10
	0.2 N NaOH/80°C/1 hr.	2		8.5
Wheat Gluten	pH 13.0/70°C/4 hr.	2	11.2	6.9
Fish Protein Conc.	pH 13.7/90°C/8 hr.	2	68.3	54.8
Sericine		2	21	14.1
β Lactoglobulin	pH 6.2/80 min./97.5°C	3	30.3	22.7
Wheat Gluten	pH 9.6/65°C/3 hr.	4	1.33	1.40
	pH 11.2/65°C/3 hr.	4		0.96
	pH 13.9/65°C/3 hr.	4		0.94
Lactalbumin	pH 9.6/65°C/3 hr.	4	8.94	8.57
	pH 11.2/65°C/3 hr.	4		7.45
	pH 13.9/65°C/3 hr.	4		7.19
Casein	pH 10.6/65°C/3 hr.		6.84	6.46
	pH 11.2/65°C/3 hr.			6.03
	pH 12.5/65°C/3 hr.			4.48
Phosvitin	0.123 N NaOH/60°C	3	23.1	18.9
	0.123 N NaOH/60°C	3		12.9
	0.123 N NaOH/60°C	3		5.33

[a](1) gm/16 gmN; (2) MM/100 g; (3) moles/mole protein; (4) mole percent

of Various Alkaline Treated Proteins

Serine Untreated	Serine Treated	Cystine Untreated	Cystine Treated	Arginine Treated	Arginine Untreated	Lysinoalanine Treated	Lysinoalanine Untreated	References
5.6	5.5	0.87	0.40	8.0	7.7	0.42	6.0	deGroot and Slump (32)
	5.5		0.37	8.0		0.68		
	5.8		0.40	7.9		0.83		
	5.7		0.40	7.7		1.09		"
	5.0		0.25	7.5		2.08		"
27	28	2.5	20	35	38	35	28	Provansal et al. (33)
27	27		TR	33		3.0		
27	23		0	31		5.5		
42.3	28.1	8.6	1.5	11.8	20.2	4.9	0	Fujimaki et al. (29)
44.8	20.1	4.8	2.8	16.3	30.4	12.0	0	
34.9	20.6	--	--	22.0	25.5	7.5	0	Ziegler (12)
--	--	3.92	0.60	5.4	5.6	3.8	0	Watanabe (93) Klostermeyer
6.81	6.75	0.98	0.69	2.70	2.75	0	0	Friedman (94)
	6.55		0	2.68		0.42		
	2.24		0	1.79		0.88		
6.18	6.11	0.95	0.56	2.22	2.14	0.26	0	Friedman
	6.08		0	2.12		1.52		
	2.26		0	1.32		3.87		
7.15	7.09	--		2.53	2.56	0.49	0	
	6.94			2.50		0.78		
	4.60			2.21		2.43		
11.5	90.2	--	--	ND	ND	4.20	0	Sen et al. (17)
	70.1	--	--	ND	ND	8.83		
	36.4	--	--	ND	ND	17.9		

LAL formation in products such as isolated soy protein may relate to the intensity of alkali and the ionic strength of the solvent system used in sample preparation. However, it also may be influenced by the extent of oxidation of the cystine in the protein and the incorporation of air during processing.

Figure 2 summarizes some of the compounds that can be formed through the addition of dehydroalanine to a variety of amino acids in proteins. Although there are no reports in the literature of such reactions, one is tempted to raise the question as to whether dehydroalanine reacts with nucleic acids containing reactive amino groups. More complete discussion of the dehydroalanine addition reactions have been made earlier by Friedman (25), Asquith et al. (26) and Feairheller et al. (27).

The reaction of lysine with dehydroalanine was studied by Snow et al. (21) using the N-α-acetyl-dehydroalanine methyl ester as a model. The studies with the model compound are difficult to compare with reactions that occur in proteins because proteins are such complex molecules and analysis is difficult. The comparison of the variety of proteins which form LAL suggests that although dehydroalanine may be formed by a variety of pathways, the Michael addition between lysine and dehydroalanine is rapid, particularly at higher pHs.

The overall effects of processing conditions on LAL formation have been investigated in a wide variety of proteins and foods. Hayashi and Kameda (28) investigated a broad range of conditions which influence LAL formation in lysozyme and ribonuclease. It was suggested earlier by Bohak (10) that intramolecular features of the protein influence the formation of LAL. Hayashi and Kameda (28) supported this suggestion with their results. LAL appears to reach a maximum value during alkaline treatment and increasing treatment time or addition of cystine or lysine does not appear to increase the LAL formation. Maximum LAL formation was achieved with treatment with 0.2N sodium hydroxide for 4 hrs at 40°C for ribonuclease and lysozyme. Fujimaki et al. (29) investigated the conditions to maximize LAL formation in wheat gluten and fish protein concentrate. They reported that conditions for the maximum formation of LAL differed significantly between the two proteins: maximum LAL formation in gluten was achieved by holding the protein at pH 13.0 for 14 hrs at 70°C and maximum LAL formation in fish protein concentrate was achieved at pH 13.7 at 90°C for 8 hrs. In addition, when gluten was oxidized with performic acid to convert the cystine to cysteic acid prior to alkaline treatment, more rigorous conditions were required to obtain LAL formation. The results suggest that with gluten, dehydroalanine formation was from cystine and when the cystine was destroyed the other sources of dehydroalanine formed the dehydroalanine more slowly.

Serassi-Kyriakou et al. (30) investigated the effect of various anions on LAL formation in silk. They observed that LAL formation was dependent on ionic strength, time, temperature and

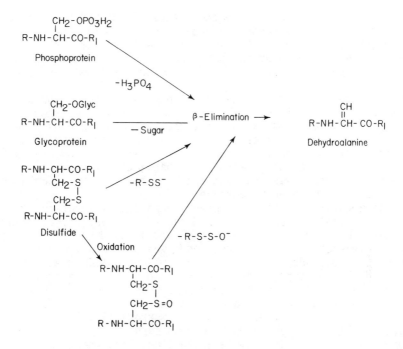

Figure 1. Postulated pathways for the formation of dehydroalanine in proteins.

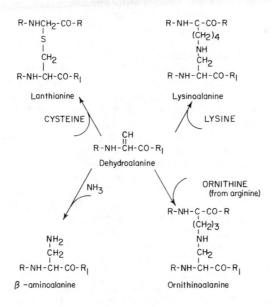

Figure 2. Reaction products between dehydroalanine and various side chains in proteins.

pH, and was also dependent on the nature of the anions present in solution. It was reported that the LAL formation was greatest when carbonate was present. Intermediate levels of LAL were formed when phosphate or tetrapyrophosphate were added. When tripolyphosphate was the anion, much lower levels of LAL formation were observed.

Considerable research has been done on the formation of LAL in a variety of proteins. Table 2 summarizes some of these investigations. The results suggest that various proteins have differing susceptibilities to LAL formation. Most workers use slightly differing reaction conditions so accurate comparisons are difficult. It should also be emphasized that conditions used in many of these investigations are much harsher than encountered in normal food or feed processing.

In addition to the LAL contents reported for proteins summarized in Table 2, LAL has been detected in a variety of other proteins and foods. Sternberg et al. (31) found LAL to be present in a variety of home cooked foods which were not exposed to alkaline conditions. Protein sources which contained significant levels of LAL were egg white (which could be slightly alkaline depending on age), chicken, steak, and frankfurters. Alkaline exposure of food proteins has been shown to cause considerable LAL formation in foods by a number of workers (28, 32-41). Traditionally, certain foods have been exposed to alkali during processing. A classic example is the tortilla, where corn is mixed with water containing 1% lime and is heated at temperatures up to 80°C for up to 45 minutes (42-45). Alkaline treatments improve the availability of niacin and the in vitro release of amino acids. It is interesting that only low levels of LAL are formed under these conditions. Tovar (46) investigated a wide variety of conditions and found that traditional conditions for production of tortillas produced only minor levels of LAL, although racemization was also observed in the protein. In samples of corn receiving alkaline treatment, particularly with lime, the formation of LAL was less than might be expected. The presence of the calcium ion does not appear to cause higher LAL formation in the corn proteins where cystine would be the likely source of the LAL precurser. In alkaline treated corn, slight losses are observed in cystine, lysine and arginine (46-48).

Several approaches have been attempted for the inhibition of LAL formation in alkanine treated proteins. Dworschak (39) observed that addition of ascorbic acid had both an inhibiting and an enhancing effect on LAL formation. The difference appeared to be related to the cystine content of the protein. It might be suggested that partial reduction of cystine to cysteine by the ascorbic acid was in part responsible for the results. When protein was low in cystine, the ascorbic acid inhibited LAL formation, but ascorbic acid was a less effective inhibitor at higher concentrations. The argument would suggest that at low concentration most of the cystine was reduced to cysteine and at

Table 2
Lysinoalanine Content of Proteins and Foods Alkaline Treated Proteins

Protein	LAL Content ppm	Treatment	Reference
Lysozyme	490	pH 13.1/40°C/2 hr	Bohak, 1964
Papain	241	pH 13.1/40°C/2 hr	Bohak, 1964
Phosvitin	830	pH 13/1/40°C/2 hr	Bohak, 1964
Lycozyc	670	0.1 N NaOH/65°C/4 hr	Finley, 1982
BSA	240	0.1 N NaOH/65°C/4 hr	Finley, 1982
α-Lactalbum	550	0.1 N NaOH/65°C/4 hr	Finley, 1982
ISP	390	0.1 N NaOH/65°C/4 hr	Finley, 1982
Leaf pruten core	320	0.1 N NaOH/65°C/4 hr	Finley, 1982
Safflower isuaic	600	0.1 N NaOH/65°C/4 hr	Finley, 1982
Sodium Caseinate	310		Raymond, 1980
Sodium caseinate	100-1400	Isolation	Erberstabler and Holstein, 1980
Sodium caseinate	80-970	Isolation	Petrus et al., 1982
Potassium Caseinate	<25		
Calcium caseinate	0-2820		
Hominey	2700	0.33 N NaOH/100°C/50 min	Sanderson et al., 1979
Hominey	0	Commercial	Sanderson et al., 1979
Masa	200	Commercial	Sanderson et al., 1979
Tortilla	810	Commercial	Sanderson et al., 1979
Isolate yeast protein	4900	pH 10.5/85°C/4 hr	Shatty and Kinsella, 1979
Isolate yeast protein	35900	pH 12.5/65°C/2 hr	Shatty and Kinsella, 1979
Infant for D	90-150	--	Haagsma and Slump, 1978
Condensed milk	210-270		Haagsma and Slump, 1978
Egg white solids	120		Haagsma and Slump, 1978
Infant formula	150-640		Sternberg et al., 1975
Tortilla	200		Sternberg et al., 1975

higher cystine levels the reduction was incomplete. Under these
conditions the partially oxidized ascorbic acid could act as a
prooxidant to promote oxidation of cystine to cystine monoxide
which forms dehydroalanine more rapidly. Murase (49) and Dworshak
(39) both reported that glucose inhibited LAL formation, presumably due to competition from the browning reaction and the formation of antioxidants by the browning reaction. Meyer (40) de-
phosphorylated casein and improved its resistance to LAL formation. Such a reduction would be expected by elimination of the
phosphoserine which Sen et al. (17) demonstrated as an excellent
dehydroalanine former.

A variety of sulfur-type reducing agents have been investigated for their potential in inhibiting LAL formation. Finley
and Kohler (50) and Friedman (51) reported that bisulfite or
bisulfide would inhibit LAL formation. The compounds worked
through a variety of mechanisms. First, the cystine was reduced
to cysteine which is resistant to alkali. Secondly, the compounds
(including the newly formed cysteine) reacted rapidly with any
dehydroalanine formed to competitively inhibit LAL formation, and,
thirdly, the reducing agents reduced cystine monoxide back to
cystine or cysteine. Cystine monoxide is a more rapid dehydroalanine former than the cystine or cysteine as was later shown
(50, 52, 53). Reduced glutathione and cysteine were effective,
but levels as high as 3% of the protein were required to obtain
inhibition.

Acylation of the protein has been proposed by Friedman (51)
as a means of inhibiting LAL formation by blocking the ε-amino
group of lysine with acetate or succinate. When gluten was 10%
acetylated or 1% succinylated, LAL formation was almost completely
blocked. Results with isolated soy protein were less impressive,
affording only limited inhibition of LAL formation. The results
reinforce the concept that each protein or modified protein has a
certain inherent susceptibility to LAL formation. Modification
of a few amino groups caused significant changes in this susceptibility to LAL formation. Clearly, control of LAL susceptibility
with minor changes could be of great benefit in developing new
modifications of protein at high pH. It is also important to
recognize that acetylation and succinylation of the protein is
likely to compromise the nutritional quality of the protein.

Modification of processing techniques has resulted in reduced LAL formation. Finley and Kohler (50) reported that reduction of air incorporation during alkaline treatment significantly
reduced LAL content of the treated proteins. The results were
supported by later work of Finley et al. (13) which demonstrated
the importance of oxidized cystine in LAL formation.

Of all the efforts to reduce LAL formation, careful control
of processing conditions is the most satisfactory approach at
this time. Careful control of pH, temperature, air incorporation,
and ingredient quality will allow manufacture of products with
minimum LAL content. The safety and nutritional quality of pro-

ducts must be clearly established before rigorous modifications such as acylation can be considered by the food industry.

The relative ease of LAL formation suggests that LAL content may be an excellent indicator of alkaline damage to protein. In routine analysis of amino acids, if LAL levels are below 50 ppm, the protein can be considered undamaged by alkali.

Methods of Analysis for LAL

In addition to being detected in routine amino acid analysis, several specific methods have been developed for determination of LAL in food or feed proteins. Since LAL is most frequently bound in the peptide, all analytical procedures start with an acid hydrolysis of the protein. The hydrolysis conditions most frequently used are 6N hydrochloric acid at 110°C for 24 hrs. From the hydrolysis step on, a variety of chromatographic procedures have been attempted.

Bohak (10) first observed LAL in alkaline treated proteins. The LAL was measured as a new peak migrating with the basic amino acids during ion exchange chromatography. The LAL peak is clearly separated from lysine and the other basic amino acids. The generally small LAL peak is sharp enough to allow measurement of levels as low as 50 ppm to be detected. Sensitivity for these determinations are best accomplished by modified procedures (67). Sensitivity is accomplished by loading sufficient sample and operating the amino acid analyzer at a high sensitivity. The technique will frequently require a separate chromatographic run from routine profile determinations. In Raymond's work, he points out the importance of separating the LAL from other basic amino compounds such as glucosamine, galactosamine, and tryptophan which occur in the same region during ion exchange chromatography. Other chromatographic modifications based on ion exchange chromatography have been proposed (32, 34, 54-59).

In all chromatographic procedures, interferences or potential interferences are a problem. Slump (58) proposed a single sodium citrate buffer (0.61N in sodium pH 4.50) which separated LAL from hydroxylysine and ornithinoalanine. The same paper reported a four buffer system for complete amino acid analysis. In the four buffer system, hydroxylysine and ornithinoalanine interfered with LAL. Most other workers have observed similar interferences to varying degrees depending on the specific buffers and resins being used.

Sternberg et al. (31) reported a thin layer chromatographic procedure which afforded separation and quantitation of LAL. Sternberg's technique allowed the detection of as little as 3 ng of LAL. High standard deviations and relatively long separation times tend to limit practical application of the thin layer technique (60-62), imporved the technique and shortened the time to 4 hrs.

Sakamoto et al. (63, 64) reported a method which measures

LAL and other crosslinking amino acids in wool by gas liquid
chromatography and mass spectrometric detection of the products.
The Sakamoto technique offered the advantage that identification
was based not only on chromatography but also on fragmentation
patterns of the compounds. The disadvantage is that derivation
is required to form the trifluoroacetylbutyl esters prior to the
gas chromatographic separation. Hasegawa and Okamoto (37) employed a similar gas chromatographic technique using the same
derivatives. Schwass et al. (8) obtained excellent separation of
LAL on an optically active column which also separated the d and
l isomers of the amino acids. High voltage electrophoresis was
used by Asquith and Carthew (65) for separation and identification
of LAL. Provansal et al. (33) utilized paper electrophoresis
after ion exchange chromatography to identify LAL in various fractions. Fritsch and Klostermeyer (41) reported improved sensitivity in LAL analysis by using o-phthalaldehyde and fluorometeric
measurement of the LAL derivative. Wood-Rethwill and Warthesen
(66) developed an HPLC technique for LAL determination which
could serve as an excellent method for rapid screening of LAL
content in foods or feeds.
   From the literature one finds that LAL can be detected in a
variety of ways. When dealing with levels commonly found in
foods, some special efforts must be taken for detection as proposed by Raymond (67) or adaptation of one of the HPLC techniques (41, 66). For analysis of alkaline treated proteins the
more routine approaches to amino acid analysis can be utilized.

Biological Effects of Lysinoalanine

   Several changes which can adversely influence the nutritional
quality occur in proteins that are subjected to severe alkaline
treatments. Losses in the amino acids (lysine and cystine,
particularly), drops in digestibility, and reduction in net protein utilization all increase as the severity of the alkaline
treatment increases (32). Increases in either temperature or pH
of treatment caused similar results. Decreased intestinal absorption amino acids was attributed to LAL-like cross-links and
racemization. Kraus and Schmidt (68) also observed a reduction
in digestibility of milk proteins as treatment temperature increased from 30 to 90°C at pH 12.
   The toxic effects of alkaline treated fish protein and
casein were reported by Carpenter and Duckworth in chicks (69).
The alkaline treatment effects resulting in LAL formation cannot
be separated completely from the racemization effects on the
amino acids in the protein (8, 70).
   Newborne and Young (71) reported that feeding rats alpha
protein (an alkaline treated soy protein isolate intended for
industrial uses) resulted in microscopic lesions in the inner
cortex of the kidney, along with noncalcified mucoid structures
in the urinary bladder. Woodard's group (72-77) confirmed that

the renal lesions in rats fed alkaline treated soy protein were cytomegalic changes in the pars recta of the proximal tubule. Woodard et al. (78) attributed the toxic effect of alkaline treated soy protein to LAL which was formed during the alkaline treatment of the protein. Complete and accurate description of the cytomegalic changes were made by Woodard et al. (78) in a review article.

The difficulties in obtaining an accurate analysis of LAL complicated the efforts to quantitate the levels of LAL which caused the lesion. Woodard et al. (78, 79) fed 250 to 3000 ppm synthetic LAL to rats and observed nephrocytomeglia at all levels. The higher doses did produce more severe lesions. It is interesting that animals injected intraperitoneally showed no qualitative or quantitative difference in the lesion from animals dosed by stomach tube with 30 mg/day free LAL. The stomach tube dosing was equivalent to 2000 to 2500 ppm dietary LAL. Female rats appeared somewhat more susceptible to the lesion than male rats. When feeding alkaline treated soy protein, deGroot's group observed nephrocalcinosis in female rats, but the lesion was overcome by increasing dietary calcium (32, 35). In these experiments, alpha protein containing LAL levels as high as 0.34% was fed to Wistar rats. VanBeek et al. (80) fed alkaline treated soy isolate at levels as high as 20% in the diet for 90 days and found no nephrocytomeglia but did find nephrocalcinosis in the rats. The nephrocalcinosis was attributed to the high phosphorus content of the diet. When free LAL was fed to rats, the lowest level that induced nephrocytomeglia was 100 ppm in the diet. deGroot et al. (35, 81) observed that bound LAL did not produce nephrocytomegly and free LAL appeared to cause the lesions. Next they fed acid hydrolyzed alkaline treated protein. The protein, which had not caused cytomegly before hydrolysis, produced significant cytomegly after hydrolysis. It is evident that the free amino acid (LAL) is much more likely to cause the lesion than when it is protein bound. Struthers et al. (82) calculated the effect level to be 80 to 100 fold greater for protein bound LAL. Struthers et al. also reported that the Sprague-Dawley strain of rats was more susceptible to renal calcification. Woodard's group studied the Sprague-Dawley strain, deGroot's group studied the Wistar strain; the difference in rat strains may explain the differences between Woodard's and deGroot's results.

deGroot et al. (81) reported feeding studies of LAL with several mammalian species. The results indicated that rats were uniquely susceptible to the lesion. Feeding of up to 1000 ppm free LAL to mice, hamsters, rabbits, quail, dogs and monkeys failed to produce renal changes. Similar results were reported by Leegwater (83) and Finot et al. (84). Apparently only the rat is susceptible to LAL at these levels.

Karayiannis et al. (85) reported no quantitative or qualitative difference in responses of Wistar and Sprague-Dawley rats to dietary levels of LAL as high as 2630 ppm bound in alkaline

treated isolated soy protein. It was suggested, therefore, that
the differences in sensitivity may lie in a particular line of
rats. It was also concluded that protein bound LAL did not induce nephrocytomeglia in mice, whereas free LAL produced nephrocytomeglia at a lower frequency than reported in rats (53, 86).
Finley et al. (87) observed that kidney homogenates from susceptible strains of rats hydrolyzed LAL at a much greater rate than
kidney homogenate from mice. The products of the hydrolysis were
l-lysine and d,l-serine. Finot (84) reported a number of potential pathways by which LAL could be metabolized. In the gut, a
considerable portion of ingested LAL is converted to carbon dioxide by the bacteria. When labeled LAL is given intravenously,
it appeared in the intestines and in the cecum of the rats. In
the urine, 10 labeled metabolites were found including at least
five acetylated LAL derivatives. It is interesting that Finot's
group found the same metabolites in the urine of mice and hamsters
that do not respond with cytomegly.

In addition to acylation, there appear to be other modes by
which LAL is metabolized in the kidney. Engelsma et al. (88) reported the oxidation of LAL by l-amino acid oxidase. The oxidation of L,D-lysinoalanine resulted in the formation of 3-(piperi-
donyl)-alanine. It was suggested, but not proven, that 2-(piperi-
donyl)-acetic acid would be the product of the oxidation of L,L-
lysinoalanine. Later, Leegwater and Tas (89) suggested that when
L,L- and L,D- LAL are treated with l-amino acid oxidase in the
presence of catalase the products are the 6S, 8S and 6R, 8R
enantiomers of 1,7-diazabicyclo-[3.3.0]nonane-6,8-dicarboxylic
acid.

Tas and Kleipool (90) studied the various optical isomers of
LAL and observed that they exhibit different activities in producing the lesion. They concluded that l,d-LAL was 10- to 3-
fold more active in producing the lesion than the l,l or d,d
forms. When combined with the kidney homogenate work of Finley
et al. (87), the results suggest that the concentration of d-
serine in the kidney homogenates after hydrolysis of the LAL.
The l-amino acids are rapidly metabolized by the homogenate and
the d-serine (which is a product of the hydrolysis of the secondary amine of LAL) accumulates in the homogenate.

Gould and MacGregor (91), in an excellent review, proposed
several nutritional factors that may influence LAL toxicity. Important factors appear to be the methionine level of the diet,
carbohydrate source, and salt concentration. The protein source
appears to be the major factor, but it is difficult to separate
variations in susceptibility and nutritional factors due to variation in amino acid profile of the protein.

Recently, Hayashi (92) suggested that the chelating characteristics of LAL could be involved with its toxicity. Since LAL
is a strong chelator, LAL could potentially remove metal ions
from metaloenzymes, thereby inhibiting the enzyme. Inhibition of
carboxypeptidase-B and alcohol dehydrogenase were demonstrated as
examples.

From the current literature it appears that free LAL is significantly more toxic than protein bound LAL. A number of factors are involved in the toxicity of LAL and its possible implications for humans. There is no current evidence to suggest that the human is susceptible to the cytomegly caused by LAL in rats. The decrease in digestibility of the protein is without a doubt the most significant factor in alkaline treatment. Milk alkali treatments as used by the food industry do not appear to yield toxic levels of LAL. Careful control of processing conditions appears to be the most satisfactory approach to prevent LAL from becoming a health hazard for humans.

Literature Cited

1. Circle, S. J.; Smith, A. K. in "Soybeans: Chemistry and Technology"; Avi Publishing Co., Westport, CT, 1972, Vol. 1.
2. Hermansson, A. M.; Sivik, B.; Skjoldebrand, L. Lebensm. Wissen. und Tech., 1971, 201, 4.
3. Shetty, J. K.; Kinsella, J. E. J. Agric. Food Chem. 1980, 28, 798.
4. Tannenbaum, S. R.; Bates, R. P.; Brodfield, L. Food Tech. 1970, 24, 607.
5. Betschart, A. A. J. Food Sci. 1974, 39, 1110.
6. Otterburn, M. S. This volume, 1983.
7. Lee, T. C.; Chichester, C.O. This volume, 1983.
8. Schwass, D.E.; Tovar, L. R.; Finley, J. W. This volume, 1983.
9. Patchornik, A.; Sokolovsky, M. J. Am. Chem. Soc. 1964, 86, 1026.
10. Bohak, Z. J. Biol. Chem. 1964, 239, 2878.
11. Patchornik, A.; Sokolovsky, M. J. Am. Chem. Soc. 1964, 86, 1860.
12. Ziegler, K. L.; Melchert, I.; Lurken, C. Nature 1967, 214, 404.
13. Finley, J. W.; Wheeler, E. L.; Walker, H. G., Jr.; Finlayson, A. J. Agric. Food Chem. 1982, 30, 818.
14. Mellet, P. Textile Res. J. 1968, 38, 977.
15. Whitaker, J. R.; Feeney, R. E. in "Protein Crosslinking: Nutrition and Medical Consequences"; Friedman, M., Ed.; Plenum Press, New York, 1977, Vol. B, p. 155.
16. Lee, H. S.; Osuga, D. T.; Nashef, A. S.; Ahmed, A. I.; Whitaker, J. R.; Feeney, R. E. J. Agric. Food Chem. 1977, 25, 1153.
17. Sen, L. C.; Gonzalez-Flores, E.; Feeney, R. E.; Whitaker, J. R. J. Agric. Food Chem. 1977, 25, 632.
18. Eiger, I. Z.; Greenstein, J. P. Arch. Biochem. 1948, 19, 467.
19. Cavins, J. F.; Friedman, M. Biochemistry 1967, 6, 3766.

20. Finley, J. W.; Friedman, M. in "Protein Crosslinking: Nutri-
     tional and Medical Consequences"; Friedman, M., Ed.; Plenum
     Press, New York, 1977, p. 123.
21. Snow, J. T.; Finley, J. W.; Friedman, M. Int. J. Peptide
     Protein Res. 1976, 8, 57.
22. Gross, E.; Kiltz, H. H. Biochem. Biophys. Res. Commun.
     1973, 50, 559.
23. Walsh, R. G.; Nashef, A. S.; Feeney, R. E. Int. J. Peptide
     Protein Res. 1979, 14, 290.
24. Carter, C. E.; Greenstein, J. P. J. Natl. Cancer Inst.,
     1946, 7, 51.
25. Friedman, M. in "Protein Crosslinking: Nutritional and
     Medical Consequences"; Friedman, M., Ed.; Plenum Press, New
     York, 1977, p. 1.
26. Asquith, R. S.; Otterburn, M. S.; Sinclair, W. J. Angew.
     Chem. 1974, 13, 514.
27. Feairheller, S. H.; Taylor, M. M.; Bailey, D. G. Adv. Exp.
     Med. Biol. 1977, 86B, 177.
28. Hayashi, R.; Kameda, I. Agric. Biol. Chem. 1980a, 44, 175.
29. Fujimaki, M.; Haraguchi, T.; Abe, K.; Homma, S.; Arai, S.
     Agric. Biol. Chem. 1980, 44, 1911.
30. Serassi-Kyriakoa, K.; Hadjichistidis, N.; Touloupis, C.
     Chimika Chronika, New Series 1978, 7, 161.
31. Sternberg, M.; Kim, C. Y.; Plunkett, R. A. J. Food Sci.
     1975a, 40, 1168.
32. deGroot, A. P.; Slump, P. J. Nutr. 1969, 98, 45.
33. Provansal, M. M. P.; Cuq, J. L. A.; Cheftel, J. C. J. Agric.
     Food Chem. 1975, 23, 938.
34. Chu, N. T.; Pellet, P. L.; Nawer, W. W. J. Agric. Food Chem.
     1976, 24, 1084.
35. deGroot, A. P.; Slump, P.; van Beek, L.; Feron, V. J. in
     "Proteins for Humans: Evaluation and Factors Affecting
     Nutritional Value"; Bodwell, C. E., Ed.; Avi Publishing Co.,
     Westport, CT, 1977, p. 270.
36. Karayiannis, N. J.; MacGregor, J. T.; Bjeldanes, L. F. Food
     Cosmet. Toxicol. 1979a, 17, 585.
37. Hasegawa, K.; Okamoto, N. Agric. Biol. Chem. 1980, 44, 649.
38. Hasegawa, K.; Okamoto, N.; Ozawa, H.; Kitajima, S.; Takado,
     Y. Agric. Biol. Chem. 1981, 45, 1645.
39. Dworshak, E.; Orsi, F.; Zsigmond, A.; Trezl, L.; Rusznak, I.
     Die Nahrung 1981, 25, 441.
40. Meyer, M.; Klostermeyer, H.; Kleyn, D. H. Zeit. Lebns.
     Untersuch. und Forsch. 1981, 172, 446.
41. Fritsch, R. J.; Klostermeyer, H. Zeit. Lebns. Untersuch. und
     Forsch. 1981, 172, 435.
42. Cravito, R. O.; Anderson, R. K.; Lockhart, E. E.; Miranda,
     F. P.: Harris, R. S. Science 1945, 102, 91.
43. Bressani, R.; Scrimshaw, N. S.: J. Agric. Food Chem. 1958,
     6, 774.

44. Bressani, R.; Pay y Paz, R.; Scrimshaw, N. S. J. Agric. Food Chem. 1958, 6, 770.
45. Katz, S. H.; Hediger, M. L.; Valleroy, L. A. Science 1974, 184, 765.
46. Tovar, L. R., Ph.D. Thesis, University of California, Berkeley, California, 1981.
47. Sanderson, J.; Wall, J. S.; Donaldson, G. L.; Cavins, J. F. Cereal Chem. 1978, 55, 204.
48. Tovar, L. R. In this publication, 1983.
49. Murase, M. Nippon Nogeikagaku. Kaishi 1981, 54, 13.
50. Finley, J. W.; Kohler, G. O. Cereal Chem. 1979, 56, 130.
51. Friedman, M. in "Nutritional Improvement of Food and Feed Proteins"; Friedman, M., Ed.; Plenum Press, New York, 1978, p. 613.
52. Finley, J. W.; Snow, J. T.; Johnston, P. H.; Friedman, M. J. Food Sci. 1978, 43, 619.
53. Sternberg, M.; Kim, C. Y. in "Protein Crosslinking: Nutritional and Medical Consequences"; Friedman, M., Ed.; Plenum Press, New York, 1977, Vol. B., p. 73.
54. Nashef, A. S.; Osuga, D. T.; Lee, H. S.; Ahmed, A. I.; Whitaker, J. R.; Feeney, R. E. J. Agric. Food Chem. 1977, 25, 245.
55. Robson, A.; Williams, M. J.; Woodhouse, J. M. J. Chromatogr. 1967, 31, 284.
56. Sternberg, M.; Kim, C. Y.; Schwende, F. J. Science 1975b, 190, 992.
57. Woodard, J. C.; Short, D. D. J. Nutr. 1973, 103, 569.
58. Slump, P. J. Chromatogr. 1977, 135, 502.
59. Erberstobler, H. F.; Holstein, B.; Lainer, E. Zeit Lebns. Untersuch. und Forsch. 1979, 168, 6.
60. Haagsma, N.; Gortemaker, B. G. M. J. Chromatogr. 1979, 168, 550.
61. Haagsma, N.; Slump, P. Zeit Lebns. Untersuch. und Forsch. 1978, 167, 238.
62. Aymard, C.; Cuq, C. L.; Cheftel, J. C. Food Chem. 1978, 3, 1.
63. Sakamoto, M.; Kajiyama, K. I.; Teshirogi, T.; Tonami, H. Textile Res. J. 1975, 45, 145.
64. Sakamoto, M.; Nakayama, F.; Kajiyama, J. J. in "Protein Crosslinking: Nutritional and Medical Consequences"; Friedman, M., Ed.; Plenum Press, New York, 1977, Vol. A, p. 687.
65. Asquith, R. S.; Carthew, P. Biochem. Biophys. Acta 1972, 278, 346.
66. Wood-Rethwill, J. C.; Warthesen, J. J. J. Food Sci. 1980, 45, 1637.
67. Raymond, M. L. J. Food Sci. 1980, 45, 56.
68. Kraus, W.; Schmidt, K. Nahrung 1974, 18, 833.
69. Carpenter, K. J.; Duckworth, J. J. Agric. Sci. 1950, 40, 44.

70. Masters, P. M.; Friedman, M. in "Chemical Deterioration of Proteins"; Whitaker, J. R., Fujimaki, M., Ed.; ACS Symposium Series No. 123, ACS, Washington, D. C., 1980, p. 165.
71. Newberne, P. M.; Young, V. R. J. Nutr. 1966, 89, 69.
72. Woodard, J. C.; Alverez, M. R. Arch. Pathol. 1967, 84, 153.
73. Woodard, J. C. Am. J. Path. 1971a, 65, 253.
74. Woodard, J. C. Am. J. Path. 1971b, 65, 269.
75. Reyniers, J. P.; Woodard, J. C.; Alverez, M. R. Lab. Invest. 1974, 30, 582.
76. Woodard, J. C.; Short, D. D.; Alverez, M. R.; Reyniers, J. in "Protein Nutritional Quality of Foods and Feeds"; Friedman, M., Ed.; Marcel Dekker, New York, 1975.
77. Woodard, J. C.; Short, D. D. Food Cosmet. Toxicol. 1977, 15, 117.
78. Woodard, J. C. Vet. Path. 1975, 12, 65.
79. Woodard, J. C.: Short, D. D.; Strattan, C. E.; Duncan, J. H. Food Cosmet. Toxicol. 1977, 15, 109.
80. van Beek, L.; Feron, V. I.; deGroot, A. P. J. Nutr. 1974, 104, 1630.
81. deGroot, A. P.; Slump, P.; Feron, V. J.; van Beek, L. J. Nutr. 1976, 106, 1527.
82. Struthers, B. J.; Dahlgren, R. A.; Hopkins, D. T. J. Nutr. 1977, 107, 1190.
83. Leegwater, D. C. Food Cosmet. Toxicol. 1978, 16, 405.
84. Finot, P. A.: Bujard, E.; Aurand, M. in "Protein Crosslinking: Nutritional and Medical Consequences"; Friedman, M., Ed.; Plenum Press, New York, 1977, p. 51.
85. Karayiannis, N. J.; MacGregor, J. T.; Bjeldanes, L. F. Food Cosmet. Toxicol. 1979b, 17, 591.
86. Feron, V. J.; van Beek, L.; Slump, P.; Beems, R. B. in "Biochemical Aspects of New Protein Food"; Pergamon Press, 1978, p. 139.
87. Finley, J. W., unpublished.
88. Engelsma, J. W.; van der Meulen, J. D.; Slump, P.; Haagsma, N. Lebnsm. Wissn. Tech. 1979, 12, 203.
89. Leegwater, D. C.; Tas, A. C. Lebnsm. Wissn. Tech. 1980, 14, 87.
90. Tas, A. C.: Kleipool, R. J. C. Lebnsm. Wissn. Tech. 1976, 9, 360.
91. Gould, D. H.; MacGregor, J. T. in "Protein Crosslinking: Nutritional and Medical Consequences"; Friedman, M., Ed.; Plenum Press, New York, 1977, Vol. B, p. 29.
92. Hayashi, R. J. Biol. Chem. 1982, 257, 13896.
93. Watanabe, K.; Klostermeyer, H. Zeit Lebensm Unters Forsch. 1977, 164, 77.
94. Friedman, M. in "Functionality and Protein Structure"; Pour-El, A., Ed.; Acs Symposium Series 92, Washington, D.C., 1979, 19.

RECEIVED June 16, 1983

Isopeptides: The Occurrence and Significance of Natural and Xenobiotic Crosslinks in Proteins

MICHAEL S. OTTERBURN

Department of Chemical Engineering, The Queen's University of Belfast, 21 Chlorine Gardens, Belfast BT9 5DL, Northern Ireland

Proteins are biopolymers having a molecular weight arbitrarily greater than 5,000 daltons. They are essential for functions in cellular structure, catalysis, metabolic regulation and contractile processes. They also play an important part in the defensive and protective mechanisms in animals.

Protein chains are built up of monomeric units, the α-amino acids linked together by amido groups (peptide links). This polymerisation occurs through the α-amino and α-carboxyl groups of adjacent residues. The result is a complex random copolymer with many different functional groups and consequently complex chemical and physical properties. Whilst it is self-evident that the protein reactivity and many of its physical properties depend on the primary sequence, the secondary and tertiary structures are also important in defining the molecules functions. Many inter- and intrachenic forces and crosslinks are responsible for maintaining these structures and it is the purpose of this review to emphasize the importance of such crosslinks in protein structure, function and reactivity.

Bonding and Crosslinking in Proteins

Bonding forces which occur in proteins fall into two groups, physical and chemical, the latter being of particular interest in this review. Physical forces include ionic interactions between oppositely charged residues (1), hydrogen bonds which are vital in stabilizing the α-helical conformations and interchenic attractions in the secondary and tertiary structures (2, 3). The role of hydrophobic interaction is also particularly important in the stabilization process (4-6). The common feature of such physical stabilization is that the attractions can be broken and reformed by various chemical and physical changes in the proteins' environment.

An alternative method of stabilization in proteins is that

brought about by covalent interactions between residues of adjacent polypeptide chains. The most widely distributed of all
known crosslinks is cystine. This molecule allows two chains
(or a single folded chain) to be covalently linked together by a
disulphide bridge. The importance of this moiety and its inherent reactivity has led to a considerable amount of work being reported in the scientific literature (7, 8).

Other crosslinks of a more specialized origin have also been
noted in the literature. Such crosslinks tend to be specific to
a particular protein rather than being ubiquitous like cystine.
Thus in collagen and elastin the aldol and aldolimide crosslinks
occur. Precursors for crosslinking in these proteins are the
lysine and hydroxylysine derived aldehydes which are formed
enzymically. The crosslinks of collagen are formed by a series
of spontaneous aldol and aldimide condensations. In elastin the
crosslinks are formed by similar reactions leading in this case
to the highly stable pyridinium compounds demosine and isodemo-
sine. In the case of collagen, the function of the crosslinks
seems to be to confer order on the aggregated protein chains with
a resulting increase in strength and dimensional stability. In
the case of elastin, the crosslinks function appears to be that
of restricting the extensibility of the polypeptide chain (9-11).

Another group of crosslinks involving tyrosyl residues has
been demonstrated to exist in the protein resilin (12). This
crosslink has been shown to be formed from dimeric and trimeric
residues of tyrosine (13). The mechanism of formation of these
compounds is believed to be initiated by a peroxidase. The enzyme catalyzes the oxidative coupling of the tyrosine residues
through the three positions of the aromatic rings. Table 1
illustrates some of the crosslinks known to occur in proteins.

Isopeptide Links

Isopeptide crosslinks are formed by the covalent reaction of
the ε-amino group of lysine reacting with either the β-carboxyl
group of aspartic acid or the α-carboxyl group of glutamic acid.
Thus the general notation of these links is to refer to them as
ω-ε isopeptide crosslinks to differentiate them from the normal
peptide link.

The idea that such crosslinks might occur in proteins was
raised by Fischer (14) and more forcefully by Astbury (15).
Pauling and Nieman also alluded to such amide crosslinks (16).
However, little or no work was carried out on these early suggestions, possibly because of the protein chemistry obsession with
cystine and the intractable crosslinks of collagen. In spite of
this hiatus, much indirect evidence was amassed for the involvement of the ε-amino group of lysine in binding reactions. This
circumstantial evidence has been adequately reviewed by Loewy
(17), Pisano et al. (18), Finlayson (19) and Asquith et al. (20).
As a consequence of this, the crosslinks (and others) were in-

Table 1

Naturally Occurring Crosslinks in Proteins

ferred from binding experiments. This unsatisfactory situation
was resolved when an adequate enzymic digestion procedure was
developed which enabled ε-(-γ-GLUTAMIC)LYSINE (G-L) to be identified for the first time. This breakthrough occurred in 1968 with
the identification of G-L in bovine and human fibrin. This work
showed that a crosslink of G-L was formed as the first step in
the fibrinogen→fibrin transformation in blood clotting. The
steps leading up to the crosslink formation were identified and
characterized (21, 22). The presence of G-L in this system
opened a new era in crosslink investigation and from that time
many workers have found the moiety in a wide variety of organisms.
This led Loewy et al. to conclude that the isopeptide occurs
universally in all living systems (23). Subsequent research
yielded the crosslink in an impressive array of cells, organisms
and tissues. The occurrence of G-L and its significance in biological materials was the subject of an excellent review by Folk
and Finlayson (24).

     Following the work on fibrin, the next protein to be exten-
sively studied as far as the isopeptide was concerned was the
heterogeneous structural protein keratin. In their work, Asquith
et al. (25) identified and isolated G-L from native wool keratin
and subsequently isolated the aspartyl analogue ε-(-β-ASPARTIC)
LYSINE (A-L) from the same source (26). Other workers went on to
identify the isopeptides in human hair, guinea pig hair, porcu-
pine quills and protein from hair follicles (27, 28). Other tissues where isopeptides have been located include avian and mouse
muscle (29), human stratum corneum (30), erthyrocyte membranes
(31), cell membranes (32) and bovine colostrum (33).

     The mechanisms of formation of G-L in all these diverse tis-
sues, whether slime moulds or human tissue, is believed to be
similar. The crosslinking being brought about enzymically via a
transglutaminase, in some cases the enzyme system, has been identified (24).

     The function of the isopeptides in the various tissues is
not clear, although they may contribute directly to the structure
of the particular protein. For example, prior to keratinization
or by simply increasing the molecular weight of a protein system
confers enhanced stability, decreased solubility and increased
resistance to enzymic hydrolysis.

Isolation and Analysis of Isopeptides

     The major problem in all work carried out on isopeptides was
related to the fact that the isopeptide bond is chemically an
amide bond and as a consequence of this is susceptible to attack
by acids or alkalis, thus destroying the isopeptide. The only
possible methods were microbiological or enzymic, both of which
obviate the problem of random hydrolysis. Methods of enzymic
digestion had previously been known and adequately used; however,
such methods, although suitable for globular proteins, proved to

be insufficient for proteins with a high crosslink density due to high concentrations of cystine. In the late 1960's and early 1970's, new methods involving reducing and blocking of cystine followed by enzymic digestion were developed. These proved to be successful enough to allow identification and isolation of the isopeptides (22, 34). Since then, other methods have been suggested which modify the reduction and blocking stages and also introduce pre-digestion stages into the schemes (35).

In all these methods, particularly with the keratins, the efficiency of reduction, blocking and digestion is in question and consequently the true concentration of isopeptide. If the reduction state is not 100% efficient, areas of the protein will be unable to be digested and thus any isopeptides present in such regions will not be monitored. Thus there are fruitful areas of research available into enzymic digestion of crosslinked proteins and, until a totally efficient system is developed, the true significance of isopeptides in proteins will not be revealed.

The original method of analyses of the isopeptides in protein digests was to use ion exchange chromatography using sodium buffers (22-25). However, alternatively lithium buffers were used in order to obtain better separation and resolution (36). More recently Griffin et al. (37) have developed HPLC to quantify G-L, whilst other workers have developed rapid ion exchange methods (38, 39).

Formation of Isopeptides in Heated Proteins

The fact that the isopeptides could be formed as a consequence of thermal treatment of proteins was first demonstrated by Asquith and Otterburn who also showed that the isopeptides had crosslinking functions and that their concentrations increased with increasing severity of heating (40). The mechanism of formation could either be via a condensation or transamination reaction depending on whether the free carboxylic acid or the amide is involved (Figure 1) (20).

Later, other workers confirmed these findings which are summarized in Table 2. Thus isopeptides to date have been found to be formed during heating in keratin (40), milk proteins (41), muscle proteins (42), ribonuclease (43) and other proteins of nutritional interest (44). The ease of formation of the isopeptide in any specific protein should be dependent on two factors: firstly, the concentration of glutamic and aspartic acids in relation to the concentration of lysine and, secondly, the proximity of the lysyl and carboxylic residues which will be determined by the conformation of the protein chain.

It has been shown by Otterburn et al. (44) that there is no obvious correlation between the quantity of isopeptides formed and the concentration of the involved residues in the protein. These authors also showed that in one specific case, viz. lysozyme, the stereostructure of the protein could be used as a guide

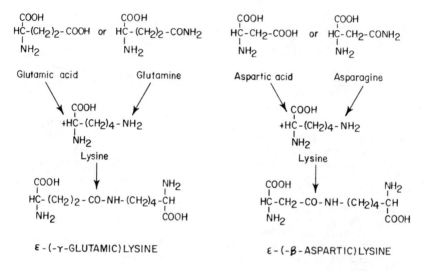

Figure 1. *Proposed reaction scheme for the formation of ω-ε isopeptides in heated proteins.*

Table 2

Isopeptides in Heated Proteins (g/16 gN)

Protein	Time of Heating (h)	Temp. °C	Aspartic	Glutamic	Lysine	A-L	G-L
Bovine haemoglobin	27	121	9.73	7.14	9.85	0.75	0.19
Blood meal	low temperature		9.20	8.92	9.50	0.33	0.32
Blood meal	high temperature		9.62	9.16	7.56	0.25	0.44
Egg albumen	57	115	9.24	13.05	6.82	0.27	0.12
Zein	57	115	5.06	22.16	0.05	0.11	0
Lactalbumin	27	85	10.07	15.46	10.37	0.04	0.06
Lactalbumin	57	115	10.07	15.46	10.37	1.04	0.74
Lysozyme	27	121	16.80	4.92	5.75	0.43	0
Casein	27	115	6.80	19.99	7.88	0.14	0.48
Chicken muscle	4	121	10.50	14.70	9.70	0.30	0.20
Chicken muscle	8	121	10.50	14.70	9.70	0.40	0.40
Chicken muscle	27	121	10.50	14.70	9.70	0.80	0.90

to the type of crosslink most likely to be formed. Weder et al.
(43) have recently shown a similar example with ribonuclease
where they showed that intermolecular bonding occurred between
dimers and oligomers of ribonuclease. The absolute vindication
of this argument awaits more work being carried out on proteins
with known secondary structures.
      The presence of reducing sugars and lipids militates against
the formation of isopeptides: in the former case, because of competitive Maillard reactions, and in the latter, by competition to
form esters or by acting as a hydrophobic barrier between the
lysyl and glutamyl or aspartyl residues (44).
      Thus there is now considerable evidence that isopeptides are
formed during the heating of proteins, the amounts formed depending on the purity of the starting material and the severity of
heating.

Nutritional Consequences of Isopeptide Formation

      It has been known for some time that heat induces changes in
the physical properties of proteins and that such changes influence the proteins digestibility and hence its nutritional value
as a food (45, 46). The nutritional value of heat sterilized
proteins was investigated by Carpenter et al. (47) and others
(48, 49). This work established that the decrease in nutritional
value was related to the involvement of reactive lysine groups.
From this work it became apparent that the ε-amino group of the
lysine residues were being blocked by physical inhibition or chemical combination (40, 50) to form moieties which were unattacked
by enzymes in the gut, thus effectively reducing the intake of
lysine by the animal. Bjarnason and Carpenter (51, 52) showed
that simple acylation of the ε-amino group was in itself insufficient to cause the effect. Indeed, acylated lysine was shown to
have growth promoting properties when fed to young rats on a lysine deficient diet.
      These observations led to the speculation that the ε-amino
group of lysine was involved in crosslink formation which either
prevented or inhibited the digestive processes. The possible
crosslinks were the isopeptides and lysinoalanine. This latter
crosslink can be formed via a Michael addition reaction of the
ε-amino group of lysine across the double bonds of dehydroalanine,
the latter being the degradation product of alkali or heat degraded cystine (53-55). Lysinoalanine is known to be stable to
acid and enzymic hydrolysis and was subsequently identified in
heated proteins (40). The concentration of lysinoalanine increases considerably in alkali/heat combinations (55). The biological stability of the isopeptides has also been investigated.
Thus Otterburn et al. (44) showed that G-L was stable to the
reduction/blocking and enzyme systems used to isolate the compound in proteins. Carpenter and Waible (56) investigated the
stability and utilization of free isopeptides as a source of

lysine. They were able to show with chicks that the free isopeptide G-L was metabolized and had some growth promoting effect. These workers also showed that none of the free isopeptide could be detected in the urine, although traces were found in the plasma. This observation indicated that some isopeptide had been absorbed through the intestinal wall although not all the G-L was accounted for.

Raczynski et al. (57) observed that the supernatant fraction of kidney homogenates caused greatest enzymic hydrolysis of G-L. However, Otterburn and Healy (58, 59) found that supernatant fractions of small intestinal homogenates exhibited maximum enzymic activity towards the isopeptides. These results were substantiated by results obtained in studying the transference of G-L across the wall of the small intestines of rats using the everted sac-technique (59). These latter results showed that G-L was hydrolyzed to a considerable degree (71.03%) in the jejunal region of the gut and to a lesser extent (24.4%) in the duodenal and ileal (8.72%) regions. Again, these results are at variance with those of Raczynski et al. (57) whose in vitro studies with everted intestinal sacs showed that radio labelled G-L passed across the gut wall unchanged.

The results of Otterburn and Healy, however, agree with the suggestions of Waible and Carpenter (56) that hydrolyses of ingested G-L can occur within the intestinal wall as a consequence of which only traces of G-L are found in the blood plasma.

Very little work has been carried out on the nutritional significance of severely heated proteins which are known to contain isopeptide crosslinks. One such study was carried out by Hurrell et al. (42) using severely heated chicken muscle protein fed as part of the diet to rats. These workers anticipated that the inaccessible lysine and lysine residues involved with isopeptides would have significantly reduced digestibility values compared with the overall protein. Thus it was expected that such high lysine fractions would accumulate in the ileal and faecal contents. However, it was found that although protein digestibility was greatly reduced after heat treatment, the isopeptides themselves were at least as digestible as the total protein component, total lysine and FDNB reactive lysine. The reduction in ileal protein digestibility only partly accounted for the much larger reduction in nutritive value as measured by the Net Protein Ratio (NPR). One explanation for this result may be found in the fact that if isopeptides are not absorbed through the ileum they will pass to the colon where intestinal bacteria and microflora are able to hydrolyze them (44).

Thus there is evidence to show that both G-L and A-L are found in proteins which have been subjected to heat treatments - the quantity of isopeptides formed being related to the severity of treatment. Further, it seems that the isopeptides are implicated to some extent in the resulting fall in nutritional value as monitored by NPR.

Conclusion

The presence of isopeptide crosslinks in heated proteins is interesting from a scientific viewpoint as it is a rare example of the formation of a xenobiotic substance which is also found in native proteins. Other examples are lanthionine and lysinoalanine which can be formed xenobiotically and have been shown by Gross to occur naturally in cinnamycin (60).

To date there is no evidence that the isopeptides have any toxicological manifestations in heated foods, although little or no work has been carried out in this area. The only evidence of any deleterious effects of the xenobiotics is the reduction they cause in nutritional value as measured by NPR. In order to fully understand the role and importance of the isopeptides in protein foodstuffs and nutrition, more work should be undertaken into their nutritional and toxicological properties.

Literature Cited

1. Speakman, J. B.; Hirst, M. C. Nature 1931, 128, 1073.
2. Mirsky, A. E.; Pauling, L. Proc. Nat. Acad. Sci. (U.S.A.) 1936, 22, 439.
3. Pimentel, G. C.; McClellan, A. L. "The Hydrogen Bond"; W. H. Freeman: San Francisco, 1960.
4. Klotz, I. M. Brookhaven Symp. Biol. 1960, 13, 25.
5. Zahn, H. Palette 1965, 21, 19.
6. Crewther, W. G.; Fraser, R. D. B.; Lennox, F. G.; Lindley, H. Adv. Protein Chem. 1965, 20, 191.
7. Friedmann, M. "The Chemistry and Biochemistry of the Sulfhydral Group in Amino Acids, Peptides and Proteins"; Pergamon Press, 1973.
8. Asquith, R. S.; Leon, N. H. "Chemistry of Natural Protein Fibres"; Asquith, R.S., Ed.; Plenum Press, New York, 1977, Chap. 5.
9. Piez, K. A. Annu. Rev. Biochem. 1968, 37, 547.
10. Traub, W.; Piez, K. A. Adv. Protein Chem. 1971, 25, 243.
11. Feeney, R. E.; Blankenhorn, G.; Dixon, H. B. F. Adv. Protein Chem. 1975, 29, 135.
12. Weis-Fogh, T. J. Exp. Biol. 1960, 37, 889.
13. Andersen, S. O. Biochim. Biophys. Acta 1964, 93, 213.
14. Fischer, E. Ber. Desch. Chem. Ges. 1906, 39, 510.
15. Astbury, W. T.; Woods, H. J. Phil. Trans. Roy. Soc. (London) Series A 1934, 232, 333.
16. Pauling, L.; Niemann, C. J. Am. Chem. Soc. 1939, 61, 1860.
17. Loewy, A. G. "Fibrinogen"; Laki, E., Ed.; Dekker, New York, 1968, p. 185.
18. Pisano, J. J.; Finlayson, J. S.; Peyton, M. P. Thromb. Diath. Haemorrh. Suppl. 1970, 39, 113.
19. Finlayson, J. S. Sem. Thromb. Haemostasis 1974, 1, 33.

20. Asquith, R. S.; Otterburn, M. S.; Sinclair, W. J. Angew. Chem. Internat. Edit. 1974, 13, 514.
21. Matacic, S. S.; Loewy, A. G. Biochem. Biophys. Res. Commun. 1968, 30, 356.
22. Pisano, J. J.; Finlayson, J. S.; Peyton, M. P. Science 1968, 160, 892.
23. Loewy, A. G.; Matacic, S. S.; Showe, M. Fed. Proc., Fed. Am. Soc. Exp. Biol. 1971, 30, 1275.
24. Folk, J. E.; Finlayson, J. S. Adv. Protein Chem. 1977, 31, 1.
25. Asquith, R. S.; Otterburn, M. S.; Buchanan, J. H.: Cole, M.; Fletcher, J. C.; Gardner, K. L. Biochim. Biophys. Acta 1970, 221, 342.
26. Asquith, R. S.; Otterburn, M. S.; Gardner, K. L. Experientia 1971, 27, 1388.
27. Harding, H. W. J.; Rogers, G. E. Biochim. Biophys. Acta 1972, 257, 37.
28. Harding, H. W. J.; Rogers, G. E. Biochemistry 1972, 11, 2858.
29. Loewy, A. G.; Matacic, S. S. Biochim. Biophys. Acta 1981, 668, 167.
30. Abernethy, J. L.; Hill, R. L.; Goldsmith, L. A. J. Biol. Chem. 1977, 252, 1837.
31. Lorand, L.; Siefring, G. E.; Lowe-Kilentz, L. J. Supramol. Struct. 1978, 9, 279.
32. Haugland, R. B.; Lin, T. I.; Dowben, R. M.; Birckbichler, P. J. Biophys. J. 1982, 37, 191.
33. Klostermeyer, H.; Rabbel, K.; Reimerdes, E.-H. Hoppe-Seyler's Z. Physiol. Chem. 1976, 357, 1197.
34. Cole, M.; Fletcher, J. C.; Gardner, K. L.; Corfield, M. C. Appl. Polym. Symp. 1971, 18, 147.
35. Schmitz, I.; Baumann, H.; Zahn, H. Proc. 5th Inter. Wolltextil-Forschungskonf., Aachen 1975, 2, 313.
36. Otterburn, M. S.; Sinclair, W. J. J. Sci. Food Agric. 1976, 27, 1071.
37. Griffin, M.; Wilson, J.; Lorand, L. Anal. Biochem. 1982, 124, 406.
38. Weder, J. K. P.; Scharf, U. Z. Lebensm. Unters-Forsch. 1981, 172, 9.
39. Sugawara, K.; Ouchi, T. Agric. Biol. Chem. 1982, 46, 1085.
40. Asquith, R. S.; Otterburn, M. S. Appl. Polym. Symp. 1971, 18, 277.
41. Schmitz, I.; Zahn, H.; Klostermeyer, H.; Rabbel, K.; Watanabe, K. Z. Lebensm. Unters-Forsch. 1976, 160, 377.
42. Hurrell, R. F.; Carpenter, K. J.; Sinclair, W. J.; Otterburn, M. S.; Asquith, R. S. Br. J. Nutr. 1976, 35, 383.
43. Weder, J. K. P.; Scharf, U. Z. Lebensm. Unters-Forsch. 1981, 172, 104.
44. Otterburn, M. S.; Healy, M. G.; Sinclair, W. J. Adv. Exp. Med. Biol. 1977, 86B, 239.

45. Mecham, D. K.; Olcott, H. S. Ind. Eng. Chem. 1947, 39, 1023.
46. Beuk, J. F.; Chornock, F. W.; Rice, E. E. J. Biol. Chem. 1948, 60, 291.
47. Carpenter, K. J. Biochem. J. 1960, 77, 604.
48. Lea, C. H.; Hannah, R. S. Biochim. Biophys. Acta 1950, 4, 1950.
49. Asquith, R. S.; Chan, D. K.; Otterburn, M. S. J. Chromatogr. 1969, 43, 312.
50. Asquith, R. S.; Speakman, J. B.; Tolgyesi, A. Nature 1957, 180, 502.
51. Bjarnason, J.; Carpenter, K. J. Br. J. Nutr. 1969, 23, 859.
52. Bjarnason, J.; Carpenter, K. J. Br. J. Nutr. 1970, 24, 313.
53. Bohak, Z. J. Biol. Chem. 1964, 239, 2878.
54. Ziegler, K. J. Biol. Chem. 1964, 239, P.C. 2713.
55. Asquith, R. S. "Fibrous Proteins: Scientific, Industrial and Medical Aspects"; Parry, D. A. D.; Creamer, L. K., Eds.; Academic Press, 1979, I, p. 371.
56. Waible, P. E.; Carpenter, K. J. Br. J. Nutr. 1972, 27, 509.
57. Raczynski, G.; Snochowski, M.; Buraczewski, S. Br. J. Nutr. 1975, 34, 291.
58. Otterburn, M. S.; Healy, M. G. Unpublished Results.
59. Healy, M. G. M.Sc. Thesis, The Queen's University of Belfast, 1980.
60. Gross, E. Adv. Exp. Med. Biol. 1977, 86B, 131.

RECEIVED June 21, 1983

14

Mode of Formation of Aflatoxin in Various Nut Fruits and Gross and Histologic Effects of Aflatoxins in Animals

RICHARD J. COLE, TIMOTHY H. SANDERS, and PAUL D. BLANKENSHIP
National Peanut Research Laboratory, Dawson, GA 31742

ROBERT A. HILL
Georgia Coastal Plain Experiment Station, Tifton, GA 31793

Aspergillus flavus Link and the closely related
fungus A. parasiticus Speare are two species of
fungi that are capable of invading various food and
feed commodities and causing extensive economic
losses by contamination of these commodities with
highly toxic aflatoxins, thus, posing a threat to
animal health. The specific conditions that result
in containation of peanut, pecans, almonds, and
pistachio nuts with the aflatoxins are discussed
in detail. The primary target organ of the aflatoxins in domestic animals is the liver. A
discussion of the gross and histological effects
of aflatoxin poisoning in rainbow trout and swine
is presented.

A considerable amount of research effort has been expended
since the discovery of the highly toxic aflatoxins contaminating
Brazilian peanut meal in Great Britain in the early 1960's.
Recently some of this effort has been expanded to define the
etiology of aflatoxin contamination in peanuts. The preharvest
and storage phases of peanut production are most often associated with significant aflatoxin contamination.

The most extensive aflatoxin contamination of peanuts occurs
during preharvest following drought stress. Environmental conditions affect the nature and degree of microbial interaction
with peanuts. Despite the omnipresence of Aspergillus flavus
propagules in the soil during peanut fruit development, the
fungus is innocuous except during periods of environmental stress.
Recent studies have shown that dry soil conditions and an elevated soil temperature in the geocarposphere during the latter
4-6 weeks of the growing season are the major factors responsible
for preharvest aflatoxin contamination (1,2)(Table I). The
apparent effect of dry soil conditions is to reduce microbial
activity and, therefore, antagonism by competitors of A. flavus.
The major fungal antagonists of A. flavus are probably A. niger

Table I. Moisture Tension, Mean Geocarposphere Temperatures, and Aflatoxin Content During The Treatment Period for the Six Treatment Regimes

	Irrigated Treatment	Drought-Heated Treatment	Drought Treatment	Drought-Cooled Treatment #1	Drought-Cooled Treatment #2	Drought-Cooled Treatment #3
Soil Moisture in Bars Tension						
overall mean under rows	1.29	15.4	21.8	18.0	17.2	20.4
between rows	0.35	12.6	22.5	16.6	14.7	15.7
Temperatures During Treatment Period, °C						
overall mean under rows	23.8	30.5	25.7	19.8	21.3	22.9
between rows	24.0	30.5	27.0	20.5	22.7	23.6
Aflatoxin Concentration (ppb)						
overall mean edibles (jumbo, medium, #1, and other edible)	0	471	19	0	0	0
overall mean other (oil stock, LSK, and damaged)	0	10,516	2553	66	542	2309

and Trichoderma sp., which cannot tolerate low environmental moisture conditions as can A. flavus. The lower limit of water activity (Aw) capable of sustaining growth is approximately 0.88 Aw for A. niger, whereas 0.78 is considered the lower limit for A. flavus (3).

In conjunction with drought stress, an elevated geocarposphere temperature during the latter 4-6 weeks of the growing season is necessary for preharvest aflatoxin contamination of peanuts (1,2). Experiments in which peanuts were grown under drought stress at selected geocarposphere temperatures, showed that an overall mean geocarposphere temperature between 26.7-32.2°C was required in addition to dry soil conditions for pre-harvest aflatoxin contamination to develop (Table I). Elevated geocarposphere temperatures presumably break down some resistance mechanism in the developing peanut fruit, enabling A. flavus to grow and produce aflatoxin.

Peanut plants that grow with adequate moisture overlap the row middles during the latter third of the growing season in such a fashion that the soil surface under, and between, the rows is shaded from direct sunlight. It has been shown that the mean geocarposphere temperature under these conditions (approximately 24°C) is not affected greatly by ambient temperatures (1,2). Peanut plants grown under severe drought stress, during the latter 4-6 weeks of the growing season, recede so as to partially expose the soil surface to direct sunlight, which causes an increase in geocarposphere temperature. Thus, the two major requirements (dry soil and elevated geocarposphere temperature) for preharvest afla-toxin contamination are achieved.

It has been reported that the aflatoxin content of insect-damaged peanuts is considerably higher than contaminated undamaged peanuts (1,2). The lesser cornstalk borer, which is the most important soil insect responsible for peanut kernel damage, favors hot, dry environmental conditions similar to those favored by A. flavus. In addition, insecticide applications must be wetted into the soil to be effective. Thus, insect treatments during drought periods are largely ineffective.

The other phase of peanut production in which aflatoxin con-tamination may occur is storage. The primary concern in main-taining peanuts aflatoxin-free during storage is moisture control (4). Required temperatures may be biologically generated in a mass of peanuts by microbial action. The source of moisture may be from a lot of improperly dried peanuts (stored with greater than 10% moisture). Condensation of moisture within the ware-house, because of an inadequate flow of air through the peanuts and the overspace, is also a cause. This occurs when the moisture condenses before it is exhausted from the warehouse. Another source of excessive moisture is a leaky warehouse roof. Peanuts moistened from a leak can become highly contaminated with afla-toxin and these can, in turn, contaminate a considerable amount of uncontaminated peanuts when they are mixed. Two additional

sources of moisture in warehouses are high moisture foreign
material, such as wild cucumbers and aqueous insecticide applications (4).

In addition to peanuts (which are not botanically true nuts),
aflatoxins have been found in many of the tree nuts including
pistachios, almonds, pecans, and other tree nuts (5).

Pistachio nuts are formed in clusters and enclosed in a hull.
They are either hand-harvested (imported nuts) or mechanically
harvested (domestically produced nuts). Conventional methods of
processing harvested nuts are used abroad. This procedure
involves sun drying in the hull. The dried nuts are stored either
in bulk or in burlap bags. Before marketing the nuts are dehulled
after soaking them in water for 4-6 hrs. The nuts are then re-
washed and dried with sun, or hot air dryers. The use of artificial drying of pistachios, as compared to sun drying, is more
desirable and provides less chance for mold growth and aflatoxin
development (6).

Storage of pistachio nuts in the hull necessitates rewetting
before dehulling; therefore, storage of nuts after dehulling
would provide less opportunity for aflatoxin contamination. Also,
the presence of the hull favors mold growth under favorable conditions (7).

Since nuts that are split are more readily invaded by A.
flavus than sound nuts, the split nuts should be separated from
intact nuts after dehulling and should be stored separately (8).

A survey conducted in 3 areas of the Gajiantep province of
Turkey, representing extremes of geography and climate, showed
that A. flavus was a common contaminant of harvested stored nuts
at all stages after dehulling, but there was no evidence of significant aflatoxin contamination of immature or freshly harvested
nuts (9). In contrast, in a study of Iranian pistachio nuts,
Rahnema (10) observed contamination of immature nuts (endosperms)
while still on the tree. Based on parallel observations in peanuts, the explanation may be that A. flavus is more competitive in
the hotter, more arid climate. In addition, the higher temperatures may predispose the developing fruit to aflatoxin development in a way similar to that observed in peanuts (1,2).

Aspergillus flavus invasion and aflatoxin contamination in
almonds are usually associated with damaged kernels (8,11,12,13).
The most significant source of damage to almond kernels is caused
by the navel orangeworm larvae, Amyelois transitella (Walker).
The insect attacks the almond kernel in the orchard, after natural
splitting of the fruit, as it matures. Apparently, the insect
provides an invasion route for A. flavus by injuring the kernel
rather than serving as a vector of the fungus (14). The source of
A. flavus propagules is from the environment, where they are
disseminated by natural factors, such as wind and rain. Studies
have shown that A. flavus invasion and aflatoxin development in
almonds occur in the orchard following the natural splitting of
the hull before harvest (12). Normally, the moisture content of

the almond kernel at harvest is insufficient to support growth of
A. flavus. Although it is somewhat unclear at this time whether
A. flavus invasion and aflatoxin development can occur in the
absence of insect damage, results suggest that sound almond
kernels are relatively free of aflatoxin contamination. However,
surveys over a three-year period established that aflatoxin may
occur in tree nuts, such as almond, throughout the growing area
and that only a relatively few kernels in a large population were
contaminated (8).

The pecan nut may be invaded by numerous fungi including the
A. flavus group. There is no clearly defined evidence that aflatoxin contamination in pecans is a preharvest problem similar to
peanuts. The problem, as currently understood, occurs when pecans
are damaged by insects or when they lie on the ground several days
after normal drop (15). In addition, the benefits of timely harvest of pecans may be lost, if they are not adequately dried and
stored. This is due to damage incurred to the shells during
mechanical harvesting (16). Furthermore, it was concluded that
resistance due to the shell apparently is a varietal characteristic that is related to shell structure. Selection of varieties
on the basis of shell structure and resistance to splitting
should provide adequate protection from A. flavus invasion and
subsequent aflatoxin contamination. This, in conjunction with
prompt harvesting and good storage practices, should insure nuts
that are aflatoxin-free.

Histologic effects of aflatoxins in animals

A typical gross clinical sign of chronic aflatoxicosis in
animals is general unthriftiness resulting from reduced feed consumption and feed conversion efficiency. The major target organ
of aflatoxin B_1 is the liver, with variable adverse effects
depending on the animal species involved. The potent hepatocar-
cinogenicity of aflatoxin B_1 is seen in the Shasta strain of rainbow trout (17) and in the Fischer strain of rat (Table II)(18).

Table II. Carcinogenic Effects of Dietary Levels of Aflatoxin B_1
              in Rats

Aflatoxin Levels (ppb)	Number of Animals With Carcinoma	Total Animals Tested
0	0	18
1	2	22
5	1	22
15	4	21
50	20	25
100	28	28

This is in contrast to the Wister strain of rat, which is not
nearly as susceptible to the carcinogenic effects of aflatoxin B_1
(19).

The rainbow trout is known to be one of the most sensitive animals to the toxic effects of dietary aflatoxin, especially the hepatocarcinogenic effects. The LD_{50} of pure aflatoxin B_1 in trout is 0.5 mg/kg for a single dose, and 0.3 mg/kg for a dose given over a 5-day period. Trout fed levels as low as 0.4 μg/kg in the diet showed a significant incidence of hepatoma after 12 months' exposure. In the latter case, the total intake of aflatoxin B_1 over the one-year period would be 0.1-0.2 μg. In trout fed aflatoxin at 20 μg/kg for 20 days, incidence of hepatoma was 40% after 12 months. Recently, it was reported that when embryonated trout eggs were placed in an aqueous solution of aflatoxin B_1 (0.5 μg/ml) for only 1 hour, the incidence of hepatoma was 40% after 10 months [20]. Table II shows that the Fischer strain of rat is also very susceptible to the hepatocarcinogenic effects of aflatoxin B_1 [18].

Induction of liver carcinoma has been less consistent in animals other than the Shasta trout and Fischer rat. For example, there are few, if any, definitive accounts of aflatoxin-induced liver cancer in swine [21]. Aflatoxicosis in most animals appears to be similar to that observed in swine. The carcass of a pig suffering from aflatoxicosis appears yellow or jaundiced due to impaired liver function and the resultant accumulation of bilirubin in the tissues. The peritoneal cavity and pericardium contain excessive fluid. The gross appearance of the liver is often yellow due to accumulation of fat. The bile is typically a straw color rather than the normal dark color. On gross observation, the lobular pattern may be accentuated due to the accumulation of fat and an increase of fibrous tissue around the lobule. Microscopically, there is fatty change, proliferation of bile ductules within the lobule, karyomegaly (enlarged nuclei), megalocytocis (enlarged hepatocytes), nodular regeneration (hyperplasia), and perilobular fibrosis developing ultimately into a dissecting fibrosis reminiscent of the condition of advanced cirrhosis seen with alcoholism in humans [21]. In aflatoxicosis, necrosis of the liver is centrolobular in swine and typically periportal in other animals, such as the rat.

Although aflatoxin has been shown to be toxic to humans [22], the role of these toxins in human primary liver cancer remains obscure. Epidemiological studies in humans conducted in portions of Africa show a correlation between increased incidence of human primary liver cancer and increase in aflatoxin intake [23]. However, epidemiological studies in the U.S. do no indicate a correlation between incidence of primary human liver cancer and aflatoxin consumption. In the Southeast, the average intake of aflatoxin is estimated to be nine times greater than the national average [24]. However, according to unpublished data from the U.S. National Center for Health Statistics, the number of deaths from liver cancer is lower in each of the eight population groups in the Southeast as compared to the national average [24].

In summary, the environmental conditions that appear to be

critical for aflatoxin contamination of nuts in general are damage, elevated temperature, and in peanuts, dry soil conditions. The latter condition is related to microbial competition and may be unique to peanuts, since they develop in a subterranean environment.

Literature Cited

1. Hill, R. A.; Blankenship, P. D.; Cole, R. J.; Sanders, T. H. Appl. Environ. Microbiol., in press.
2. Blankenship, P. D.; Cole, R. J.; Sanders, T. H.; Hill, R. A., in preparation.
3. Hill, R. A., personal communication.
4. Smith, J. S., Jr.; Davidson, J. I., Jr. Trans. ASAE 1982, 231-236.
5. Stoloff, L. J. Assoc. Off. Anal. Chem. 1978, 63, 1067-1073.
6. Sommer, N. R., personal communication.
7. Denizel, T. Archieves de L'Institut Pasteur Die Tunis 1977, 54, 433-440.
8. Fuller, G.; Spooner, W. W.; King, A. D., Jr. J. Am. Oil Chem. Soc. 1977, 231A-235A.
9. Denizel, T.; Jarvis, B.; Rolfe, E. J. J. Sci. Food Agric. 1976, 27, 1021-1026.
10. Rahnema, R. I.U.P.A.C. Symposium, Göteborg, Sweden, 1972, Abstract.
11. Stoloff, L. Proc. Am. Phytopathol. 1976, 3, 156-172.
12. Phillips, D. J.; Uota, M.; Monticelli, D.; Curtis, C. J. Am. Soc. Hort. Sci. 1976, 100, 19-23.
13. Shade, J. E.; McGreevey, R.; King, A. D., Jr. Appl. Microbiol. 1975, 29, 48-53.
14. Phillips, D. J.; Purcell, S. L.; Stanley, G. I. U. S. Department of Agriculture ARM-W-20, 1980; 12 pp.
15. Schroeder, H. W. HortScience 1976, 11, 53-54.
16. Schroeder, H. W. Archives de L'Institut Pasteur de Tunis 1977, 54, 479-485.
17. Halver, J. W. in "Aflatoxin"; Goldblatt, L. A., Ed.; Academic Press: New York, 1969; Chap. 10, p. 265.
18. Wogan, G. N.; Palialunga, S.; Newberne, P. M. Fd Cosmet. Toxicol. 1974, 12, 681.
19. Stoloff, L. A. in "Mycotoxins in Human and Animal Health"; Rodricks, J. V.; Hesseltine, C. W.; Mehlman, M. A.; Eds.; Pathotox Publ., Inc.: Park Forest South, Ill., 1977; p. 7.
20. Wales, J. H.; Sinnhuber, R. O.; Hendricks, J. D.; Nixon, J.E.; Eisel, T. A. J. Nat. Cancer Inst. 1978, 60, 1137.
21. Cole, Richard J. Public Health Lab. 1979, 37, 57-68.
22. Van Rensburg, S. J. in "Mycotoxins in Human and Animal Health"; Rodricks, J. V.; Hesseltine, C. W.; Mehlman, M. A., Eds.; Pathotox Publ. Inc.: Park Forest South, Ill., 1977; p. 699.
23. Shank, R. C. in "Mycotoxic Fungi, Mycotoxins, Mycotoxicoses"; Wyllie, T. D.; Morehouse, L. G.; Eds.; Marcel Dekker, Inc.: New York, 1978; Vol. 3; p. 1.
24. "Aflatoxin and Other Mycotoxins: An Agriculture Perspective," Council Agric. Sci. Technol. (CAST) Report No. 80, 1979.

RECEIVED May 13, 1983

The Vomitoxin Story

THOMAS R. ROMER

Romer Labs, Inc., Washington, MO 63090

Vomitoxin or deoxynivalenol (Figure 1) is a mycotoxin that has been receiving much attention lately. In fact, vomitoxin is receiving as much attention in the 1980s as aflatoxin did in the 1970s. While aflatoxin has been found to cause sickness and death in animals and humans in real situations, vomitoxin is only known to cause some animals to lower their feed consumption or vomit at the concentrations found in naturally contaminated grain. Why, then, is there so much interest in vomitoxin at this time? The answer to this question is at least fourfold: 1) Lowered feed consumption (refusal) is an economic problem for the animal industry; 2) Vomitoxin is a potential adulterant which may fall under the Food, Drug and Cosmetic Act, which prohibits interstate commerce of an adulterated food; 3) Vomitoxin has been found in the United States and Canada every year since 1980 when analytical methods were first available for routine testing; and 4) Vomitoxin has been shown to cause serious toxic effects to laboratory animals and is suspected of causing other human and animal diseases.

Of the above four factors, the most significant is number three, the high incidence of vomitoxin in grains. If vomitoxin were seldom found in natural samples, it would not be a significant problem. However, since vomitoxin is often found in grain samples, the fact that the only toxic effects of vomitoxin known to occur in real situations are refusal and vomiting only alerts us to the fact that vomitoxin is present in natural samples at concentrations high enough to exhibit some toxic effects.

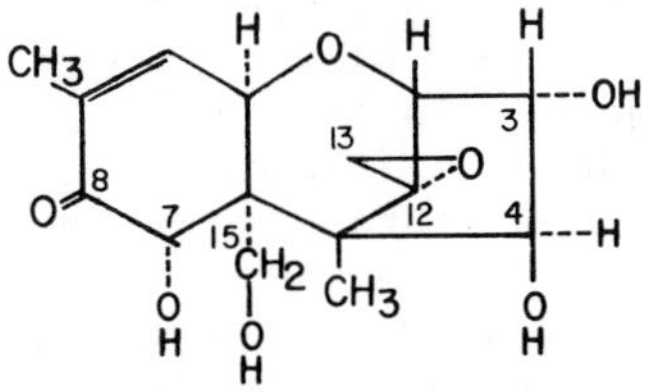

Figure 1. Structure of deoxynivalenol (vomitoxin).

0097–6156/83/0234–0241$06.00/0

The first crop in North America to be surveyed for vomitoxin was the 1980 wheat from eastern Canada (1). Soft winter wheat harvested in Ontario was noticed to contain pink kernels; this is one of the signs that the Fusarium mold which produces vomitoxin causes when it invades the kernels. Forty-four of 45 samples analyzed contained vomitoxin in concentration ranging from 0.01 to 4.3 parts per million (ppm). In Quebec, the contamination was worse. One hundred per cent contamination of the hard spring wheat crop was found based on analyses of 27 samples. Eighty five per cent of the samples contained greater than 0.3 ppm.

These same wheat crops were analyzed again in 1981 (2). A sampling plan was used in Ontario which included 60% of the entire crop. The average level of vomitoxin found was 0.18 ppm. This level was not considered to pose a health hazard to consumers since this wheat is used only in the preparation of non-staple foods (cakes, biscuits, etc.). However, because of the sampling limitation and to ensure that this average level was maintained, an upper limit of 0.3 ppm vomitoxin was recommended for Ontario soft wheat to be used in non-staple foods. The hard spring wheat of Quebec is used in the manufacture of staple foods such as bread. Because of the potential vomitoxin intake from wheat used in breadmaking, an interim guideline of 0.1 ppm vomitoxin in hard wheat was recommended. Analyses of the 1981 crop of Quebec hard wheat determined that the levels of vomitoxin were much higher than 0.1 ppm (some samples contained 5 ppm). As a result of these findings, it was recommended that 1981 Quebec hard wheat should not be used in the production of foods for human consumption. These guidelines of 0.1 ppm for wheat flour to be used in staple foods and 0.3 ppm for wheat flour used in non-staple foods are still in effect today and affect the shipping of wheat into Canada. Levels of vomitoxin in the 1980 and 1981 dried corn, which is used for flour, grits, meal and breakfast cereals, were slightly higher than that of wheat grown in the same area, but since the consumption of corn products in Canada is much lower than that of wheat products, no guidelines were placed on corn products.

In the U.S., routine analysis of grains for vomitoxin didn't begin until 1981, about a year after the Canadians' first surveys. In 1981, the U.S. cornbelt was heavily contaminated with vomitoxin from Iowa to New York. In Illinois, 274 of 342 samples of grain (mostly corn, but some wheat and oats) and animal feeds were found to contain from 0.1 to 22 ppm with a mean of 3 ppm vomitoxin (3). In 1982, the winter wheat crop of Kansas, Nebraska, Missouri and Iowa was contaminated with vomitoxin. A million acres of land in southeast and southcentral Nebraska (one third of the Nebraska wheat producing area) contained scabby wheat, a condition caused by the Fusarium mold that produces vomitoxin. A survey of 87 samples of wheat heads, grain, chaff, and straw found 76 (87%) to contain over 0.3 ppm, 63 (72%) over 1 ppm and 11 (13%) over 5 ppm vomitoxin (4). The scabby wheat area extended into north-

central and northeastern Kansas, southwest Iowa and northwest
Missouri. A survey of 43 grain samples from 30 Missouri counties
found 39 (91%) to contain over 0.1 ppm, 32 (74%) over 1 ppm and
8 (19%) over 10 ppm vomitoxin, with the highest level found being
61 ppm (5). These two surveys of the 1982 U.S. wheat crop were
conducted in areas where scabby wheat was prevalent and, thus, do
not represent the total wheat crop of the two states surveyed.
A third survey in which 55 samples were collected from scappy
wheat areas of all of the above four states found three samples
(5%) containing no detectable vomitoxin, 41 (75%) containing over
1 ppm and 15 (27%) containing over 5 ppm (6).

　　From the above surveys we can see that vomitoxin contamination of grains is common in North America. However, frequent
contamination is not a sufficient reason to label a mycotoxin a
hazard. Animal studies need also be conducted to determine if a
mycotoxin is a potential health hazard for humans or an economic
hazard for the animal industry.

　　In a study performed by Health and Welfare, Canada (7), pure
vomitoxin was administered to female mice on days 8 to 11 of
pregnancy. Doses ranged from 0.5 to 15 mg/kg/day. Fetal effects .
were observed at doses of 2.5 mg/kg/day and above. At the 2.5
mg/kg dose, 72% of the fetuses at term were missing one or more
ribs and exhibited many other bone-type effects such as fused
arches and fused ribs. Resorptions accompanied by vaginal bleeding occurred in frequencies of 100% at the 15 and 10 mg/kg and
80% at the 5 mg/kg doses. The 2.5 mg/kg dose is equivalent to
about 12 ppm vomitoxin in the mouse diet. This means that each
dam consumed about 20% of her body weight in feed per day. Since
a pregnant woman consumes about 1.5% of her body weight in food
per day, the concentration of vomitoxin in her total diet would
need to be 160 ppm in order for her to consume 2.5 mg/kg body
weight/day. However, since only part of a pregnant woman's diet
is likely to be composed of materials susceptible to vomitoxin
contamination, these food proudcts (e.g., bread) would have to
contain about 500 ppm in order for her total diet to contain
160 ppm vomitoxin.

　　In another study (8), pregnant rats were fed up to 5 ppm
pure vomitoxin in their diet for the full term of pregnancy. Although all of the results from this study have not been collected
and analyzed, the data on the fetal bone effects have been analyzed. No statistically significant bone defects were noted; however, some anomalies were observed in the 5 ppm fetuses that were
not observed in the control group. These anomalies included
asymmetrical cervical centra, curved spine, cleft palate, and
microphthalmia (uni- or bilateral). Since a pregnant woman consumes 5 to 10 times less food per day relative to her body weight
than does a pregnant rat, the concentration of vomitoxin in the
woman's diet needs to be 25 to 50 ppm in order for her to receive
the equivalent amount of vomitoxin as did the rats on the 5 ppm
diet.

One of the main concerns regarding vomitoxin is whether it causes any chronic toxic effects, that is, effects when low concentrations are consumed over a long period of time. One typical chronic effect is cancer. So far, no studies have shown that vomitoxin can cause cancer; however, no chronic studies have been performed with vomitoxin. Vomitoxin has been related to cancer of the esophagus in humans in Transkei, Africa (9), but this study only involved a few samples and no animal studies have corroborated this relationship. Another chronic effect that is a concern with vomitoxin is that of immunosuppression, that is, an effect which lowers the body's ability to resist disease. A Japanese study (10) has demonstrated that when small amounts of T-2 toxin, a trichothecene similar to vomitoxin, were administered to cats, a significant decrease in the white blood cell count resulted. If vomitoxin is found to have a similar immunosuppressive effect at low concentrations, it may become regarded as a human health hazard.

What, then, should feed and food companies do with respect to vomitoxin? They should keep abreast of the latest toxicity information, especially chronic toxicity studies. Feed and grain companies need to keep abreast of the latest information on tissue residue research on vomitoxin and its metabolic break-down products (some residue research is in process at the present time, both in the U.S. and Canada). At the same time, companies can test their ingredients and final products using available procedures (11, 12, 13, 14, 15). Several procedures are available ranging from the highly sophisticated mass spectrometric (14) to a simple rapid "go or no go" test that can be used at the plant or elevator site (15). Many U.S. and Canadian companies are already testing for vomitoxin, some as part of their own quality control program, others because of the Canadian guidelines which allow a maximum level of 0.1 ppm vomitoxin in wheat flour or bran used to make staple food products (e.g., bread) and 0.3 ppm in the flour or bran used to make non-staple food products (e.g., cakes, cookies, pretzels, etc.). At the present time, there are no U.S. guidelines as such, but the Food and Drug Administration has developed "advisory" levels for vomitoxin in wheat and wheat products. The advisory level for wheat and wheat products intended for human consumption is 2 ppm in the wheat before milling and 1 ppm in the finished wheat products. For wheat and wheat products which are used as animal feed ingredients, the advisory level is 4 ppm with the added recommendation that these ingredients not exceed 10% of swine and pet diets or 50% of the diets of ruminants and poultry. The reason for the lower recommended level for swine, cats, and dogs compared to ruminants and poultry is that the former are more susceptible to the known effects of vomitoxin (refusal and vomiting). Since vomitoxin can also be found in corn at concentrations as high or higher than is found in wheat and since corn is normally used at higher than a 10% level in swine feed and pet foods, it is advisable to consider a

final level of 1 ppm vomitoxin in high-corn swine and pet diets
as a maximum concentration and monitor the corn accordingly.
Several feeding studies have been performed on swine using, in
most cases, corn or wheat naturally contaminated with vomitoxin
(4, 16, 17). In general, the only effect noticed was lowered
feed consumption with swine when 0.3 ppm or more vomitoxin was
incorporated into the diet via naturally contaminated wheat or
corn. The lowered feed consumption was noticed mainly during
the first week of the studies which results in a depression in
final weight compared to controls. When pure vomitoxin was
incorporated into swine diets, the feed consumption decrease
ranged from 20% at 3.6 ppm to 90% at 40 ppm. The minimum emetic
dose was 0.1 to 0.2 mg/kg body weight when administration was
oral (gavage) (18). It is necessary to remember that some of the
lowered feed consumption in diets containing naturally contaminated ingredients may be caused by trichothecene mycotoxins
other than vomitoxin which have not yet been identified.

　　Poultry have been found to be highly resistant to the effects
of vomitoxin. A diet containing sufficient naturally contaminated corn to provide a 50 ppm vomitoxin concentration was fed
to 6 day old broiler cockerels for 6 days with no effect on growth
or feed consumption. The only observed effects of the contaminated diet were plaques in the mouth and gizzard erosion (19).
When a diet containing 15 ppm pure vomitoxin was fed to broilers
for 6 weeks, no deleterious effects were noticed (20).

　　A diet containing sufficient naturally contaminated corn to
provide a final concentration of 50 ppm vomitoxin was fed to
laying hens for 4 weeks with no effects on production, consumption, body weight, egg weight or shell strength. Sample chicks
were necropsied at hatch and grown to one week of age; no treatment effects were found (21). However, in another study (22),
when diets containing 0.3 to 0.7 ppm vomitoxin from naturally
contaminated wheat were fed to laying hens for 3 weeks, there was
a 2% decrease in egg weight and egg shell thickness. This latter
result points out a significant factor that always needs to be
considered when feeding grain containing vomitoxin. Just because
the level of vomitoxin in the grain is not sufficient to cause a
problem in the animals being fed (e.g., laying hens) does not
mean the grain is not harmful. Even if all of the mold toxins
for which there are analytical methods have not been detected,
grain could still contain unidentified mold toxins. More than
30 compounds have been discovered that belong to the trichothecene
family of mycotoxins which include vomitoxin, T-2 toxin and diacetoxyscirpenol. However, these three are the only trichothecenes
for which there exist routine analytical methods. The fact that
vomitoxin is found in a sample of grain is proof that at least
one mold has been growing in the grain. More than one mold may
have been growing and more than one toxin may have been produced.

　　Cattle, like poultry, seem to be unaffected by vomitoxin.
Steers and heifers were fed diets containing 11 ppm vomitoxin for

18 weeks with no ill effects noticed (4). However, neither the
serum chemistry nor the histopathology portion of this research
has been completed. In another study (23), dry dairy cattle were
fed a diet containing 4.7 ppm vomitoxin for 30 days. No effects
on feed consumption or other performance factors were noticed.
In both of these cattle studies, naturally contaminated wheat was
the source of vomitoxin in the feed.

We need to realize that none of the vomitoxin toxicity
studies discussed above tested for immunosuppression. Also, none
of the swine or cattle studies tested for reproductive effects.
One of the studies cited above (7) found that vomitoxin can produce reproductive effects in laboratory animals. Zearalenone, a
mycotoxin known to produce reproductive effects on swine (24) and
lengthen their estrus cycle (25), is often found along with vomitoxin in contaminated grain. Thus, it is important that vomitoxin
be tested both alone and in combination with zearalenone to determine if it adversely effects the reproductive system of swine
and/or cattle.

When the results of subchronic and chronic studies on the
reproductive, immunosuppressive, and other possible adverse effects of vomitoxin have been completed, it will be easier to
judge how much of a hazard vomitoxin poses for the feed and the
food industries.

Literature Cited

1. Scott, P. M. Joint Mycotoxin Committee Report, Association
    of Official Analytical Chemists Convention, Washington, D.C.,
    October 23, 1980.
2. Scott, P. M. Joint Mycotoxin Committee Report, Association
    of Official Analytical Chemists Convention, Washington, D.C.,
    October 22, 1981.
3. Buck, W. University of Illinois, Urbana, Illinois, Personal
    Communication.
4. Schneider, N. R.; Carlson, M. University of Nebraska,
    Lincoln, Nebraska, Personal Communication.
5. Rottinghaus, G. University of Missouri, Columbia, Missouri,
    Personal Communication.
6. Eppley, R. M. Bureau of Foods, Food and Drug Administration,
    Washington, D.C., Personal Communication.
7. Khera, K. S.; Whalen, C.; Angers, G.; Vesonder, R. F.;
    Kuiper-Goodman, T. Bull. Environ. Contam. Toxicol., 1982,
    29, 487.
8. Morrissey, R. E. To be published in April, 1983, Teratology.
9. Marasas, W. F. O.; van Rensburg, S. J.; Mirocha, C. J. J.
    Agric. Food Chem., 1979, 27, 5, 1108.
10. Sato, N.; Ueno, Y.; Enomoto, M. Japan. J. Pharmacol., 1975,
    25, 263.
11. Scott, P. M.; Lau, P. Y.; Kanhere, S. R. JAOAC, 1981, 64,
    1364 (A GLC Method).

12. *Romer, T.R.; Greaves, D. E.; Gibson, G. E.   A GLC method presented at the AOAC spring workshop, Ottawa, Ontario, 1981.
13. *Romer, T. R.; Langford, W. F.   A GLC method presented at the AOAC fall meeting, Washington, D.C., 1981.
14. Rothberg, J. M.; MacDonald, J. L.; Swims, J. C.; Romer, T. R.   Proceedings of the 29th Annual Conference of Mass Spectrometry and Allied Topics, Minneapolis, Minnesota, May 24-29, 1981.
15. *A modification of 12.
16. Trenholm, H. L.; Friend, D. W.; Hamilton, R. M. G.; Thompson, B. K.   Publication 1745/E, available from Communications Branch, Agriculture, Canada   K1A 0C7, 1982.
17. Pollman, D. S.; Koch, B. A.   Progress Report 422 - Ag. Exper. Sta., Kansas State University, Manhattan, Kansas, 66506, 1982.
18. Forsyth, D. M.; Yoshizawa, T.; Morooka, N.; Tuite, J.   Appl. and Environ. Microbiol. 1977, 34, 5, 547.
19. Moran, E. T., Jr.; Hunter, B.; Ferket, P.; Young, L. G.; McGirr, L. G.   Poultry Science 1982, 61, 1828.
20. Cole, R.; Vesonder, R.; Lomax, L.   Personal Communication.
21. Moran, E. T., Jr.; Hunter, R. B.; Ferket, P. R.; Young, L. G.   Proceedings of the Poultry Industry School. Ontario Agricultural College, University of Guelph, 1983, 13-14.
22. Hamilton, R. M. G.   Poultry Science Annual Meeting, University of British Columbia, Vancouver, British Columbia, Canada, August 3-7, 1981.
23. Trenholn, H. L.   Animal Research Center, Ottawa, Ontario, Canada, Personal Communication.
24. Mirocha, C. J.; Christensen, C. M.   Ann. Rev. Phytopathology 1974, 12, 303.
25. Cantley, T. C.; Redmer, D. A.; Osweiler, G. D.; Day, B. N.   Fifteenth meeting Midwestern Section ASAS, March 22-24, 1982, Abstract #67.

*Available from the author.

RECEIVED June 16, 1983

Aflatoxins in Corn

U. L. DIENER and N. D. DAVIS

Department of Botany, Plant Pathology, and Microbiology, Auburn University, Auburn, AL 36849

Certain fungi (molds) synthesize chemicals, called mycotoxins, that are poisonous and produce symptoms of toxicity when food and feed containing them is eaten by humans and animals. The aflatoxins are mycotoxins produced by two fungi, Aspergillus flavus and A. parasiticus, which are distributed worldwide in air and soils and may contaminate corn, peanuts, cottonseed, tree nuts and other crops with aflatoxin. Animal products may contain aflatoxins where contaminated feeds have been ingested. Aflatoxin B_1 is the most potent, naturally-occurring, cancer-producing substance known, causing liver cancer in most experimental and domesticated animals and man. Preharvest infection by A. flavus may occur via colonization of corn silks followed by invasion of the glumes and surface of developing kernels. Internal seed infection occurs later during kernel denting. Commonly, ear-damaging insects transport fungal spores both externally and internally, and may provide infection sites and disperse the fungus within the ear. Stress induced by water deprivation, above normal temperatures, inadequate fertilization, and weed competition appears to exacerbate susceptibility of developing kernels to infection by A. flavus and subsequent aflatoxin biosynthesis. Aflatoxin can develop in storage; rapid drying of corn to safe storage moisture after harvest and dry storage facilities with aeration are essential to prevent contamination. Although control with fungicides and/or resistant varieties has been notably unsuccessful to date, considerable progress has been made in preventing and reducing contamination of human foods as well as losses in animal feeds by detoxifying aflatoxin-contaminated products, particularly by ammoniation.

0097–6156/83/0234–0249$06.25/0

Certain fungi (molds) synthesize chemicals that are poisonous and produce symptoms of toxicity when food or feed containing them is eaten by humans and animals. These chemicals are called mycotoxins, a term derived from the Greek words "myces" meaning fungus and "toxikon" meaning poison. Mycotoxic effects, such as ergot poisoning, can be traced to civilizations of 5,000 years ago. Ergotism (St. Anthony's Fire) reached epidemic proportions in the Middle Ages in Central Europe from the consumption of contaminated rye bread. In Russia in the 1940s, stachybotryotoxicosis caused illness and death to horses and humans, as did alimentary toxic aleukia in humans, which was associated with Fusarium infection of overwintered wheat and millet (1).

The impetus that stimulated scientific interest in mycotoxins evolved from the death of 100,000 turkey poults at 500 locations in England in 1960, which led to the discovery by British scientists of aflatoxin (a toxic metabolite of the fungus Aspergillus flavus Link ex Fr.) in the peanut meal fraction of the feed (2,3). Research soon demonstrated that aflatoxin B_1 is possibly the most potent, naturally occurring carcinogen ever utilized in animal studies (4). In addition, it can cause acute aflatoxicosis in animals and humans; a case of the latter was cited in a CAST report (5).

"Perhaps the single, most impressive, aflatoxin-related episode reported in recent scientific literature is an acute poisoning in an area of India in 1974 involving over 400 people and resulting in 106 deaths. The circumstances were typical of those highly conducive to excessive mycotoxin exposure, i.e., a poor, rural subsistence economy, where the people were virtually totally dependent on a single food crop (corn, Zea mays L.) that they produced themselves, and conditions were favorable for aflatoxin formation as a result of unseasonable rains that drenched the crop at harvest in the warm subtropical climate of the area. Only corn-eating ethnic groups and individuals were affected. No new cases occurred after the locally grown corn supplies were exhausted. Several members of some rural households were affected. Dogs eating the same food suffered a similar fate. Medical features of the syndrome were consistent with experimental data on aflatoxicosis. Aflatoxin-contaminated corn was consumed in affected households but not in unaffected households. Aflatoxin concentrations were relatively high with samples containing from 250 to 15,600 parts per billion" (5).

Three years later in 1977 and again in 1980, outbreaks of aflatoxin in corn in Southeastern United States caused extensive crop losses and in animals that ingested contaminated corn. This occurrence instigated the development of a Regional Technical Committee of corn researchers in the Southeast, which sponsored a symposium in Atlanta, Georgia, in January 1982 on "Aflatoxin and Aspergillus flavus in Corn" (6).

Biology of Aspergillus Flavus and Aspergillus Parasiticus

Aspergillus flavus and A. parasiticus Speare, closely
related fungi, occur world-wide in the soil and contaminate a
wide variety of crops in the field, during harvest, in storage,
or during processing. They are seed-inhabiting fungi of important food crops such as corn, peanuts, cottonseed, and tree nuts.
Aflatoxins are produced only by these two fungi. Far less is
known about the basic physiology and nutrition of A. flavus than
A. parasiticus. Researchers have seldom distinguished between
the two species and referred to A. parasiticus as A. flavus.
Some morphological characteristics of these two species are given
in Table I.

Table I.   Morphological and Growth Comparisons of the
Aflatoxin-producing Fungi

Characteristic	A. parasiticus	A. flavus
Conidia	Distinctively verruculose	Almost smooth to lightly roughened
Conidiophore heads	Mostly uniseriate, sometimes mixed	Consistently biseriate
Color	Ivy green	Yellow-green
Colony	Compact	Irregular

A. flavus typically produces only the toxic metabolites aflatoxin B_1 (AFB_1) and aflatoxin B_2 (AFB_2), whereas toxigenic A. parasiticus isolates produce AFG_1 and AFG_2 as well
as AFB_1 and AFB_2. Over 90% of the analyses of contaminated
corn samples show only AFB_1 and AFB_2, whereas AFG_1 is common in contaminated peanuts. A. flavus is considered dominant in
cottonseed, pecans, and other tree nuts as well as corn.
     Several trace elements are required for aflatoxin formation
by A. flavus, particularly zinc (7). The necessity for zinc,
magnesium, and other mineral elements for aflatoxin production by
A. flavus (A. parasiticus) is illustrated in Table II (8).
Zinc, magnesium, iron and molybdenum were essential, whereas manganese appeared to stimulate aflatoxin formation.

Table II.   Essentiality of Certain Mineral Elements to Aflatoxin
            Production by Aspergillus flavus

Element omitted	Mycelial dry wt. g/100 ml	B_1	Aflatoxin mg/100 ml G_1	Total (B+G)
Magnesium	1.60	0	0	0
Zinc	0.60	0	0	0
Iron	1.33	0.13	0.16	0.29
Molybdenum	2.86	0.17	0.30	0.47
Copper	2.85	0.82	1.76	2.58
Boron	2.91	0.69	2.00	2.69
Manganese	2.12	1.24	2.64	3.88
None of above	2.77	0.69	2.00	2.69
All of above	0.65	0	0	0

Lillehoj et al. (9) found that the addition of low levels
of zinc, copper, and manganese stimulated aflatoxin production by
A. flavus growing on corn germ, as others had discovered with
nutrient solutions (8,10). Other investigators have found otherwise, but apparently the concentration of metal salt determines
whether it is stimulatory or inhibitory (11,12), as can be noted
for zinc in Table III (8). Thus, some of the contradictions in
the literature probably are due to concentration differences in
non-comparable experiments.

Table III.   Influence of Zinc Level on Aflatoxin Production by
             Aspergillus flavus

$ZnSO_4$ ppm	Mycelial dry wt. g/100 ml	B_1	Aflatoxin mg/100 ml G_1	Total (B+G)
None	0.21	0	0	0
1	2.77	0.32	0.56	0.88
3	2.67	0.69	1.20	1.89
5	3.48	0.85	2.40	3.29
7	3.04	0.34	0.60	0.94
10	3.51	0.21	0.38	0.59

The influence of various carbohydrates supplied as sole carbon sources on growth and aflatoxin production by A. flavus, actually A. parasiticus, is shown in Table IV (8). The fungus grew and produced some aflatoxin on all of the carbohydrates tested except lactose. The highest yields of aflatoxin were produced from glucose and sucrose.

Table IV.   Influence of Carbohydrate Source on Production of Aflatoxin by Aspergillus flavus

Carbohydrate (66 g/1 of carbon)	Mycelial dry wt. g/100 ml	Aflatoxin mg/100 ml B_1	G_1	Total (B+G)
Glucose	2.25	0.76	1.92	2.68
Sucrose	2.28	0.76	1.62	2.38
Fructose	2.96	0.38	0.88	1.26
Raffinose	2.66	0.42	0.48	0.90
Mannitol	3.13	0.03	0.08	0.11
Galactose	2.27	0.02	0.05	0.07
Lactose	No Growth	0	0	0
Glucose + Fructose	2.03	0.76	1.84	2.60
Glucose + Galactose	2.51	0.48	0.93	1.41

The effect of sucrose concentration on aflatoxin production by A. flavus is shown in Table V (13). The highest yields were produced with 15 and 20% sucrose in a 2% yeast extract medium.

Table V.   Influence of Sucrose Concentration on Aflatoxin Production by Aspergillus flavus

Sucrose %	Mycelial dry wt. g/100 ml	Aflatoxin mg/100 ml B_1	G_1	Total (B+G)
0	0.3	0.1	0.1	0.2
1	1.0	0.5	0.7	1.2
5	1.6	0.7	0.9	1.6
10	3.0	1.4	1.7	3.1
15	3.0	2.7	3.5	6.2
20	2.8	2.8	3.6	6.4
30	3.2	2.7	2.3	5.0
50	3.2	2.6	2.0	4.6

The influence of nitrogen source on growth and aflatoxin production by A. flavus (A. parasiticus) is shown in Table VI (8). Note that the complex organic sources of nitrogen, such as yeast extract and peptone, gave tremendous yields as compared to the best single amino acid. Inorganic nitrogen sources, such as potassium nitrate, were totally inadequate for aflatoxin production.

Table VI. Influence of Nitrogen Source on Growth and Production of Aflatoxin by Aspergillus flavus in a Chemically Defined Medium

Nitrogen (0.42 g/l Nitrogen)	Mycelial dry wt. g/100 ml	Aflatoxin mg/100 ml B_1	G_1	Total (B+G)
None	No Growth	0	0	0
Yeast extract	3.87	2.47	3.20	5.67
Peptone	2.60	1.71	1.56	3.27
Aspartate	3.96	0.76	0.64	1.40
Glycine	4.09	0.44	0.74	1.18
Glutamine	3.62	0.63	0.53	1.16
Glutamate	3.94	0.57	0.58	1.15
Asparagine	3.59	0.19	0.18	0.37
Alanine	3.73	0.12	0.15	0.27
Methionine	3.61	0.12	0.09	0.21
Valine	3.04	0.06	0.05	0.11
Leucine	2.88	0.03	0.03	0.06
KNO_3	3.66	0.02	0.02	0.04
$NaNo_3$	3.71	0.01	0.01	0.02

The effect of yeast extract concentration on aflatoxin production by A. flavus is shown in Table VII (13). The highest yields were produced with 2% yeast extract in 20% sucrose medium. Yeast extract provided most of the major and minor elements needed for growth and toxin production and technical grade sucrose provided carbon and iron.

Amino acids mixtures stimulate aflatoxin biosynthesis, particularly asparagine and aspartic acid. Proline has been reported to stimulate conidial germination in a culture that was probably A. parasiticus, although reported as A. flavus (14). These investigators reported the greatest toxin formation with a mixture of amino acids followed by a mixture of proline plus glutamate or proline plus aspartate. The effect in the latter instances may have been due to the effect on conidial germination rather than a direct effect on aflatoxin biosynthesis.

The cardinal temperatures for vegetative growth for A. flavus are: minimum 6 to 8° C; optimum 36 to 38° C; and maximum 44 to 46° C (15). However, optima and limiting temperatures for aflatoxin production on media and natural substrates vary. The optimum for A. flavus in liquid (SMKY) medium and on peanuts was 25° C, whereas A. parasiticus showed highest aflatoxin production at 35° C and high total aflatoxins at 30° C over incubation periods of 5 to 21 days (16). Precise limiting temperatures and relative humidity for aflatoxin production by A. parasiticus were determined for wet-heat, pasteurized peanuts, freshly-dug peanuts and stored peanuts (17-19). Limiting temperatures were 12 and 41° C and limiting relative humidity was 83% for sound mature kernels, broken mature (damaged) kernels, immature kernels, and kernels in intact pods incubated for 84 days at 30° C. Similar data are presently being obtained for aflatoxin formation in corn by A. flavus.

Table VII.   Influence of Yeast Extract Concentration on Aflatoxin Production by Aspergillus flavus Growing in 20% Sucrose Medium

Yeast extract %	Mycelial dry wt. g/100 ml	Aflatoxin mg/100 ml B_1	G_1	Total (B+G)
None	0	0	0	0
0.7	3.3	2.4	3.8	6.2
2.0	4.1	3.6	4.3	7.9
3.0	4.2	4.3	3.2	7.5
5.0	5.2	3.0	2.7	5.7

The effect of temperature on linear growth rates of A. flavus and A. parasiticus was determined on potato-dextrose and cornmeal agars by Davis and Diener (unpublished data). A. flavus grew slightly faster than A. parasiticus at 20, 27, and 35° C. Other workers measuring growth in grams of mycelium produced reported no difference in the two species (20,21). At best, data are meager for valid conclusions.

Wicklow et al. (22) view the A. flavus sclerotium as primary inoculum in regions where aflatoxin contamination of corn is a recurrent problem. Germination of the sclerotium results in production of conidia that represent infective inoculum. Dispersal of inoculum by arthropods and wind may be facilitated by strongly roughened or echinulate conidial walls. Wicklow and Cole (23) detected aflatrem, cyclopiazonic acid, and dehydroxyflavinine only in the sclerotia from 85% of the isolates examined and never in the culture medium of fungus mycelium. They argue that the sclerotium is important as a survival structure and contains the chemical defense systems of the fungus as the evolutionary outcome of selective forces determining the intrafungus distribution of compounds toxic to potential predators and parasites (6).

Epidemiology of Aflatoxin Formation by Aspergillus Flavus

Preharvest contamination of corn with aflatoxin is a serious problem. Aspergillus flavus can colonize corn silks and invade developing kernels. The most susceptible stage for colonization appears to be just after pollination when the silks are yellow-brown in color. At this stage, A. flavus conidia germinate readily and rapidly colonize silks and pollen grains on the silks. In contrast, conidia germinate poorly and little growth occurs on unpollinated silks or dry brown silks. Fungus infection of corn silks is favored by high temperatures (Table VIII) (24).

Table VIII. Effect of Temperature and Time of Silk Inoculation on Seed Infection by Aspergillus flavus

Time of Inoc.[a]	Percentage of Kernels Infected at each Temperature Regime			
	34/30	26/30	34/22	26/22
1	30	6	30	3
2	46	4	5	6
3	49	15	1	2
5	14	3	1	1

[a] Weeks after silk emergence.

In a phytotron, the percentage of infected kernels was 49, 15, and 2, respectively, for day/night temperature regimes of 34/30, 26/30, and 26/22 C. Growth of the fungus from the external silks into the kernels and the accompanying infection process are not well understood. The fungus can grow from external silks into the ear in four days. Shortly thereafter, the surface of the kernels and the glumes of the kernel are colonized. Internal infection of the kernel, however, occurs later apparently during the period of kernel denting. Infection at this stage has been reported for other seed infecting fungi. Payne indicates that insects probably play an important role in providing infection sites by injuring the kernels, in spreading the fungus with the ear, and in bringing fungus spores into the ear (6).

In general, levels of contamination of insects by A. flavus ranged from 2 to 50% of the insects observed in preharvest corn including the corn earworm, Heliothis zea (Boddie), European corn borer, Ostrinia nubilalis (Hubner), and rice weevil, Sitophilus oryzae (L) according to McMillian (6). Corn-ear-inhabiting insects have been contaminated much more with A. flavus than A. parasiticus and the fungus has been isolated fom all stages of the life cycle of H. zea and from all except the egg in S. oryzae. H. zea can also transmit A. flavus from one life-cycle stage to the next. Spore-contaminated feces have been collected from H. zea larvae, 24 hours after the ingestion of A. flavus conidia. The biology of several corn insects is detrimentally affected by A. flavus, A. parasiticus, and/or their metabolites and they have been suggested as control agents. A direct cause-and-effect relationship has been demonstrated between A. flavus contaminated maize weevils (S. zeamais Motschulsky) and A. flavus contamination in corn ears damaged by weevils. Generally, insecticide applications and the planting of tight-husked, insect-resistant hybrids have resulted in reduced insect damage to grain and lower aflatoxin levels.

The colonization of developing corn kernels by A. flavus has been associated with the early milk stage (25), aflatoxin has been detected in kernels at late milk stage (26), and maximum aflatoxin formation has been reported when A. flavus invaded kernels at late milk-early dough stage (27,28). The interaction between kernel moisture content (KMC) and aflatoxin accumulation was studied by inoculation with A. flavus about 20 days after silking in corn grown in Illinois, Missouri, and Georgia (29). Ears were harvested 15, 30, 45, and 70 days after inoculation. Data in Table IX show that in Illinois the KMC remained high for 70 days with formation of negligible levels of AFB. In Missouri, AFB_1 levels became significant when KMC dropped below 30%. In Georgia, AFB_1 levels were significant at 51%, 31% (220 ppb), and reached 440 ppb at KMC of 14%. Some of these differences are obviously related to temperature effects resulting from the three distinct regional locations. Except under controlled experimental conditions, researchers often cannot measure differences resulting from only one variable in the field.

Table IX. Kernel Moisture Content and Aflatoxin B_1 in Corn
Kernels Harvested at Various Intervals after
Inoculation with Aspergillus flavus in 1974

Post Inoc. days [a]	Illinois KMC %	AFB$_1$ ppb	Missouri KMC %	AFB$_1$ ppb	Georgia KMC %	AFB$_1$ ppb
15	65	1	46	3	51	63
30	48	1	29	61	31	203
45	43	5	27	105	23	307
70	34	9	24	63	14	440
Means	48	4	32	58	30	253

[a] Inoculated 20 days after flowering.

Most data on the relation of temperature to aflatoxin formation have been obtained with A. parasiticus. Aflatoxin contamination of cottonseed by A. flavus in the field occurs primarily
in low-altitude areas of Arizona and the Imperial Valley of California and not in the hot and humid Southeastern States. Chronic
field contamination of cottonseed apparently requires daily mean
temperature of 34° C or above (T.E. Russell, personal communication). The significant difference between Arizona and the Southeast cotton areas is the high night temperatures of 32-34 C in
Arizona.

The relation of temperature to aflatoxin contamination in
corn kernels from inoculation at the early dough, medium dough,
and late dough stages of development was studied in a phytotron
(30). Aflatoxin levels were significantly higher in kernels from
plants grown at the highest combination of daily temperatures
(Table X).

Table X. Aflatoxin B_1 Levels in Corn Inoculated with
Aspergillus flavus at Three Developmental
Stages and Grown under Four Different
Postinoculation Temperature Regimes

Kernel Develop. at Inoc.	Aflatoxin B_1 (ppm) Day/Night Temperature C			
	22/18	30/18	22/26	30/26
Early Dough	12.6	12.4	13.0	12.7
Medium Dough	11.2	22.0	26.5	29.4
Late Dough	13.1	18.0	25.8	31.4

These data and those in Table IX emphasize the critical role of temperature in aflatoxin formation in developing corn kernels.

Fungi are aerobic organisms and small changes in gaseous environment can cause dramatic changes in metabolic cellular processes (31,32). When CO_2 was removed from the atmosphere, spore germination of A. flavus was inhibited (14). In high-moisture stored corn, growth and aflatoxin production by A. flavus was blocked at oxygen levels below 0.5% (33). The sensitivity of aflatoxin-producing fungi to atmospheric gases, particularly oxygen and carbon dioxide, suggests research to determine the level of gases in the microenvironment of developing corn kernels.

Although A. flavus will grow on almost any natural or processed substrate, aflatoxin occurs naturally primarily in corn, peanuts, cottonseed, grain sorghum, tree nuts, millet, copra, and figs (34). Substrate factors must be involved in contamination, since it is limited to a relatively small number of agricultural commodities. The restricted access of zinc has been proposed as an explanation for the inability of A. flavus to elaborate aflatoxin in soybeans (35). The availability of zinc for aflatoxin biosynthesis appears to be blocked by the presence of phytic acid in soybeans (36).

Production of aflatoxin by A. flavus is relatively independent of vegetative growth. An elevated carbon-to-nitrogen ratio has been linked to aflatoxin formation and high toxin production is dependent of high concentrations of specific carbohydrates in the substrate as well as specific organic nitrogen sources. Glucose concentrations of 20–30% (37) and sucrose levels of 10–20% (13,38) have produced maximum aflatoxin yields. Amino acids, such as aspartate, glycine, glutamate, and glutamine, appear to promote elevated aflatoxin formation (8,39).

Plant stress was involved in the corn-aflatoxin outbreak in Iowa in 1975. That region of the state had experienced drought and above-normal temperatures, whereas other areas in Iowa with no toxin contamination had normal rainfall and temperatures (40). In 1976, corn test plots in six southern and three Corn Belt states were sampled and monthly average temperature and rainfall were recorded (41). No aflatoxin positive samples were taken in Iowa, Illinois, and Ohio, which had lower temperatures than the six southern states. The location with the highest 3-month average temperature (Florida) had 75% of its samples aflatoxin-positive. Florida had much above normal rainfall in June (+4.6") and much below normal in July (-3.4) and August (-5.4). Thus, distinct drought stress was present in these last two months.

Other research has been summarized (42) by a proposal that elevated temperatures and water stress are responsible for increased parasitic ability of A. flavus, associated infection processes, and higher aflatoxin concentration in developing kernels (Table XI).

Table XI. Effect of Water Stress on Kernel Infection and
           Aflatoxin Production by Aspergillus flavus

Treatment	Infected kernels %	Aflatoxin B_1 ppb
No Stress	40	28
Preinoculation Stress	38	291
Postinoculation Stress	35	392

Jones et al. (43) also found aflatoxin was less severe in
the high corn-yielding Tidewater region than in the sandy Coastal
Plain soils. Stress was linked to reduced water holding capacity
of the soil and drought related interference with nutrient uptake
by corn plants. A controlled irrigation study during 1977 and
1978 showed 23.6% aflatoxin-positive samples (7.3 ppb AFB_1)
from irrigated plots as compared to 54.9% positive samples (61.9
ppb AFB_1) from non-irrigated plots. This convincing evidence
of an association between water stress on developing corn plants
and enchanced vulnerability of the kernels to aflatoxin contamination paralleled the findings of Pettit et al. (44) in 1971 on
the effect of irrigation on aflatoxin accumulation in peanuts.
    Fertility stress from reduced fertilization and dense popu-
lations of plants contributes to aflatoxin development in preharvest corn (26). A definite relationship between increased
aflatoxin levels in kernels from plants grown under nitrogen
stress has been reported (45). The competition of weeds for
available nutrients and water also has been linked to presence of
aflatoxin in corn (46).

Sampling and Analysis

    In aflatoxin-contaminated lots of corn, a small percentage
of kernels may contain very high concentrations of aflatoxin making accurate determinations of aflatoxin levels difficult (6).
This factor makes getting a representative sample for chemical
analysis the critical step. Research indicates that the variance
and skewness of the distribution of aflatoxin concentrations of
samples about a lot mean are inversely proportional to sample
size and to toxin concentration in the lot. The distribution of
sample concentrations about the lot mean is practically normal
when lot concentration is greater than 20 ppb aflatoxin and sample weight is 4.45 kg or greater. Probe sampling may be used
when a lot of corn has been recently blended in harvesting, handling, or other operations; otherwise, stream sampling should be
used.

A number of reliable effective methods of detection and determination of aflatoxin in corn are available (6).

(1) the bright greenish-yellow fluorescence (BGYF) presump-
tive test or black light test is widely used by farmers, elevator
operators, and industry to identify suspect lots of corn that may
contain aflatoxin. It alone does not demonstrate the presence of
aflatoxin, but requires a chemical analysis for confirmation.

(2) For laboratories with minimal equipment and requirements
for results in a minimum amount of time, the Holaday-Velasco
minicolumn method has been adopted for aflatoxin in corn by the
Association of Official Analytical Chemists (AOAC) as well as the
American Association of Cereal Chemists (AACC).

(3) The official method is by the CB method, but an improved
method is needed that is less expensive and uses less toxic solvents. Modified and alternate methods abound but are untested
except by their creator.

There are several promising quantitative methods that need
evaluation in collaborative studies by the AOAC and the AACC.
High performance liquid chromatography (HPLC), the fluorometric-
iodine method (FL-IM), the enzyme-linked immunosorbent assay
(ELISA), the solid-phase radioimmunoassay (RIA), and the tandem
mass spectrometer, all have great potential. Research is needed
to determine the extent, limitations, and applications for each
method.

Biological Effects of Aflatoxin in Domestic Animals

Bovine. Although acute aflatoxicosis in cattle results in
overt symptoms, such as reduced feed consumption, severely depressed milk-yield, weight loss, and liver damage, the insidious
biological effects resulting from chronic exposure to sub-acute
levels of aflatoxin may be of greater economic importance (6).
Low to moderate intakes of aflatoxin-contaminated rations by
dairy and beef cattle have been associated with reduced feed efficiency, immunosuppression, increased susceptibility to stress,
and reduced reproductive performance. These low level effects
are difficult to recognize; thus, the incidence of chronic aflatoxicosis in cattle as well as other livestock may be greater
than reported. Not only is animal health affected during chronic
aflatoxicosis, but also a portion of ingested AFB_1 is converted
to a hydroxylated metabolite, AFM_1, and excreted in milk. Because the conversion rate is approximately 0.9%, a dairy cow may
produce milk containing some AFM_1 without manifesting symptoms
of intoxication. Research concerning the biological effects of
AFB_1 in the bovine has been principally designed for testing
acute toxicological response. Little definitive data are available on the effects of aflatoxin on physiological processes, such
as nutrient (particularly trace mineral) metabolism or cell-
mediated immune response.

Porcine. Data from veterinary diagnostic laboratories

indicate that porcine aflatoxicosis was common in 1981 in Southeastern and Midwestern United States (6). Twenty to 60% of corn
and feed samples suspected of toxicity contained aflatoxin and
concentrations exceeding 200 ppb were common. Suckling piglets,
growing and finishing swine, and breeding stock are susceptible
to aflatoxicosis, but clinical and pathological alterations vary
greatly depending upon age, diet, dosage, and duration of exposure. Decrease in the rate of weight gain and impaired feed
conversion efficiency are among the mildest effects, and lethal,
acute, severe, toxic hepatitis, nephrosis, and systemic hemorrhages are among the most severe. Aflatoxins are carcinogenic in
pigs, but toxin-induced neoplasia in pigs have not been recognized to occur naturally. Spontaneous porcine aflatoxicosis is
associated with increased susceptibility to disease and experimental aflatoxicosis may cause immunosuppression in pigs (6). The
conditions under which this occurs however are incompletely defined. Aflatoxins are absorbed rapidly from the porcine gastrointestinal tract and are concentrated largely in the liver and
kidney. Excretion occurs mostly in the feces and in lesser
amounts in the urine. Aflatoxins B_1, B_2, G_1, G_2, M_1,
M_2 and aflatoxicol are metabolites now identified in pigs.

   Avian. Aflatoxin (AFB_1) from peanut meal caused significant losses of turkeys, ducklings and pheasants in England, 1960
(2,3). Research demonstrated that exposure to AFB_1 resulted in
hepatic cell damage with necrosis, congestion, and bile duct proliferation (2). There were macroscopic hemorrhages, icterus, and
the livers were firm and pale. Large, focal areas of lymphoid
hyperplasia and mitotic figures were observed. Aflatoxin is recognized as an important carcinogen. Aflatoxin (0.25-0.5 $\mu g/g$
B_1) consumed during periods of immunization against Pasteurella
multocida interfered with the development of acquired resistance
in 20-67% of turkey poults and chicks (47). Decreased immunity
persisted even when an aflatoxin-free diet was substituted. This
immunosuppression resulted from impairment of the reticuloendo-
thelial system. Aflatoxin B_1 (0.2 $\mu g/g$) in commercial feed for
New Hampshire and broiler chicks decreased weight gains, and
increased susceptibility and mortality from cecal coccidiosis
(48). In another trial, vaccinated and nonvaccinated groups of
chickens exposed to AFB_1 were more susceptible to challenge
inoculation with Marek's virus than similar AFB_1 free groups
(49). In further trials in turkey poults (50), inclusion of
AFB_1 in the diet at 0.5 $\mu g/g$ reduced leukocyte counts as well
as serum complement titers. Also, serum γ-globulins increased
during the AFB_1 exposure period. Toxic effects were diminished
by the addition of 2 $\mu g/g$ Selenium (Se) in the diet (50). Selenium, at concentrations that increased liver glutathione peroxidase (GSH.Px) actvity, probably detoxified the AFB_1-2,3 oxide
to reduced GSH. Phagocytic activity was markedly suppressed in

the AFB_1 exposed groups; this suppression of activity was prevented in poults exposed to AFB_1 and receiving dietary Se at
2.0 μg/g. Hepatotoxicity in turkeys poults from AFB_1 exposure
probably resulted in Se deficiency, reducing bile flow with
diminished absorption of vitamin A resulting in increased membrane permeability, edema, and hemorrhage.

Equine. Clinical signs and symptoms of equine aflatoxicosis
are variable and do not offer a clear pathognomonic picture of
the disease (6). Of the hematologic values examined, prolonged
clotting time appeared to be significant. Elevations of blood-
biochemical enzymes, such as glutamic oxaloacetic transaminase,
lactate dehydrogenase, iditol dehydrogenase, gamma glutamyl
transferase, and arginase during the toxicities were reported.
Liver necrosis and hemorrhagic lesions were found in most of the
animals necropsied along with histopathologic damage to the
liver, kidney, heart, and brain. Toxic levels of aflatoxin reported in clinical cases ranged from 54.8 ppb to 6,500 ppb.
Aflatoxin B_1 and M_1 were isolated from feed, feces, and liver
tissues.

Economic Effects of Aflatoxin in Corn

Corn is important to the grain and livestock economy of the
Southeast. In recent years, grain infection and aflatoxin contamination have become serious problems and unless these problems
are solved, future growth of the grain and livestock industries
in the region could be adversely affected (6).

Losses from aflatoxin occur at all levels in the production,
marketing, and utilization process. Contaminated grain causes
serious marketing problems for producers and grain buyers. Some
elevators refuse to buy corn if it tests positive above FDA action guidelines of 20 ppb. Other buyers may purchase corn at
higher levels of aflatoxin, but discount the price paid according
to the amount of aflatoxin in the sample analyzed. Livestock and
poultry producers have become acutely aware of the potential
problem related to contaminated feeds. Many problems with animal
performance, disease, and death have been attributed to
aflatoxin-contaminated feed, although it has frequently been
impossible to determine the actual cause of the problems. Nearly
30 lawsuits, totaling over $8 million in damages, have been filed
against grain and feed firms by livestock feeders in the
Southeastern States during the past three years. Additional
costs resulting from aflatoxin contamination of corn include (a)
surveillance and assays by state departments of agriculture and
(b) legislative appropriations for research and extension efforts. Summary of losses are shown in Table XII totaling over
$400 million for the two epidemic years of 1977 and 1980.

Table XII.   Cost of Aflatoxin in Corn in Southeast

Data in $1,000	1977	1980
Private cost: a/		
Corn producer	79,939	97,157
Handler	7,592	13,997
Swine	58,691	100,360
Milk	--	2
Poultry	50,000	25,000
Cornmeal	--	145
Public costs:		
Surveillance and assay	545	673
Research and extension b/	800	500
TOTAL	197,567	237,834

a/ Milk and cornmeal estimate from NC only.
b/ Data from NC & GA in 1977; NC only in 1980.

While the short-run costs are substantial for the individual and for society, they may be greater in the long run if recurrent aflatoxin contamination in corn cannot be eliminated or
detoxified.   Farmers, who are unable to market the corn, will ultimately shift acreage to other crops, which have less year-to-
year risks and considerably less net returns.   Fewer buyers may
be needed to handle the crops that are produced and marketed.
Some feeders, particularly poultry integrators, are already pur-
chasing Midwestern grain in preference to local grain. Others are
considering bringing grain from the Midwest in unit trains to
lower their costs.   Absence of corn production in the Southeast
could alter some of the comparative advantage of the area in
feeding certain species, such as broilers and hogs.   However,
some of the effect on poultry producers may be dampened by further downward adjustments in grain freight rates from the Midwest.   These changes could impact adversely on both producers and
consumers.

Prevention and Control of Aflatoxin in Corn

Screening Methods.   Screening to detect resistance in corn
to kernel infection by A. flavus and/or aflatoxin production have
been conducted in the field and to a lesser extent in the laboratory (6).   To date, screening for genotypic differences has
focused primarily on level of aflatoxin production rather than on
frequency of kernel infection.   Inoculation methods have generally included some form of wounding of the kernels to establish the

fungus in ears, although recent studies show that infection and subsequent aflatoxin production can occur in the absence of wounding. In screening for resistance to the fungus or toxin production, researchers are facing problems that are more formidable than those usually encountered. Future progress in screening will be facilitated by: 1) identification of at least one resistant check; 2) improvements in uniformity of treatment response among replications, location, and years; 3) development of inoculation methods that yield infection levels of sufficient magnitude to differentiate among genotypes; and 4) development of a rapid and inexpensive method for aflatoxin assessment. Identification of plant characters (morphological or biochemical) that reduce infection or aflatoxin synthesis may provide a significant step forward.

Plant Breeding. Differences in aflatoxin levels in preharvest commercial corn hybrids have been reported in isolated instances (6). However, inability to repeat differences among hybrids over locations and years has been a major obstacle to recommending one hybrid over another for reducing aflatoxin contamination. Studies have shown that maize parents can be classified as donors of low, intermediate, and high aflatoxin production to their respective progenies. These results may indicate that aflatoxin contamination is under genetic control, but differences among genotypes have been so erratic that recurrent selection is not currently warranted. In genetic studies, a large interaction between genotype and environment has been observed; this interaction probably has masked differences in aflatoxin associated with inherited response. Many factors may contribute to the large errors encountered including: sampling technique, aflatoxin analysis, inoculation method, number of samples, a lack of knowledge of the host-pathogen relationship, and varying environmental conditions. Elucidation of the chemical basis for genetic control of the infection and contamination process would probably help reduce the large experimental errors. Genetically controlled, indirect methods of reducing preharvest aflatoxin contamination include planting hybrids with adaptation to location and a high degree of resistance to ear-damaging insects, diseases, and stress during the grain filling period. In addition, the choice of 1) planting date, 2) optimum plant density, and 3) good cultural practices, such as weed control and fertility balance to alleviate stress during the grain filling period, should be useful in controlling the aflatoxin problem.

Natural Metabolites. An innovative area of research is the effect of corn metabolites on A. flavus, A. parasiticus, and aflatoxin production. Metabolites from several plants have been reported to inhibit A. flavus or aflatoxin synthesis. A number of chemicals consisting of volatile oils from corn husks, kernels, and silks were extracted by several investigators (51,52) and tested in culture by Wilson et al. (53). Several alcohols

and aldehydes were inhibitory to A. flavus with β-ionone dramatically restricting growth, sporulation, and aflatoxin production
by A. flavus and A. parasiticus. Naturally occurring compounds
may be useful in plant breeding or in chemical control of A.
flavus in the field or in storage.

Pesticide Control. Numerous antimicrobial compounds have
been studied in the last 10 to 15 years seeking means of controlling growth of Aspergillus flavus and aflatoxin production in
corn (6). A number of chemicals, including pesticides, inhibit
aflatoxin production in the laboratory, but only the propionates
and some acetates have been found effective in stored corn. Over
30 pesticides have been tested for their ability to inhibit
growth and aflatoxin production by A. flavus, but only five have
been applied to corn during the growing season to determine if
preharvest development of aflatoxin can be reduced or prevented.
The insecticide Gardona when sprayed three times per week reduced, but did not eliminate aflatoxin B_1 accumulation on preharvest corn (54). Preharvest corn that was naturally contaminated by A. flavus after kernel damage contained 28.9 ppb aflatoxin
B_1. Application of the insecticides bux, carbaryl, and dyfon-
ate reduced aflatoxin B_1 levels to 4 ppb, 1 ppb, and 2 ppb, respectively (55).

Detoxification. Outbreaks of aflatoxin in corn occur spo-
radically in different sections of the United States. In recent
years, incidence has centered largely in the Southeastern States.
When these outbreaks occur, some means of salvaging the contaminated corn must be considered. Numerous approaches have been
suggested, largely falling in the broad categories of physical
separation, chemical inactivation, and biological inactivation.
Research conducted on peanut and cottonseed meals has provided a
basis for the selection of methods to be applied to the detoxification of corn. A review of the literature indicates that the
most practical method for salvaging aflatoxin-contaminated corn
is ammoniation. Extensive work at the Northern Regional Research
Center resulted in development of a procedure whereby introduction of ammonia reduced aflatoxin in corn from in excess of 1,000
ppb to less than 10 ppb (56,57,58). Although toxicological studies have not yet been completed to qualify the process for FDA
approval, indications are that the method is feasible and offers
promise to farmers and buyers, who may otherwise face financial
disaster as a result of aflatoxin contamination of corn.

Literature Cited

1. Forgacs, J.; Carll, W. T. Adv. Vet. Sci. 1962, 7, 273-382.
2. Lancaster, M. C.; Jenkins, F. P.; Philp, J. M. Nature 1961,
    192, 1095-1096.
3. Sargeant, K.; Sheridan, A.; O'Kelly, J.; Carnaghan, R. B. A.
    Nature 1961, 192, 1096-1097.

4. Wogan, G. N.; Newberne, P. M. Cancer Res. 1967, 27, 2370-2376.
5. Council for Agricultural Science and Technology "Aflatoxin and Other Mycotoxins: An Agricultural Perspective"; CAST: Ames, Iowa, 1979, 56 pp.
6. Diener, U. L.; Asquith, R. L.; Dickens, J. W. "Aflatoxin and Aspergillus flavus in Corn"; Ala. AES, Auburn, AL, 1983, 112 pp.
7. Nesbitt, B. F.; O'Kelly, J.; Sargeant, K.; Sheridan, A. Nature 1962, 195, 1062-1063.
8. Davis, N. D.; Diener, U. L. Mycopathol. Mycol. Appl. 1967, 31, 251-256.
9. Lillehoj, E. B.; Garcia, W. J.; Lambrow, M. Appl. Microbiol. 1974, 28, 763-767.
10. Eldridge, D. W. M.S. Thesis, Auburn University, Alabama, 1964.
11. Marsh, P. B.; Simpson, M. E.; Trucksess, M. W. Appl. Microbiol. 1975, 30, 52-57.
12. Rabie, C. J.; Meyer, C. J.; Van Heerden, L.; Lubben, A. Can. J. Microbiol. 1981, 27, 962-966.
13. Davis, N. D.; Diener, U. L.; Eldridge, D. W. Appl. Microbiol. 1966, 14, 378-380.
14. Pass, T.; Griffin, G. J. Can. J. Microbiol. 1972, 18, 1453-1461.
15. Semeniuk, G. in "Storage of Cereal Grains and their Products"; Anderson, J. A.; Alcock, A. W., Eds.; Am. Assoc. Cereal Chem., St. Paul, 1954, p.
16. Diener, U. L.; Davis, N. D. Phytopathology 1966, 56, 1390-1393.
17. Diener, U. L.; Davis, N. D. J. Am. Oil Chem. Soc. 1967, 44, 259-263.
18. Diener, U. L.; Davis, N. D. Trop. Sci. 1968, 10, 22-28.
19. Diener, U. L.; Davis, N. D. J. Am. Oil Chem. Soc. 1970, 47, 347-351.
20. Bennett, J. W.; Horowitz, P. C.; Lee, L. S. Mycologia 1979, 71, 415-422.
21. El-Gendy, S. M.; Marth, E. H. Arch. Lebensmittelhyg. 1980, 31, 189-220.
22. Wicklow, D. T.; Horn, B. W.; Cole, R. J. Mycologia 1982, 74, 398-403.
23. Wicklow, D. T.; Cole, R. J. Can. J. Bot. 1982, 60, 525-528.
24. Payne, G. A.; Thompson, D. L.; Lillehoj, E. B. Phytopathology 1981, 71, 898.
25. Taubenhaus, J. J. TX AES Bull. 1920, 270, 38 pp.
26. Anderson, H. W.; Nehring, E. W.; Wichser, W. R. J. Agric. Food Chem. 1975, 23, 775-782.
27. Rambo, G. W.; Tuite, J.; Crane, P. Phytopathology 1974, 64, 797-800.
28. Widstrom, N. W.; Wilson, D. W.; McMillian, W. W. Appl. Environ. Microbiol. 1981, 42, 249-251.

29. Lillehoj, E. B.; Kwolek, W. F.; Vandegraft, E. E.; Zuber,
     M. S.; Calvert, O. H.; Widstrom, N.; Futrell, M. C.;
     Bockholt, A. C. Crop Sci. 1975, 15, 267-270.
30. Thompson, D. L.; Lillehoj, E. B.; Leonard, K. J.; Kwolek,
     W. F.; Zuber, M. S. Crop Sci. 1980, 20, 609-612.
31. Detroy, R. W.; Lillehoj, E. B.; Ciegler, A. "Microbial
     Toxins"; Ciegler, A.; Kadis, S.; Ajl, S. J., Eds.;
     Academic: New York, 1971, Vol. VI, p. 3-178.
32. Shih, C. N.; Marth, E. H. Biochem. Biophys. Acta 1974, 338,
     286-296.
33. Wilson, D. M.; Jay, E. Appl. Microbiol. 1975, 29, 224-228.
34. Stoloff, L. "Mycotoxins in Human and Animal Health";
     Rodricks, J. V.; Hesseltine, C. W.; Mehlman, M. A., Eds.;
     Pathotox: Park Forest South, Ill., 1977, p. 7-28.
35. Gupta, S. K.; Venkitasubramanian, T. A. Z. Lebensm. Unters.
     Forsch. 1975, 159, 107-111.
36. Gupta, S. K.; Venkitasubramanian, T. A. Appl. Microbiol.
     1975, 29, 834-836.
37. Shih, C. N.; Marth, E. H. Appl. Microbiol. 1974, 27,
     452-456.
38. Llewellyn, G. C.; Jones, H. C.; Gates, J. E.; Eadie, T.
     J. Assoc. Off. Anal. Chem. 1980, 63, 622-625.
39. Mateles, R. I.; Adye, J. C. Appl. Microbiol. 1965, 13,
     208-211.
40. Lillehoj, E. B.; Hesseltine, C. W. "Mycotoxins in Human and
     Animal Health"; Rodricks, J. V.; Hesseltine, C. W.;
     Mehlman, M. A., Eds.; Pathotox: Park Forest South, Ill.,
     1977, p. 107-119.
41. Lillehoj, E. B.; Kwolek, W. F.; Zuber, M. S.; Calvert, O.
     H.; Horner, E. S.; Widstrom, N. W.; Guthrie, W. D.; Scott,
     G. E.; Thompson, D. L.; Findley, W. R.; Bockholt, A. J.
     Cereal Chem. 1978, 55, 1007-1013.
42. Jones, R. K.; Duncan, H. E.; Payne, G. A.; Leonard, H. J.
     Plant Dis. 1980, 64, 859-863.
43. Jones, R. K.; Duncan, H. E.; Hamilton, P. B. Phytopathology
     1981, 71, 810-816.
44. Pettit, R. E.; Taber, R. A.; Schroeder, H. W.; Harrison,
     A. L. Appl. Microbiol. 1971, 22, 629-634.
45. Jones, R. K.; Duncan, H. E. Plant Dis. 1981, 65, 741-744.
46. Cobb, W. Y. Quart. Bull. Assoc. Food Drug Off. 1979, 43,
     99-107.
47. Pier, A. C.; Heddleston, K. L. Avian Dis. 1970, 14, 797-809.
48. Edds, G. T.; Simpson, C. F. Am. J. Vet. Res. 1976, 37,
     65-68. 49.
49. Edds, G. T.; Nair, K. P. C.; Simpson, C. F. Am. J. Vet.
     Res., 1973, 34, 819-826.
50. Goldstein, S. L. M.S. Thesis, University of Florida,
     Gainesville, 1981.
51. Buttery, R. G.; Ling, L. C.; Chan, B. G. J. Agric. Food
     Chem. 1978, 26, 866-869.

52. Flath, R. A.; Forrey, R. R.; John, J. O.; Chan, B. G. J. Agric. Food Chem. 1978, 26, 1290–1293.

53. Wilson, D. M.; Gueldner, R. C.; McKinney, J. M.; Livesay, R. H.; Evans, B. D.; Hill, R. A. J. Am. Oil Chem. Soc. 1981, 58, 959A–961A.

54. Widstrom, N. W.; Lillehoj, E. B.; Sparks, A. N.; Kwolek, W. F. J. Econ. Entomol. 1976, 69, 677–679.

55. Elahi, M.; Draughon, F. A. Proc. 41st Inst. Food Technol. Mtg. 1981, p. 111.

56. Brekke, O. L.; Peplinski, A. J.; Lancaster, E. B. Trans. ASAE 1977, 20, 1160–1168.

57. Brekke, O. L.; Peplinski, A. J.; Nofsinger, G. W.; Conway, H. F.; Stringfellow, A. C.; Montgomery, R. R.; Silman, R. W.; Sohns, V. E.; Bagley, E. B. Trans. ASAE 1979, 22, 425–432.

58. Brekke, O. L.; Stringfellow, A. C.; Peplinski, A. J. J. Agric. Food Chem. 1978, 26, 1383–1389.

RECEIVED June 6, 1983

Detection of Trichothecene Mycotoxins

Quantitation of Deoxynivalenol by Negative Chemical Ionization Mass Spectrometry

JANET M. ROTHBERG, JOHN L. MACDONALD, and JOSEPH C. SWIMS

Central Research Services, Ralston Purina Company, St. Louis, MO 63164

A GC/MS technique has been developed for the detection of trichothecene mycotoxins. The technique has been used to quantitate the trichothecene deoxynivalenol in corn, wheat and mixed feeds. The trichothecenes are derivatized with heptafluorobutyrylimidazole and the derivatives are separated by gas chromatography. Methane negative chemical ionization produces characteristic fragment ions with high molecular weights which are measured by selected ion monitoring. The technique has been used to determine low levels of six trichothecene compounds: diacetoxyscirpenol, neosolaniol, T-2 toxin, HT-2 toxin, deoxynivalenol, and fusarenon-x. One hundred femtograms of deoxynivalenol has been detected by this method. The coefficients of variation of the method for quantitation of deoxynivalenol in both corn and wheat are 15% with a mean recovery of greater than 95% in spiked corn and wheat. Levels of deoxynivalenol which were measured by different laboratories using a variety of methods will be compared.

Trichothecences are a class of structurally similar mycotoxins produced principally by Fusarium molds. These cyclic compounds are of interest to feed manufacturers because they can cause feed refusal or reduced feed efficiencies in some animal species (1,2,3). Several approaches have been reported for the analysis of trichothecenes in feeds and feed ingredients. Trimethylsilyl derivatives of the trichothecenes have been formed and the derivatives measured by gas chromatography using a flame ionization detector (4,5,6,7). Other workers obtained improved

sensitivity by forming the heptafluorobutyryl (HFB) derivatives
of the trichothecenes which could then be measured by electron
capture gas chromatography (5,8,9). The use of mass spectrometry
has also been reported for confirmation and quantitation of the
trichothecenes deoxynivalenol (DON), diacetoxyscirpenol (DAS),
T-2 toxin and HT-2 toxin (10,11,12).

The technique described here uses gas chromatography
combined with negative chemical ionization (NCI) mass
spectrometry to analyze extracts of feed ingredients.
Heptafluorobutyryl derivatives of the trichothecenes are formed
by reaction with heptafluorobutyryl imidazole (HFBI) and the
derivatives are then separated by gas-liquid chromatography.
Characteristic high molecular weight (542-943 amu) negative ions
are measured using selected ion monitoring (SIM). The methods
listed above generally require some treatment of the sample
extracts prior to gas chromatographic analysis to remove
substances which interfere with quantitation of the
trichothecenes. The combination of sensitivity and selectivity
resulting from the use of NCI and selected ion monitoring permits
analysis of sample extracts without additional sample clean-up.

Detection of six trichothecenes; DON, DAS, T-2 toxin, HT-2
toxin, neosolaniol (NSL), fusarenone-x (F-X) is shown here. This
method has been used for quantitation of DON in corn, wheat,
wheat bran, and mixed feeds. The precision of the method was
measured by repetitive analysis of naturally contaminated
samples. Recovery was measured from samples spiked with DON
standards.

Experimental

Deoxynivalenol standard was purchased from Mycolabs, Inc.,
Chesterfield, Missouri. Additional deoxynivalenol,
diacetoxyscirpenol and T-2 toxin were purified from Fusarium
cultures in this laboratory. The HT-2 toxin standard was
obtained from Sigma Chemical Company, St. Louis, MO. Fusarenon-x
and neosolaniol were provided by Dr. Loshio Ueno, Tokyo
University of Science, Tokyo, Japan.

The n-heptafluorobutyrylimidazole reagent was obtained from
Regis Chemical Company, Morton Grove, Illinois. Solvents were of
a quality suitable for pesticide analysis and were obtained from
various sources.

All mass spectra were recorded using a Hewlett-Packard 5985B
mass spectrometer equipped with a dual electron impact/chemical
ionization source including negative ion capability. The source
temperature was 125°C, filament emission current was 300 uA,
and electron energy was 230 ev. The interface between the GC and
MS was a glass-lined stainless steel transfer line. Methane was
used both for carrier gas and as the chemical ionization reactant
gas. A methane flow of 11.5 mL/min. resulted in an ion source
pressure of 0.5 torr.

Samples were analyzed on a 6 ft x 2 mm ID glass column packed with 3% SP-1000 (Supelco, Bellefonte, PA.). The column temperature was programmed from 150°C to 225°C at 10°C/min. The injection port temperature was 200°C and the interface temperature was 250°C.

The instrument was operated in the selected ion monitoring (SIM) mode. This allowed groups of one to four ions to be monitored at a time. Masses to be monitored were changed prior to the retention time of each trichothecene derivative.

Samples

Corn contaminated with DON was obtained from the 1980 corn crop from Eastern Canada. The corn was selected for analysis due to the presence of mold on the kernels. Wheat contaminated with DON was taken from samples of the 1980 wheat crop from the upper midwestern United States. Wheat samples were selected for analysis due to the pink color of the grain.

Samples of naturally contaminated corn and wheat were blended to produce samples containing various levels of DON. Following grinding, samples containing high levels of DON were blended with samples which had been assayed by the method described here and found to contain low levels of DON. These blended samples were used to measure the precision of the method and provide control samples to be analyzed with each set of unknown samples.

Artificially DON contaminated samples were prepared by adding aliquots from standard solutions of DON in acetone to ground samples of corn and wheat. After addition, the solvent was allowed to evaporate before analysis. These samples were used to measure recovery of DON through the method.

Procedure

Extraction. A 25-g ground sample was extracted in 100 mL of 50% methanol/water (v/v). The mixture was blended at the highest speed of an explosion-proof blender. The sample was then centrifuged at 28,000 rpm. for 5 minutes. Sample extracts were refrigerated overnight if they could not be analyzed on the same day.

Derivatization. A 1 mL aliquot from the centrifuged sample extract was diluted to 200 mLs in a volumetric flask. A 1 mL aliquot of this diluted extract was transferred to a small screw-capped culture tube which was then placed in a 50°C water bath and dried under a stream of nitrogen. Then the sample was then dissolved in 1 mL of 95% toluene/5% acetonitrile (v/v) and mixed vigorously for at least 30 seconds. Two hundred microliters of n-heptaflourobutrylimidazole (HFBI) was added to each sample and the solution was again mixed vigorously for 15 seconds.

Except for those samples and standards containing DAS, the samples were placed in a 100°C oil bath for 15 minutes. After removal of the sample from the oil bath, 3 mL of 5% sodium bicarbonate solution was added to each sample and then mixed vigorously for 30 seconds. The sample was allowed to phase, the organic layer was removed and transferred to a culture tube containing 300 mg of anhydrous sodium sulfate crystals. This tube was then shaken briefly. Five microliters of the derivatized sample was injected into the GC/MS.

The diacetoxyscirpenol (DAS) standard and samples containing DAS were derivatized at room temperature for 15 minutes. At 100°C losses of DAS have been experienced.

GC/MS Analysis. The six trichothecenes were detected by monitoring the molecular ion (M+1) and characteristic fragment ions of each derivative. The ions monitored are shown in Table II. Quantitation of the deoxynivalenol derivative (DON-HFB) were 670, 671, 884, and 885 amu.

Results and Discussion

Confirmation of Trichothenes

The basic skeletal structure of the Fusarium trichothecenes is shown in Figure I. The six trichothecenes discussed here differ in the number and position of hydroxyl groups, acetate esters, or isobutyl esters substituted at one of four sites on the molecule. When the trichothecene is derivatized with HFBI, heptafluorobutryrl esters are formed with hydroxyl groups on the trichothecene molecule. Depending on the number of hydroxyl groups, 1,2,or 3 HFB groups may be added, thus increasing the molecular weight of the compound by 196 amu for each HFB group attached. The resulting derivatives have molecular weights in the range of 540-950 amu.

The NCI spectra are generally characterized by an abundant molecular ion, the loss of hydrogen fluoride (M-20) groups, and loss of intact HFB (M-213) groups. Table I shows the tabulated NCI spectra of six derivatized trichothecenes. For example, in the case of deoxynivalenol-HFB, the molecular ion is m/e= 884, loss of HF(M-20) results in m/e= 864, loss of intact HFB groups (M-213) gives fragment ions of m/e= 671,458.

Table I. Tabulated NCI Spectra of Six Trichothecene Derivatives

Compound	Mass Intensity
Deoxynivalenol/tri-HFB	884 (66), 671 (5), 670 (7), 630 (2)
Fusarenon-x/tri-HFB	942 (100), 943 (35), 728 (9), 922 (5)
Neosolaniol/di-HFB	692 (97), 754 (51), 774 (25), 693 (24)
HT-2/di-HFB	816 (100), 817 (36), 233 (22), 583 (6)
Diacetoxyscirpenol/HFB	480 (100), 481 (26), 562 (2), 542 (9)
T-2/HFB	580 (100), 581 (30), 662 (4), 642 (8)

One of the advantages of this GC/MS method of detection of
the derivatized trichothecenes is the reduction of the effect of
the interferences from the sample matrix. Many interferences are
small molecular weight compounds, but the large molecular weight
trichothecene derivatives can be selectively monitored at the
higher mass ions. Interferences seen in the electron capture
chromatographic determination of trichothecenes due to the excess
HFBI left in the extract after derivatization and due to the low
molecular weight compounds from the sample matrix are not
apparent in NCI mass spectrometry.

A second advantage is that attachment of the electronegative
HFB groups to the trichothecenes results in very high sensitivity
when using negative chemical ionization This sensitivity is
demonstrated by the detection of a 300 femtogram injection of
DON-HFB as shown in Figure II. A comparison of negative chemical
ionization (NCI), positive chemical ionization (PCI), and
electron impact (EI) sensitivities to derivatized DON standard is
shown in Table II. Each source technique was run on the same
instrument on the same day. The NCI technique is about 5000
times more sensitive than PCI, and 10,000 times more sensitive
than EI.

Confirmation of trichothecene contaminated samples is
performed by selected ion monitoring (SIM) mass spectrometry,
scanning the molecular ion of each trichothecene derivative.
Using SIM, coeluting peaks can be separated and quantitated
without difficulty. Figure III shows separation of six
trichothecene standards that were derivatized separately and
combined before injection. The molecular ion was monitored for
each compound in this demonstration. Even though, under the
conditions used here, NSL and DAS are not completely resolved,
they can easily be detected independently with SIM.

Table II. Limit of Detection Of Three Mass Spectral
Techniques to Deoxynivalenol Standard

Technique	Lowest DON Standard Measureable
Electron Impact	100 pg
Positive Chemical Ionization	500 pg
Negative Chemical Ionization	0.1 pg

Quantitation of Deoxynivalenol

The method has been used for the quantitation of
deoxynivalenol in corn, wheat, and mixed feeds. The precision
and recovery of the method have been established in our
laboratory. The precison study was performed on large batches of
naturally contaminated corn and wheat. Corn containing low level
of DON was ground, mixed, and riffled with high DON-level corn to
give a large homogeneous sample of contaminated corn with a level
of approximately 1500 ppb.

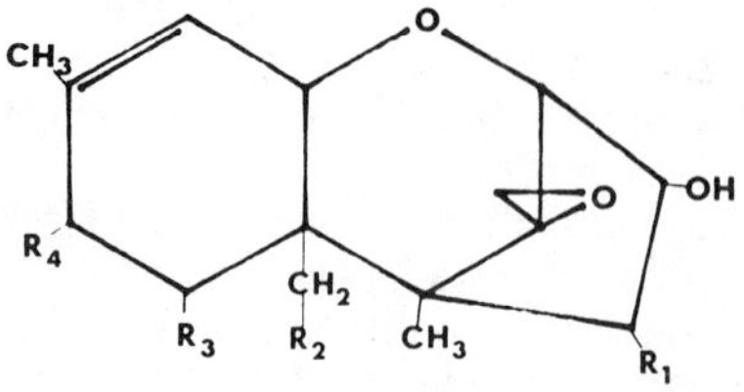

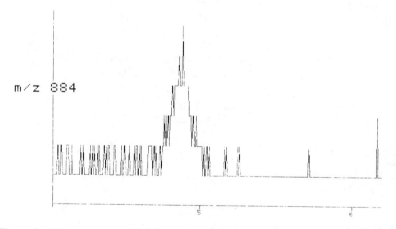

R1	R2	R3	R4	COMPOUND
OAc	OAc	H	H	DIACETOXYSCIRPENOL
OAc	OAc	H	OOCBu	T-2 TOXIN
OAc	OAc	H	OH	NEOSOLANIOL
OH	OAc	H	OOCBu	HT-2 TOXIN
OAc	OH	OH	= O	FUSARENON-X
H	OH	OH	= O	DEOXYNIVALENOL

Figure 1. Structure of six trichothecenes showing four groups for substitutions.

m/z 884

Figure 2. NCI spectrum of DON standard (100 femtograms) showing instrument sensitivity.

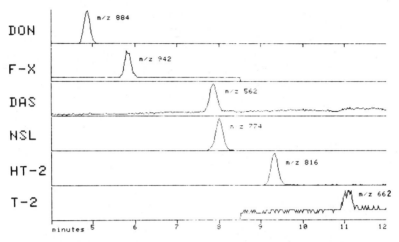

Figure 3. Separation of six combined derivatives of trichothecene standards by selected ion monitoring. A series of unique ion fragments are monitored for analysis. (Molecular ions only are shown in figure.)

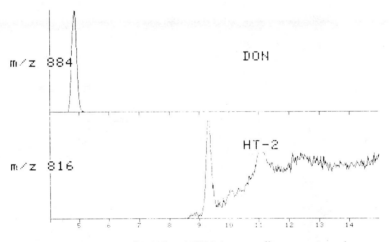

Figure 4. Confirmation of DON and HT-2 in naturally contaminated corn.

The same preparation was performed with wheat. At least
eight portions of each of the corn and wheat samples were
extracted, diluted, derivatized, and analyzed by mass
spectrometry. Quantitation of the DON in the sample matrices was
accomplished by measurement of the peak area of the molecular ion
of the DON-HFB in the sample and comparing this to the peak area
of the same ion as the standard.

Table III shows precision data on the replicate samples of
corn and wheat. The coefficient of variation of the values for
the artifically contaminated corn was less than 11%. Eight
samples of the artificially contaminated wheat samples were run,
the CV was 10%.

Table III.   Precision Data on Wheat and Corn Artificially
                Contaminated with Deoxynivalenol

	N	Mean	PPB DON Range	CV
Corn	11	1456	1187-1682	11.4%
Wheat	8	1466	1245-1720	10.3%

Table IV shows the recovery data for DON-spiked matrices of
both corn and wheat. The spike level was varied to cover the
range of values corresponding to the levels found in the
naturally-contaminated matrices. The mean recovery for both corn
and wheat samples was 97%.

Table IV.   Recoveries in DON-Spiked Matrices Data

CORN:

Spike Level	N	Average Recovery	C.V.
170 ppb	3	126%	11%
200	3	87%	17%
860	13	105%	19%
1000	2	78%	33%
2000	3	85%	25%

Mean Recovery for all corn spikes = 97%

WHEAT:

Spike Level	N	Average Recovery	C.V.
1000 ppb	3	94%	11%
2000 ppb	3	100%	8%

Mean Recovery for all wheat samples = 97%

To compare results for quantitation of DON by various
methods, samples of contaminated corn, wheat and mixed feeds were
submitted to six labs who used various methods for quantitation
of DON. The methods of analysis included gas
chromatography/electron capture (GC/EC) method, (6) a combined

thin-layer chromatography (TLC), GC, and MS analysis, (17)
Romer's GC/EC method, (15) and the method described in this
paper. The results of the correlation study are shown in Table
V. The study shows that there is considerable variation between
laboratories, regardless of the method of
analysis. The results of the analysis by the NCI-mass
spectrometric method described in this paper, are generally
slightly higher than obtained by other methods. One possible
explanation for the higher results obtained with this method may
be higher recoveries obtained by NCI-MS compared to recoveries
reported for other procedures. Table VI shows a correlation
study between two laboratories on samples of wheat bran analyzed
for deoxynivalenol. The agreement between the two laboratories
was good, the results obtained by Scott's method (6) agreed
well with the results obtained by the NCI-MS technique.

Table V: Deoxynivalenol Correlation Study

DON in ppb

Sample	Lab A	Lab B	Lab C	Lab D	Lab E	Lab F	Lab G	Mean	%CV **
Corn	1280	1000	1000	600	1710	760	1580	1160	38
Corn	40	500	10	300	200	70	20	130	20
Wheat	1310	1000	1090	800	630	990	1380	1030	28
Wheat	1250	1000	1150	800	830	830	1510	1062	27
Wheat	200	500	150	300	200	160	174	240	13
Mixed Feed	200	1000	*	300	200	130	380	240	54
Mixed Feed	4960	500	*	4800	4080	2920	7410	4110	40
Mixed Feed	7100	500	*	6400	5180	4500	10000	6640	32
Method	(5)	(17)	(5)	(11)	(15)	(5)	NCI-Mass Spec.		

* Lab chose not to run mixed feeds.
** Excludes Lab B results. Values reported as "less than" are
not included in mean/CV.

Table VI: Wheat Bran Correlation Study Deoxynivalenol Level(ppb)

Sample	Lab A	Lab B
Wheat Bran	627	620
Wheat Bran	504	497
Wheat Bran	514	600
Wheat Bran	728	754
Wheat Control	201	312
Method	NCI Mass Spec	(5)

Conclusion

Negative ion chemical ionization mass spectrometry can be used to confirm trichothecenes and quantitate DON in naturally contaminated grains and feeds. The effects of interferences are eliminated by selectively scanning the relatively high molecular weight fragments and molecular ion of the trichothecene derivatives. Separation of a mixture of trichothecene derivatives is accomplished in 15 minutes on a packed GC column.

Acknowledgment

The authors acknowledge the assistance of Thomas R. Romer, of Romer's Lab, Inc., for the early work done on gas chromatography separation of the derivatized trichothecenes, for his assistance in the procurement of samples and standards. Acknowledgment is also given to Dave Greaves, formerly of Ralston Purina Company for the extraction of the samples, and to Roland Laramore, Ralston Purina Co., and Fran Olivigni, formerly of Ralston Purina Company, for the preparation of the deoxynivalenol, diacetoxyscirpenol, and the T-2 toxin standards.

Literature Cited

1. Vesonder, R. F.; Ciegler, A.; Jensen, A. H. Appl. Microbiol. 1973, 26, 1008-1010.
2. Forsyth, D. M.; Yoshizawa, T.; Mooroka, N.; Tuite, J. Appl. Environ. Microbiol 1977, 34, 547-552.
3. Vesonder, R. F.; Ciegler, A.; Burmeister, H. R.; Jensen, A. H. Appl. Environ. Microbiol. 1979, 38,344-346.
4. Ikediobi, C. O., Hus, I. C.; Bamburg, J. R; Strong, F. M. Anal. Biochem. 1979, 43, 327-340.
5. Scott, P. M., Lau, P-4; Kanhere, S. R. Meeting of Assoc. of Official Analytical Chemists 1981.
6. Pareless, S. R.; Collins, G. J.; Rosen, J. D. J. Agric. Food Chem. 1976, 24 (4), 872-875.
7. Ikediobi, C.O., Hsu, I. C.; Bamburg, J. R.; Strong, F. M. Anal Biochem. 1970, 43, 327-340.
8. Szathmary, Cs.; Galacz, J.; Vida, L.; Alexander, G. J. Chrom. 1980, 191, 327-331.
9. Ueno, Y.; Sat, N.; Ishii, K.; Sakai, K.; Tsunoda, H.; Enomoto M. Appl. Micro 1973, 25 (4), 699-704.
10. Romer, T. R.; Boling, T. M.; MacDonald, J. L. J. Assoc. Off. Anal Chem. 1978, 61, 801-808.
11. Romer, T. R.; Greaves, D. A.; Langford, W. L. 95th Annu. Mtg Assoc. Off. Anal. Chem., October 19-22, 1981, Washington, D. C.
12. Ishii, J., Y. Ando, and Ueno, Y. Chem. Pharm Bull 1975, 23 (9), 2152-2164.

13. Rothberg, J. M.; MacDonald, J. L.; Swims, J. C.; Romer T. R. American Soc. for Mass Spec. May, 1981, Minneapolis. "Analysis of Trichothecences Using Chemical Ionization Mass Spectroscopy."
14. MacDonald, J. L.; Romer, T. R.   Proc 25th Annual Conf. Mass Spec. Allied Topics, 1977. Washington, D.C.
15. Romer, T. R.; Greaves, D. A.; Gibson, G. I. Assoc. Off. Analytical Chemists, May, 1981, Ottawa, Ontario, Canada.
16. Romer, T. R.; Boling, T. M. 93rd Annu. Mtg. Assoc. Off. Anal. Chem., October 15-18, 1979, Washington, D. C.
17. Stahr, H. M., Lerdal, D., Hyde, W., Pfeiffer, R. Amer. Assn. Veterinary Lab Diagnosticians 1981, 24th Ann. Proceedings, 277-286.

RECEIVED July 15, 1983

Antinutrients and Allergens in Oilseeds

ROBERT L. ORY, ANTONIO A. SEKUL, and ROBERT R. MOD

Southern Regional Research Center, U.S. Department of Agriculture, ARS, New Orleans, LA 70179

The presence of antinutrients and allergens in foods and feeds has prompted much research on these xenobiotics as concern for the safety of foods. Some of the more prominant adventitious components of peanuts and soybeans (allergens, trypsin inhibitors, hemagglutinins), cottonseed (allergens, gossypol, cyclopropene fatty acids), and castor seed (allergens, toxins), their effects on selected enzymes and metabolism of mammals, on the general well-being of humans, some of the chemical/biochemical methods used to identify these materials, their subcellular site in the seeds, and methods for measuring them are described.

Antinutrients and allergens have always been present in certain foods but the growing interest in oilseeds as a source of edible protein as well as oil, and current interest in xenobiotics and safety of foods is focusing more attention on the antinutrients, such as trypsin inhibitors, hemagglutinins, gossypol, toxins, etc. In 1979, however, Dr. Philip L. White, Director of the Department of Food and Nutrition for the American Medical Association, said, "Nothing has happened in the last 1, 5, 10, or 50 years that has suddenly made our food supply hazardous. If anything it is much less hazardous today than it was 75 years ago" (1). Despite such statements, people today are not sure what foods are safe or which ones contain allergens, antinutrients, carcinogens, toxins, etc. Consumers are also paying more attention to nutrient contents of both fresh and prepared foods. To keep pace with this awareness of nutritional content by consumers, research has increased on the safety, wholesomeness, and stability of both traditional foods and new food products entering the market, especially those from plant sources. This report

describes a few of these antinutrients, emphasizing their
chemistry and the analytical methods used to measure them rather
than their physiological activity in humans.

Food Allergies. The term "allergie" was introduced by von
Pirquet (2) in 1906 to describe the change in a person's capacity
to react to a second injection of horse serum. Allergens are
generally large molecular weight materials too large to dialyze
out of solution and are mostly glycoprotein in nature. Allergenic activity is most often associated with the protein moiety
of the compound. The most frequent foods that induce allergic
reactions in humans are cow's milk, chocolate, beverages made
from the Kola nut, corn, eggs, the pea family of legumes (mostly
peanuts, which are not nuts but are legumes), citrus, tomatoes,
wheat and other small grains, cinnamon and artificial food colors
(3). Extracts of peanuts frequently cross react with antibodies
to various beans and peas, especially soybeans. Cereal grains
include many staple foods prepared from wheat, such as bread and
pasta products, some which have been reported to produce allergic
reactions in humans. Wheat is probably the most frequent offender and wheat gluten hypersensitivity, called celiac disease,
induces adverse reactions in humans sensitive to wheat gluten.
       In clinical diagnosis of sensitivity to allergens in food,
the two methods used most frequently are the skin prick test
(SPT) and the radioallergosorbent test (RAST). These tests have
been used reliably for the diagnosis of allergy to peas, codfish,
peanuts, egg white, wheat and wheat flour but were only partly
reliable in detecting allergy to cow's milk, sardines, and white
beans (4).

Oilseed Allergens. Legumes and oilseeds contain large amounts of
storage and non-storage proteins. Most storage proteins are
globulins soluble in dilute salt or buffer and insoluble in
water. The non-storage proteins contain water-soluble albumins,
enzymes and glycoproteins that include trypsin inhibitors, hemagglutinins, allergens, and other xenobiotics which affect nutritional value of the protein. Many of these are often associated
with storage proteins. Some allergens found in oilseeds and tree
nuts are shown in Table 1. Allergen concentrations in oilseeds
appear to be much higher than those in tree nuts, peanuts and
soybeans (two legumes). Except for castor beans, cottonseeds,
and flaxseed, the yields of recovered allergens are generally
less than 1%. Nitrogen contents of these allergens range from
11% to 18% but carbohydrate contents show much wider variation:
3% to 39%. Peanuts appear to be more allergenic than tree nuts,
perhaps because they are consumed in larger quantities.
       Amino acid profiles of the allergens in cottonseeds, castor
seeds, and peanuts show more similarity in the former two seeds
than with the peanut (5). Castor seed and cottonseed allergens

Table I. Some Allergens in Tree Nuts, Oilseeds, and Legumes

Seed	Allergen*	% Yield	% N	% Carb.
Almonds	1A	0.46	16.9	12.6
Brazil Nuts	1A	0.81	17.6	6.9
Filberts	1A	0.30	17.1	10.5
Castor Seeds	1A	1.76	18.4	3.1
Cottonseed	1A	1.38	12.1	36.4
Flaxseed	1A	1.98	11.3	39.4
Peanuts	1A	0.07	15.4	16.7
	1B	0.18	15.2	10.6
Soybeans	1B	0.10	13.3	20.4

* Isolated by method of Spies, et al. (5); % N=nitrogen; % Carb.=carbohydrate.

have high arginine and glutamic acid concentrations (lower in peanuts), and they have low lysine (higher in peanut allergen). Glycine content in the peanut allergen, PN-1B, is 5-10 times higher than that in castor and cottonseed allergens, CB-1A and CS-1A. Neither amino acids, percent nitrogen, or percent carbohydrate contents are consistent enough to be correlated with allergenic sensitivity.

Peanuts. Peanuts are one of the world's major oilseeds. They have been reported to contain various compounds such as hemagglutinins (6), antihemophilia factors (7), trypsin inhibitors (8), and allergens (5). Spies et al (5) were the first to chemically characterize isolated peanut allergens, but when they did this research, peanut allergens were not considered a hazard. Recently several reports of allergic reaction to peanuts by humans have appeared (9,10).

Reports in the literature today concern allergens present in raw peanuts. However, people who show positive reactions to peanut allergens are generally allergic to roasted peanut products. By Spies' (5) classification, PN-1A is heat-stable whereas PN-1B is heat-sensitive and would be destroyed in the roasting process. PN-1A is present in extremely low amounts in the seed. We examined raw and roasted peanut allergen extracts using blood serum of two sensitive individuals as the source of antibody. The immunodiffusion reaction between the peanut allergen and antibodies in their blood produced a sharp precipitin arc, but the precipitin arc disappeared after saline deproteination of the gel on the glass plate. No precipitin arc occurred with blood from

nonsensitive individuals. We also compared immunodiffusion of
immunoglobulins as a more precise test for effects of peanut
allergens on immunoglobulins in their blood. This method is
based on a report by Kamat, et al (11), that blood serum
immunoglobulins from cotton mill workers in India and normal
blood sera showed striking differences in IgG levels. Normal
sera had IgG levels of 1400 mg. whereas sera of cotton mill
byssinotics averaged 1850 mg.

We employed this technique to examine blood from peanut-
sensitive individuals for IgA and IgG levels (Figure 1). The gel
contained antibodies to human IgA. Blood sera in wells were as
follows: 1,5,9, are standard IgA; 3,7,11 are serum of a non-sensi-
tive person; 2,6,10 are from sensitive patient PL; and 4,8,12 are
from sensitive patient CS. Immunodiffusion was run overnight at
40C. There were significant changes in the size of immunodiffusion rings for both sensitive individuals compared to
nonsensitive controls. Quantity of a specific immunoglobulin was
determined by measuring the diameter of the ring and substituting
this value in a chart which gives the level of immunoglobulin
present in that person's blood. In both patients examined, the
IgA levels were much lower than that of the nonsensitive person
and the IgA standard. IgG levels of the two patients were
slightly higher than the two non-allergic controls. (In our
tests on cotton dust antigens, IgG in blood of one byssinotic
patient was calculated to be 1790 mg compared to 1292 mg for
normal blood, in accord with values reported by Kamat, et al
(11).) Other antinutrients in peanuts, such as hemagglutinins
and trypsin inhibitors, are destroyed by heat during roasting.

Trypsin Inhibitors. Trypsin inhibitor activity is found in
virtually all legumes, including soybeans and peanuts. Trypsin
inhibitor activity in peanuts (PTI), like that in soybeans, can
be detected by various methods, most which measure the activity
of trypsin on hydrolysis of a protein or synthetic substrate by
spectrophotometer. We developed an indirect immunochemical
immunoelectrophoretic analysis (IEA) method which detects PTI in
microquantities of peanut meals or extracts. Instead of
measuring the inhibitor directly, as is done for soybean trypsin
inhibitor, the indirect method measures the effect of inhibitor
fractions on trypsin hydrolysis of arachin, the major peanut
protein (Figure 2). The protein source, arachin, the major peanut
peanut globulin, was placed in all wells and antibodies to
arachin was placed in the troughs. IEA in 1.5% ionagar, pH 8.2
Veronal buffer, 0.25M, was run for 2 hr at 4 V/cm. For trypsin +
PTI interaction, materials stood 20 hr before adding to arachin.
For trypsin + arachin, materials stood 2 hr. After IEA, arcs
were stained with Amido Black. The indirect method measures the
electrophoretic migration of arachin untreated (upper slide),
treated with trypsin (second slide) and treated with trypsin
which was first incubated with the peanut inhibitor extract

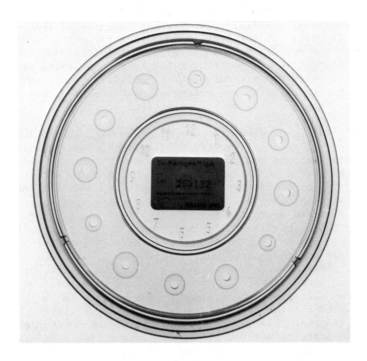

Figure 1. *Effect of peanut allergens on IgA levels in blood of sensitive individuals.*
Key: 1, 5, and 9, standard IgA; 3, 7, and 11, nonsensitive individual; 2, 6, and
10, sensitive patient PL; and 4, 8, and 12, sensitive patient CS.

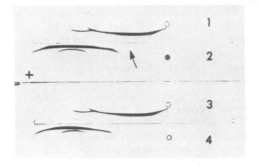

Figure 2. *Indirect measurement of peanut trypsin inhibitor activity by immuno-*
electrophoretic analysis.

(third slide). As shown here, the inhibitor-treated fraction
shows an increase in migration of arachin compared to that with
untreated trypsin. If the trypsin inhibitor is heated before
mixing with the trypsin (the lower slide), the inhibitor effect
is completely destroyed, confirming the heat sensitivity of PTI.
Comparing PTI with and without heating and adding to trypsin,
indicates the specificity and potential usefulness of this method
for simultaneous analysis of several peanut fractions.

Hemagglutinins. Hemagglutinins are found in virtually all oilseeds and cereal grains. Dechary (6) isolated a hemagglutinin
from peanuts that was nonspecific for types A, B, and O red blood
cells.   It behaved in a most unusual manner and its rather low
potency could not be increased by any of the methods available
for fractionating peanuts. We conducted similar studies on hemagglutinins purified from rice germ (RGA) by gel electrophoresis,
immunoelectrophoretic analysis (IEA), red blood cell aggluti-
nation tests, and by crossed IEA, a more sensitive test than one
phase IEA, if enough antiserum is available. Crossed IEA uses
considerably more antiserum. Figure 3 shows the effects of the
RGA on human serum proteins. Normal human serum without RGA is
shown in the left plate and mixed with RGA extract for 1 hr.
before crossed IEA in first dimension in the right plate. Second
dimension IEA (both plates) into a gel containing antibodies to
human serum proteins was run for 2 hr. On the left side human
serum proteins show the primary serum albumin (tall peak in front
of the group) and the immunoglobulins (peaks closer to the
origin). After electrophoresis in one direction the gel was
electrophoresed in the second direction into a gel containing
antibodies to human serum proteins. Several proteins, including
the front-running serum albumin and the slower immunoglobulins,
now show decreased migration indicating some type of binding of
the agglutinin to these proteins. This method can be used to
examine the effect of agglutinins on binding to specific proteins
in blood.

Cottonseed (and Castor Seed). Although cotton has been grown
since ancient times for the fiber, the seed is an important
source of vegetable oil and meal today. The meal, used for many
years as animal feed, is now being proposed as a new source of
edible protein for humans if certain harmful compounds present in
seeds can be eliminated. Cottonseed meal contains storage
proteins and allergens. Cottonseed contains three major classes
of protein; 2S, 5S, and 9S, in almost equal amounts. The 5S and
9S proteins are storage globulins whereas the 2S proteins are
albumins, sometimes classified as storage proteins because of
their amino acid composition, properties, and high concentrations
in the seed (12).

The primary allergens of cottonseed, CS-1A, and castor seed, CB-1A, were purified sufficiently from defatted meals to permit determination of their chemical structure (5). They are soluble in water and 25% ethyl alcohol but not in 75% ethyl alcohol and are immunologically distinct from other allergens in the seeds. They are not precipitated by basic lead acetate, are stable in boiling water, and resist drastic chemical treatment. The CS-1A allergen was localized in the protein bodies of cottonseed by Youle and Huang (12) using immunodiffusion of the allergen and the 2S, 5S, and 9S proteins of the protein bodies against anti-bodies to the CS-1A allergen. They showed that 2S albumins contain the cottonseed allergen, CS-1A, by cross reacting the 2S albumins with the allergen. However, since there are no recorded incidents of allergencity to cottonseed proteins by those consuming it, the presence of this allergen in the meal is not a deterrent to its acceptance as a source of protein.

Another concern today for allergens in seeds is the interest in sprouted or partly germinated seeds (e.g.: bean, alfalfa, or barley sprouts). These are not considered allergenic but we wondered about the effect of germination on allergens. In germinating oilseeds, the storage proteins are metabolized by proteases, but the allergens are not. We examined the effects of seed germination on the allergen CB-1A in castor seeds (the counterpart of CS-1A in cottonseed). Many allergens are not digested by proteases in the alimentary system, which prevents their metabolism by non-ruminants. The CB-1A allergen maintained its antigenic structure up to ten days of germination to confirm in vitro tests on the effect of proteolytic enzymes on allergens, which showed they are not metabolized by proteases (13).

While castor seeds are industrially important as a source of oil, the oil or protein is not edible because several potent allergens are present in the seed. The seed contains approximately 50% oil and 18% protein but also contains the toxalbumin ricin, the CB-1A series of allergens, and an alkaloid, ricinine. Ricin, molecular weight 40,000, is an extremely potent phytotoxin, the most potent xenobiotic yet discovered in oilseeds. Even crushing of castor seeds to separate the oil for industrial uses can be quite hazardous. Ricin is water-soluble and is present in the dust generated during crushing. Constant inhalation of the dust can cause serious problems unless air-filtering masks and other precautions are taken. Ricin, like the castor allergen, is not digested by mammalian proteolytic enzymes.

Gossypol. Gossypol is another substance in cottonseed that prevents greater utilization of the meal by non-ruminants. It is a polyphenolic greenish-yellow pigment present within glands in glanded cottonseed, that can reduce the nutritive value of the meal. The structure of gossypol is shown in Figure 4. Gossypol is not present in the newer variety of glandless seed. The

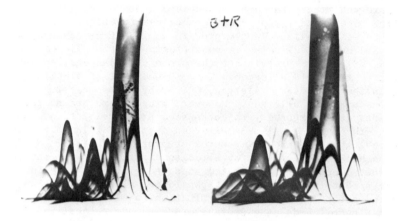

Figure 3. Crossed immunoelectrophoretic analysis of binding between rice germ agglutinin and human serum proteins.

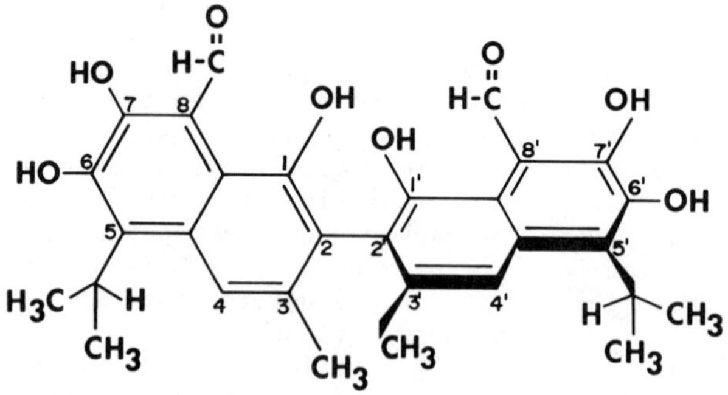

Figure 4. Chemical structure of gossypol.

pigment glands appear as dark purplish-black dots throughout the endosperm. Gossypol glands vary in size from 100 to 400 μ. From 10 to 40 glands are found in a cross section or a seed kernel. When the seeds are crushed to produce the oil, gossypol can be leached into the oil or can be retained by the meal. If retained by the meal, the meal is unsuitable as a source of feed for non-ruminants. Gossypol occurs in both free and bound forms. Inter-reaction of gossypol with proteins takes place through the aldehyde groups of gossypol and the amino groups of free amino acids or terminal amino groups of polypeptides in the protein. The most frequently bound amino acid is lysine, which lowers nutritive value of the protein.

The earliest effects of gossypol were found on hatchability of eggs and on egg discoloration (14). Chicks fed cottonseed meal containing high gossypol produced smaller eggs and eggs with decreased hatchability. Egg layers produced eggs which had discolored yolks. This effect (the Halphen reaction) was believed to be due to reaction of gossypol with iron in the egg yolk that produced a greenish yolk instead of yellow. Reaction of gossypol with iron can produce low serum levels of iron and low uptake of iron by monogastrics. Gossypol can also inhibit various enzymes. Tanksley et al. (15) found that gossypol prevented the conversion of pepsinogen to pepsin. They incubated pepsinogen with 2:1 or 3:1 molar ratios of gossypol and showed that the conversion of pepsinogen to pepsin was blocked at low pH values. This was the first report of a naturally occurring inhibitor for the conversion of an inactive zymogen to its active form. Gossypol also inhibits activity of ATPase and succinate dehydrogenase in vitro (16).

The effect of gossypol-acetic acid on plasma lipid concentration was recently studied in adult monkeys (17). Significant decreases in total plasma cholesterol, low density lipoprotein (LDL), and very low density lipoprotein-cholesterol were observed without any significant decrease in plasma high density lipoprotein chloresterol levels in monkeys given 10 mg/kg/day. This therapeutic property of gossypol has not been previously reported. It is tempting to speculate that gossypol might possibly reduce intestinal absorption of dietary cholesterol or hepatic synthesis of LDL in mammals.

In addition to its adverse effects on mammals, gossypol has also been shown to be toxic to insects. Among the pesticides shown to manifest plant resistance are certain classes of phenolic compounds, including gossypol, flavonoids, and aromatic acids (18). The roles of these compounds are difficult to elucidate because compounds toxic to one insect may not be toxic to another, but glandless cottonseed is significantly more susceptible to insect attack than glanded cottonseed. Gossypol in cotton acts as an inhibitor of insects but the resistance has not been correlated with the total gossypol. Eagle (19) concluded

that free gossypol content of cottonseed meal is not a true
measure of meal toxicity, although many others consider total
gossypol as the primary toxic agent.

Perhaps the most interesting effect of gossypol today is its
use in China as a male contraceptive. Gossypol was first noted
to affect fertility as long as twenty years ago but clinical
trials only began about 1972 (20). Up to 1972, more than 10,000
men had been studied over long periods. Each received daily oral
doses of 20 mg until sperm count was sufficiently reduced (about
two months), with maintenance doses of 75-100 mg taken twice
monthly. Side effects were minimal and sperm counts returned to
normal within a few months after use of gossypol was discontinu-
ed. The mechanism of action was found to be inhibition of lactate dehydrogenase-X, an enzyme found only in sperm and testis
cells.

Cyclopropene Fatty Acids Cyclopropene fatty acids (CPFA) are
present in cottonseed oil. They can affect lipid metabolizing
enzymes in animals by changing the oleic:linoleic fatty acid
ratio towards higher saturation (21). The absolute amounts of
oleic and linoleic acids decrease and more stearic (saturated
C-18 fatty acid) is produced. With a lipase prepared from castor
seeds, we showed that CPFA inhibited activity by forming a
covalent bond between the SH-group of cysteine at the active site
of the enzyme (22). In vitro tests with the SH-sensitive lipase
of castor seeds showed that cottonseed oil containing malvalic
acid, a CPFA, reduced lipase activity unless cysteine was added
first. Free cysteine bound to CPFA preferentially, reducing
inhibition of the enzyme (22).

In conclusion, many oilseeds and cereal grains being considered as sources of protein for future food products contain compounds with allergenic or antinutrient properties. Unless precautions are taken to remove or detoxify such compounds, undesirable
effects can occur. However, with the technology available for
food processing today, our food supply is quite safe and should
not present serious problems for consumers.

Literature Cited

1. Anon. Food & Nutrition News 1979, 50 (2), 4.
2. von Pirquet, C. Muenchen. Med. Woechenschr. 1906, 53, 1457.
3. Speer, F. Amer. Family Physician 1976, 13, 106.
4. Aas, K. Clinical Allergy 1978, 8, 39.
5. Spies, J.R.; Coulson, E.J.; Chambers, D.C.; Bernton, H.S.;
    Stevens, H.; Shimp, J.H. J. Amer. Chem. Soc. 1951, 73,
    3995.
6. Dechary, J.M.; Leonard, G.L.; Corkern, S. Lloydia 1970, 33,
    270.
7. Frampton, V.L.; Boudreaux, H.B. Econ. Bot. 1963, 17, 312.

8. Ory, R.L.; Neucere, N.J. J. Amer. Peanut Res. and Education Assoc. 1971, 3, 57.
9. Gillespie, D.N.; Nakajima, S.; Gleich, G.J. J. Allergy Clin. Immunol. 1976, 57, 302.
10. Sachs, M.I,; Jones, R.T.; Yunginger, J.N.; Gleich, G.J. J. Allergy Clin. Immunol. 1979, 63, 197.
11. Kamat, S.R.; Tasker, S.P.; Iyer, E.R.; Naik, M. J. Soc. Occup. Med. 1979, 29, 102.
12. Youle, R.J.; Huang, A.H.C. J. Agric. Food Chem. 1979, 27, 500.
13. Daussant, J.; Ory, R.L.; Layton, L.L. J. Agric. Food Chem. 1976, 24, 103.
14. Adams, R.; Geissman, T.A.; Edwards, J.D. Chem. Rev. 1960, 60, 555.
15. Tanksley, T.D.; Neumann, H.; Lyman, C.M.; Pace, C.N.; Prescott, J.M. J. Biol. Chem. 1970, 245, 6456.
16. Kalla, N.R.; Tet Wei, J.F. IRCS Med. Sci. Libr. Compend. 1981, 9, 792.
17. Shandilya, L.N.; Clarkson, T.B. Lipids 1982, 17, 285.
18. Hedin, P.A. J. Agric. Food Chem. 1982, 30, 201.
19. Eagle, E.; Davies, D.L. J. Amer. Oil Chem. Soc. 1958, 35, 36.
20. Maugh, T.H. Science 1981, 212, 314.
21. Reiser, R., Raju, P. K. Biochem. Biophys. Res. Commun. 1964, 17, 8.
22. Ory, R.L.; Altschul, A.M. Biochem. Biophys. Res. Commun. 1964, 17, 12.

RECEIVED May 13, 1983

Psoralens as Phytoalexins in Food Plants of the Family Umbelliferae

Significance in Relation to Storage and Processing

ROSS C. BEIER, G. WAYNE IVIE, and ERNEST H. OERTLI

Veterinary Toxicology and Entomology Research Laboratory, Agricultural Research Service, U.S. Department of Agriculture, College Station, TX 77841

Linear furanocoumarins (psoralens) are phototoxic, photomutagenic, and photocarcinogenic compounds that occur as natural constituents of hundreds of plant species, including some food plants of the family Umbelliferae (e.g., parsnip, celery, and parsley). Certain plant stresses, particularly diseases, induce biosynthesis of toxic natural plant products; a phenomenon referred to as a phytoalexin response. Such interactions in food plants of the family Umbelliferae may have toxicological implications for man because of the biological activity of psoralens. The linear furanocoumarin phytoalexin response in celery is discussed, with brief comments concerning carrots and parsley.

Historical

Psoralens. Many plants contain linear furanocoumarins (psoralens) (1), which were identified in the late 1940's as the cause of the photosensitization properties of these plants (2-4). Plants containing linear furanocoumarins can cause photosensitization in livestock and poultry (5-9), resulting in economic losses and, in some cases, animal death.

Man has also encountered problems with the photosensitizing properties of linear furanocoumarins. Celery handlers and field workers are frequently affected with photosensitization of the fingers, hands, and forearms (10,11). These skin disorders are referred to as celery dermatitis, celery itch, or celery blisters, and are caused by linear furanocoumarins in diseased celery (12). Some researchers (12,13) have found linear furanocoumarins only in diseased plants, whereas others (14,15) obtained them from healthy celery.

Biological   Activities   of   Linear   Furanocoumarins.   The biological activity of these compounds are extremely diverse because of their interactions with DNA (32-35), and RNA (36). Linear furanocoumarins have antifeedant activity toward various insects   (37,38)   and   are   phototoxic   to   others   (39). Interestingly, the black swallowtail butterfly has maximized its metabolic detoxification processes allowing its larva to feed on plants with a high linear furanocoumarin content (40). Psoralen, bergapten, xanthotoxin, and isopimpinellin are antibacterial when combined with UV light, whereas psoralen and xanthotoxin have some antibacterial activity without UV light (41). A mixture of pimpinellin, isopimpinellin, isobergapten, and sphondin was fungitoxic at 200 ppm or less (42). The individual   linear   furanocoumarins,   psoralen   (43),   and xanthotoxin (44,45) are also antifungal.

Toxicological Implications for Man.   Because psoralens are potent photoactive compounds, they have been used medically for treatment   of   skin   depigmentation   or   vitiligo   (16,17),   and psoriasis (18).   However, there has recently been concern associated with the medical use of these compounds (19). This concern is due to the observed phototoxicity during therapeutic use (17), the suspected photocarcinogenicity of xanthotoxin (20,21), and the latent onset of tumors in treated laboratory animals (22).   Acute gout secondary to psoriasis also was exacerbated by psoralen and UV-A (PUVA) photochemotherapy (23).

Psoralens in Healthy Celery.   Healthy celery contains at least four linear furanocoumarins (Figure 1), psoralen, bergapten, xanthotoxin, and isopimpinellin (14).   The observed quantities of linear furanocoumarins in healthy samples of three different celery cultivars grown at different locations in the U.S. are shown in Table I.

Table I.   Summary of the Linear Furanocoumarin Content in Fresh
         Celery Grown in California, Florida, and Michigan[a]

| | Cultivar[b,c] | | |
Compound	A	B	C
Psoralen	0.15 + 0.06	<0.03	0.07 + 0.03
Bergapten	0.14 + 0.04	0.04 + 0.03	0.35 + 0.05
Xanthotoxin	0.61 + 0.14	0.04 + 0.06	0.47 + 0.05
Isopimpinellin	0.08 + 0.03	0.05 + 0.03	0.41 + 0.04

[a]Data from Beier et al. (14).
[b]Cultivar A: Tall Utah 5270-R grown in California,
  Cultivar B: Florida 2192 grown in Florida,
  Cultivar C: Florida 683 grown in Michigan.
[c]Concentration is reported in ppm of fresh plant material.

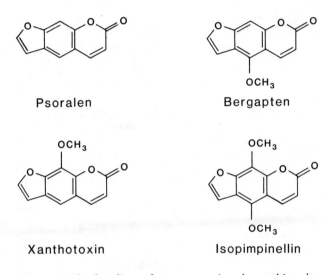

Psoralen   Bergapten

Xanthotoxin   Isopimpinellin

Figure 1. The four linear furanocoumarins observed in celery.

In general, low levels of the four psoralens were observed in
fresh healthy celery, with a maximum total of 1.3 ppm observed
in Cv. Florida 683 grown in Michigan.

During the measurement of linear furanocoumarins in fresh
celery (14), relatively high levels of psoralens were randomly
observed in some samples. It was then hypothesized that
psoralens may function as phytoalexins in celery. The linear
furanocoumarin, xanthotoxin, has been previously reported as
being a phytoalexin in parsnip root (Pastnaca sativa) (24).

Phytoalexins. Let us now review the history of the term
phytoalexin. An early definition stated that a phytoalexin
was, "a chemical compound produced only when the living cells
of the host are invaded by a parasite and undergo necrobiosis"
(25). This definition was later expanded to, "antibiotics
which are produced as a result of the interaction of two
different metabolic systems, the host and parasite, and which
inhibit the growth of microorganisms pathogenic to plants"
(26). A broader definition which seems to relate well and
encompass experimental observations is, "the term phytoalexin
serves as an umbrella under which chemical compounds
contributing to disease resistance can be classified whether
they are formed in response to injury, physiological stimuli,
the presence of infectious agents or are the products of such
agents" (27). A working definition has recently been devised
by a group of scientists: "Phytoalexins are low molecular
weight, antimicrobial compounds that are both synthesized by
and accumulated in plants after exposure to microorganisms
(28). In addition to the originally observed antifungal
activity, phytoalexins exhibit toxicity across much of the
biological spectrum, and their activity is not confined to
microorganisms (29).

Linear Furanocoumarins in Diseased Celery. There are a number
of reports of linear furanocoumarins (12,13) in diseased
celery, and the effects of diseased celery (10,30,31) on celery
workers and handlers. In these reports, only diseased celery
caused celery dermatitis; however, low levels of linear
furanocoumarins are found in healthy celery (14,15). Therfore,
it seems logical that some elevated concentration of psoralens
exists at which celery dermatitis will begin to occur.
Unfortunately, there are no quantitative data on the amounts of
psoralens in diseased celery.

Phytoalexins in Celery. Past studies support the hypothesis
that linear furanocoumarins act as phytoalexins in celery. The
infection of celery with Sclerotinia sclerotiorum has been
correlated with elevated levels of psoralens, and with the
onset of celery dermatitis (12,13). Spurious elevated levels
of linear furanocoumarins also are found during analysis of

apparently healthy celery, whereas healthy celery in general has very low levels of psoralens (14).

Elicitors of the Phytoalexin Response. The production of phytoalexins can be elicited not only by living organisms, but also by many chemical compounds and stress situations (27,46,47). Hg^{++} (48) and Cu^{++} (49) ions, fungicides (50,51), and polyamines (52) are some of the different chemical elicitors of phytoalexins. Physical stresses such as cold (53) and UV light (54,55) also stimulate the phytoalexin response. Even though these different stresses may act at different sites and in different ways, the result is always a dramatic change in metabolism of the susceptible plants.

Stimulation of Phytoalexins in Celery

Experimental. Extracts of fresh celery petioles (Apium graveolens cv. 5270-R) grown and packed in California and shipped to Texas were prepared according to the flow chart in Figure 2. Celery samples (5 g) were placed in 25 x 150 mm tubes used for simultaneous ether extraction and polytron grinding. With this sample size our minimum detection limit, obtained by HPLC, was about 0.03 ppm (14).

The linear furanocoumarins were characterized with a Varian/MAT CH-7 mass spectrometer, and their mass spectra were identical to those of the authentic psoralens (56). The isolated compounds were also co-injected with standard psoralens on normal and reverse phase HPLC to further substantiate their authenticity.

$CuSO_4$ Treatment. Celery petioles were immersed in a $CuSO_4$ solution (9 X 10^{-3} M) for 0.5 hr at room temperature. Some treated plant material was kept at 26°C and some at 2°C. Figure 3 shows some HPLC tracings of $CuSO_4$ treated celery and controls after 72 hrs at 26°C and 2°C with comparison to standard psoralens. At 26°C, the psoralen level was the lowest and bergapten the highest of the observed linear furanocoumarins. However, at 2°C the psoralen level was relatively much higher, second only to xanthotoxin (57). A plot of the increase of total psoralens over the control values at 26°C is shown in Figure 4. Although the observed ppm and fold increase vary from one experiment to the next, the shape of the curve (i.e., decrease about day three with elevated levels immediately thereafter) remains the same.

Evaluation of the onset of phytoalexin production with respect to elicitor concentration was attempted by treating celery for 0.5 hr periods with various concentrations of $CuSO_4$. Concentrations ranging from 10^{-1} to 10^{-6} M were used followed by a 72 hr incubation period at 26°C (Table 2). Results lead to the conclusion that bergapten and

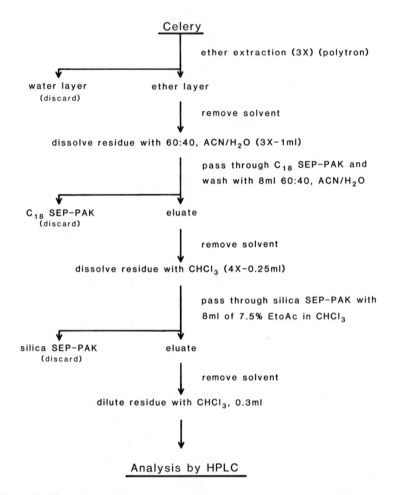

Figure 2. Flow chart of the basic extraction procedure used prior to HPLC analysis of celery.

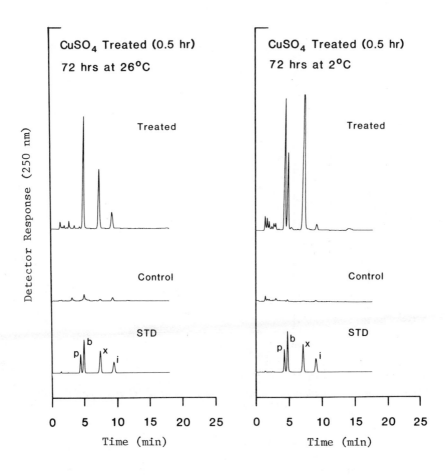

Figure 3. HPLC tracings of detector response vs. retention time for psoralen (p), bergapten (b), xanthotoxin (x), and isopimpinellin (i) standards, and CuSO₄-treated celery cv. 5270-R and controls after 72 h treatment.

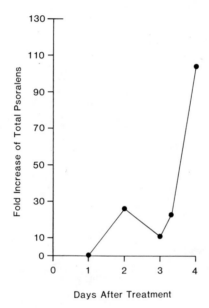

Figure 4. *Increase of total psoralens over controls at 26 °C and 24-h intervals after CuSO₄ treatment.*

xanthotoxin both changed linearly with the concentration of $CuSO_4$ after exceeding the threshold for the phytoalexin response (<u>57</u>).

Table 2. Levels of bergapten and xanthotoxin observed from celery treated for 0.5 hr with various concentrations of $CuSO_4$ (<u>57</u>)

Conc. of $CuSO_4$ (M)	(ppm) at 72 hrs	
	Bergapten	Xanthotoxin
10^{-1}	1.2	5.1
10^{-2}	0.7	3.2
10^{-3}	0.3	1.1
10^{-4}	0.03	0.1
10^{-6}	0.03	0.1
0	0.04	0.2
Fold increase at 10^{-1}M	30	25

To establish that the onset of phytoalexin synthesis is both concentration and time dependent is very important. This indeed would mimic phytoalexin responses in other plants.

<u>UV Treatment.</u> A combination of long and short wave UV light was used to treat celery petioles for a 1-hr period. The irradiated petioles and controls were kept at room temperature for 72 hrs in the dark. The HPLC tracings obtained from extracts of irradiated celery are shown in Figure 5. The response at 26°C is very similar to that observed with $CuSO_4$ treatment; however, the response at 2°C differs from the $CuSO_4$ treatment in that the level of psoralen is relatively very low, whereas the psoralen level in $CuSO_4$ treated celery at 2°C is second only to xanthotoxin.

<u>Cold Treatment.</u> Celery was placed in the freezer (-15°C) for 70 min. Treated samples and controls were kept at room temperature for 72 hrs and then analyzed (Table 3). The quantities of total psoralens increased 8.8 times over the controls.

<u>Sodium Hypochlorite Treatment.</u> This treatment was considered because sodium hypochlorite is often used to sterilize plant tissues prior to microbiological studies. Since the disease organism <u>S. sclerotiorum</u> is often implicated in the production of linear furanocoumarins in celery, sterilizing the plant tissues maybe an appropriate first step in many investigations.

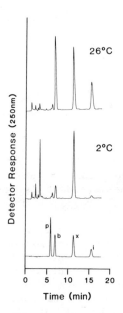

Figure 5. *HPLC tracings of detector response vs. retention time for UV-treated celery cv. 5270-R after 72 h at 2 °C and 26 °C in comparison to the linear furanocoumarin standards: psoralen (p), bergapten (b), xanthotoxin (x), and isopimpinellin (i).*

Celery petioles were immersed in 0.1% sodium hypochlorite for 20 min. and incubated for 72 hrs at 26°C.   Subsequent extraction and HPLC analysis gave the tracings shown in Figure 6.   The psoralen levels at 2°C are similar to the $CuSO_4$ treated celery, but at 26°C the levels are lower and appear qualitatively different from those observed in the $CuSO_4$-treated plant material.

A composite bar graph showing the levels of the four linear furanocoumarins in both UV-treated and sodium hypochlorite treated celery analyzed after 72 hrs at 26°C is shown in Figure 7.   The observed levels in both treated tissues were significantly higher than those in the controls.

Summary

The total quantities of psoralens and their increased concentration in celery after different treatments is described in Table 3.

Table 3.   Summary of Phytoalexin Response in Treated Celery (57)

Treatment	Time (hr)	Total Psoralens (ppm)	Fold Increase
$CuSO_4$	96	26.0	104.0
$CuSO_4$	79	21.1	23.0
UV light	72	7.4	3.4
Sodium hypochlorite	72	4.9	2.2
Cold	72	2.2	8.8
$CuSO_4$*	48	29.0	
			-23.0
4-day-old $CuSO_4$*	48	1.3	

*These experiments were carried out on celery procured at the same time. Part of the lot was immediately treated, while another portion was retained for 4 days in the refrigerator before treatment.

All of the treatments in Table 3 caused an increase in the quantities of linear furanocoumarins to some degree, with some samples containing as much as 29 ppm of total psoralens.   It is also interesting that a sample of harvested celery allowed to age 4 days in the laboratory prior to $CuSO_4$ treatment exhibited a 23 fold decrease in the total linear furanocoumarin production when compared to non-aged $CuSO_4$-treated celery (Table 3).   This result may reflect a deterioration of the cellular condition in these samples.

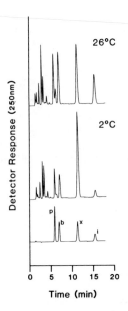

Figure 6. *HPLC tracings of the detector response vs. retention time for sodium hypochlorite-treated celery cv. 5270-R after 72 h at 2 °C and 26 °C in comparison to the linear furanocoumarin standards: psoralen (p), bergapten (b), xanthotoxin (x), and isopimpinellin (i).*

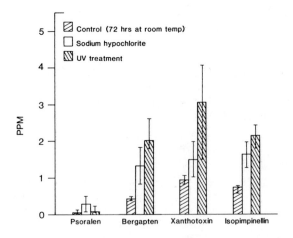

Psoralens from celery cv. 5270–R

Figure 7. *A bar graph of the observed levels of psoralen, bergapten, xanthotoxin, and isopimpinellin in celery cv. 5270-R 72 h after UV light and sodium hypochlorite treatment.*

What is the Impact of the Phytoalexin Response in Celery. Studies to date indicate that celery purchased at local markets should contain low levels of linear furanocoumarins (14). Increased levels of psoralens as a result of a phytoalexin response will probably be of little or no significance to the consumer. The major interest that arises from this phenomenon will be to the grower, field worker and celery handler. Clearly, certain chemicals and stress situations can cause up to 100 fold increases in the linear furanocoumarin content of previously excised celery petioles. Therefore, it seems possible that certain stress situations and/or chemical treatments may indeed elevate levels of psoralens in celery to a point where the risk of dermatitis is greatly enhanced.

The actual role of linear furanocoumarins in the disease resistance of celery is unknown; however, it has been concluded that the phytoalexins studied to date play an important role in resistance (47).

Phytoalexins in Other Umbelliferae?

Carrots. Previous phytochemical studies with carrot (Daucus carota L.) have been unsuccessful in demonstrating the presence of psoralens, and it is generally accepted that carrots lack linear furanocoumarins (58,59). We have recently developed techniques to look for psoralens at the sub parts-per-million level in carrot (60), and were similarly unable to see linear furanocoumarins in this plant.

Along with our celery studies, we treated carrot slices with $CuSO_4$ (9 X 10^{-3} M) for 0.5 hr, and made analyses by HPLC after 72 hrs. Even with this attempted stimulation, no linear furanocoumarins were detected.

It has been suggested (46) that phytoalexins can be used in some cases as taxonomic markers. That application may indeed be appropriate in the case of carrots.

Parsley. Parsley (Petroselinum sativum) has been known to cause dermatitis on the hands and arms. This condition was accompanied by blisters which developed on the back of the hands of schoolgirls that picked parsley. Peasants in a village near Sofia, Bulgaria, are familiar with this problem, and some cover their hands with fat before picking (61).

The first linear furanocoumarin to be isolated from parsley was bergapten (62). Later work provided quantitative data for bergapten, xanthotoxin, and isopimpinellin from dried parsley grown in greenhouse conditions (15).

We are presently investigating parsley for its linear furanocoumarins besides those previously identified. Preliminary studies with $CuSO_4$ suggests that parsley also produces psoralens as phytoalexins.

Literature Cited

1. Nielsen, B. E. "The Biology and Chemistry of the Umbelliferae"; Heywood, V. H., Ed.; Academic Press: London, 1971, p. 325.
2. Fahmy, I. R.; Abushady, H.; Schonberg, A.; Sina, A. Nature 1947, 160, 468-9.
3. Fahmy, I. R.; Abu-Shady, H. Quart. J. Pharm. Pharmacol. 1947, 20, 281-91.
4. Fahmy, I. R.; Abu-Shady, H. Q. J. Pharm. Parmacol. 1948, 21, 499-503.
5. Binns, W.; James, L. F.; Brooksby, W. Vet. Med. Small Anim. Clin. 1964, 59, 375-9.
6. Musajo, L.; Rodighiero, G. Phytophysiology 1972, 7, 115-47.
7. Stegmaier, O. C. J. Invest. Dermatol. 1959, 32, 345-9.
8. Dollahite, J. W.; Younger, R. L.; Hoffman, G. O. Am. J. Vet. Res. 1978, 39, 193-7.
9. Egyed, M. N.; Shlosberg, A.; Eilat, A.; Cohen, U.; Beemer, A. Refu. Vet. 1974, 31, 128-31.
10. Birmingham, D. J.; Key, M. M.; Tubich, G. E.; Perone, V. B. Archs. Derm. 1961, 83, 73-85.
11. Legrain, P. MM.; Barthe, R. Bull. Soc. Fr. Derm. Syph. 1926, 33, 662-4.
12. Scheel, L. D.; Perone, V. B.; Larkin, R. L.; Kupel, R. E. Biochemistry 1963, 2, 1127-31.
13. Wu, C. M.; Koehler, P. E.; Ayres, J. C. Appl. Microbiol. 1972, 23, 852-6.
14. Beier, R. C.; Ivie, G. W.; Oertli, E. H.; Holt, D. L. Food Chem. Toxicol. 1983, 21, 163-5.
15. Innocenti, G.; Dall'Acqua, F.; Caporale, G. Planta Medica 1976, 29, 165-70.
16. Scott, B. R.; Pathak, M. A.; Mohn, G. R. Mutat. Res. 1976, 39, 29-74.
17. Pathak, M. A.; Daniels, F.; Fitzpatrick, T. B. J. Invest. Dermatol. 1962, 39, 225-49.
18. Van Scott, E. J. Am. Med. Assoc. 1976, 235, 197-8.
19. "Psoralens," National Toxicology Program Technical Bulletin, 1982, 6, p. 8.
20. Reed, W. B. Acta Derm.-Venereol. 1976, 56, 315-7.
21. Stern, R. S.; Thibodeau, L. A.; Kleinerman, R. A.; Parrish, J. A.; Fitzpatrick, T. B.; 22 participating investigators. N. Eng. J. Med. 1979, 300, 809-13.
22. Zajdela, F.; Bisagni, E. Carcinogenesis 1981, 2, 121-7.
23. Burnett, J. W. Arch. Dermatol. 1982, 118, 211.
24. Johnson, C.; Brannon, D. R.; Kuć, J. Phytochemistry 1973, 12, 2961-2.
25. Müller, K.; Börger, H. Arb. Biol. Reichsanstat. Land-u Forstwirtsch. 1940, 23, 189-231.
26. Müller, K. Phytopathol. Z. 1956, 27, 237-54.

27. Kuć, J. Annu. Rev. Phytopathol. 1972, 10, 207-32.
28. Paxton, J. D. Pl. Disease 1980, 64, 734.
29. Smith, D. A. "Phytoalexins"; Bailey, J. A.; Mansfield, J. W., Eds.; John Wiley and Sons: New York, 1982, p. 218.
30. Henry, S. A.; Cantab, M. D.; Cantab, D.P.H. Br. J. Derm. 1933, 45, 301-9.
31. Marasas, W.F.O.; van Rensburg, S. J. "Plant Disease"; Horsfall, J. G.; Cowling, E. B., Eds.; Academic Press: New York, 1979, Vol. IV, p. 368.
32. Parsons, B. J. Photochemistry and Photobiology 1980, 32, 813-21.
33. Grekin, D. A.; Epstein, J. H. Photochemistry and Photobiology 1981, 33, 957-60.
34. Belogurov, A. A.; Zavilgelsky, G. B. Mutation Research 1981, 84, 11-5.
35. Cassier, C.; Moustacchi, E. Mutation Research 1981, 84, 37-47.
36. Talib, S.; Banerjee, A. K. Virology 1982, 118, 430-8.
37. Tajima, T.; Munakata, K. Agric. Biol. Chem. 1979, 43, 1701-6.
38. Muckensturm, B.; Duplay, D.; Robert, P. C.; Simonis, M. T.; Kienlen, J. C. Biochemical Systematics and Ecology 1981, 9, 289-92.
39. Berenbaum, M. Ecology 1981, 62, 1254-66.
40. Ivie, G. W.; Bull, D. L.; Beier, R. C.; Pryor, N. W.; Oertli, E. H. Science 1983 (In press).
41. Fowles, W. L.; Griffith, D. G.; Oginsky, E. L. Nature 1958, 181, 571-2.
42. Martin, J. T.; Baker, E. A.; Byrde, R.J.W. Ann. Appl. Biol. 1966, 57, 501-8.
43. Stanley, W. L.; Jund, L. J. Agric. Food Chem. 1971, 19, 1106-10.
44. Knudsen, E. A. Acta Derm. (Stockholm) 1980, 60, 452-6.
45. Oberste-Lehn, H.; Plempel, M. Dermatologica 1977, 154, 193-202.
46. Grisebach, H.; Ebel, J. Angew. Chem. Int. Ed. Engl. 1978, 17, 635-47.
47. Bell, A. A. Annu. Rev. Plant Physiol. 1981, 32, 21-81.
48. Hargreaves, J. A. Physiol. Plant Path. 1979, 15, 279-87.
49. Carlson, R. E.; Dolphin, D. H. Phytochemistry 1981, 20, 2281-4.
50. Reilly, J. J.; Klarman, W. L. Phytopathology 1972, 62, 1113-5.
51. Oku, H.; Nakanishi, T.; Shiraishi, T.; Ouchi, S. Sci. Rep. Fac. Agric., Okayama Univ. 1973, 42, 17-20.
52. Hadwiger, L. A.; Jafri, A.; von Broembsen, S.; Eddy, R., Jr. Plant Physiol. 1974, 53, 52-63.
53. Rahe, J. E.; Arnold, R. M. Can. J. Bot. 1975, 53, 921-8.
54. Hadwiger, L. A.; Schwochau, M. E. Can. J. Bot. 1971, 47, 588-90.

55. Bridge, M. A.; Klarman, W. L.   Phytopathology 1972, 63,
     606-9.
56. Ivie, G. W. J. Agric. Food Chem. 1978, 26, 1394-1403.
57. Beier, R. C.; Oertli, E. H.   Phytochemistry 1983 (In
     press).
58. Berenbaum, M.; Feeny, P. Science 1981, 212,   927-9.
59. Ivie, G.; Holt, D.; Ivey, M. Science 1981, 213, 909-10.
60. Ivie, G. W.; Beier, R. C.; Holt, D. L.   J. Agric. Food
     Chem. 1982, 30, 413-6.
61. Stransky, L.; Tsankov, N.   Contact Dermatitis 1980, 6,
     233-4.
62. Musajo, L.; Caporale, G.; Rodighiero, G.   G. Gazz. Chim.
     Ital. 1954, 84, 870-3.

RECEIVED June 28, 1983

Food, Drug, and Cosmetic Colors: Toxicological Considerations

JOSEPH F. BORZELLECA

Department of Pharmacology and Toxicology, Medical College of Virginia, Virginia Commonwealth University, Richmond, VA 23298

JOHN HALLAGAN and CAROLINE REESE

The Offices of Daniel R. Thompson, 900 17th St. N.W., Washington, DC 20006

The Food, Drug and Cosmetic (FD&C) Colors have been studied extensively. The most recent have been chronic toxicity/oncogenicity studies in Charles River CD rats and Charles River CD-1 mice. The colors evaluated and the dietary levels employed were:

	Dietary Levels (%)	
Color	Rat	Mouse
FD&C Blue 1	0.0, 0.1, 1.0, 2.0	0.0, 0.5, 1.5, 5.0
FD&C Green 3	0.0, 1.25, 2.5, 5.0	0.0, 0.5, 1.5, 5.0
FD&C Blue 2	0.0, 0.5, 1.0, 2.0	0.0, 0.5, 1.5, 5.0
FD&C Yellow 6	0.0, 0.75, 1.5, 3.0, 5.0	0.0, 0.5, 1.5, 5.0
FD&C Yellow 5	0.0, 0.1, 1.0, 2.0, 5.0	0.0, 0.5, 1.5, 5.0
FD&C Red 3	0.0, 0.1, 0.5, 1.0, 4.0	0.0, 0.3, 1.0, 3.0

Many parameters were measured during the course of these studies including reproductive performance (rats only), body weights, feed consumption, clinical chemistries (blood, urine), hematology, gross and histological examination of tissues. Data were subjected to extensive statistical analyses. There were no consistent statistically significant and biologically relevant compound related effects, including tumors. These studies were supported by the Certified Colors Manufacturers Association and were conducted by Bio-dynamics Laboratory and International Reseach and Development Corporation.

Colors have been an essential part of our existence. Nature is colorful. Colors have been used throughout history by man in at least three major areas - food, drugs and cosmetics. Colored candy has been identified in paintings in Egyptian tombs dating

back to about 1500 B.C. Artificially colored wines were
reported by Pliny the Elder in about 400 B.C. Ebers Papyrus,
the oldest record of drugs, identifies colors that were used in
drugs. About 5000 B.C., Egyptians were using green copper for
eye shadow. Also used were henna to dye hair, carmine to redden
lips, kohl (an antimony compound) to blacken eyebrows, lids and
lashes. Around 500 B.C., saffron was used to make faces yellow
and henna to dye feet red in India. Chinese used vegetable dyes
on feet, cheeks, and tips of their tongues for various reasons.
The Romans used white lead and chalk on their faces and blue and
gold dye on their hair.

The sources of dyes used by man include animal, vegetable,
and mineral. Sir William Henry Perkins, in 1856, synthesized
the first aniline dye. In 1860, a triphenylmethane dye, fuch-
sine, was used by the French to color wine. On August 2, 1886,
the U.S. Congress authorized the addition of color to butter.
On June 6, 1896, Congress approved colorants in cheese, and by
1900 colorants were added to catsup, jellies, cordials, candies,
sausage and noodles. However, there were some concerns by the
public. For example, chrome yellow, martius yellow and quick-
silver vermillion were added to foods to hide poor quality or
to increase weight. There was no control over the purity of
colorants used. For example, it has been noted that rejected
textile dyes were sometimes added to foods. Use of arsenic acid
and mercury in the manufacture of colorants also created some
concerns.

In 1899, the National Confectioners Association published a
list of unfit colorants for foods. This was the first time that
any group addressed the issue of safety of colorants. Unfortunately, this was not very effective. In August, 1904, the
U.S.D.A. issued a Food Inspection Decision which stated, "Food
is adulterated if it is colored, powdered or polished with
attempt to deceive." Another Food Inspection Decision was
issued in September 1905 in which the U.S.D.A. required that
colors must be declared on labels. In 1906 the U.S.D.A.
declared martius yellow in macaroni to be an unsafe color; and
in 1907 the F.D.A. prohibited the use of dangerous and impure
colorants in food. The Food and Drug Act was passed in 1906.
Dr. Bernard C. Hesse of the U.S. Department of Agriculture had
evaluated the chemistry and physiology of approximately 700 coal
tar dyes. Only colors of known composition were examined physiologically. Those showing non-favorable results could be used
in foods. The U.S.D.A. began to certify synthetic organic food
colors in April 1908. The cost of the certification was to be
borne by industry (and still is). The colors approved at that
time were amaranth (Red 2), ponceau 3R (Orange 1), erythrosine
(Red 3), naphthol yellow S (Yellow 7), light green SF yellowish,
and indigo disulfo acid sodium salt (Blue 2). Other colors were
added: in 1916, tartrazine (Yellow 5); in 1927, FCF green

(Green 3); and 1929 ponceau SX (Red 4), sunset yellow SCF (Yellow 6), and brilliant blue SCF (Blue 1). In 1938, the Federal Food, Drug and Cosmetic Act was passed. It stated that uncertified coal tar colors in food, drugs and cosmetics could not be shipped in interstate commerce. Use of colors was limited. All colors had to be certified and harmless. Three categories of coal tar colors were established: Food, Drug and Cosmetic colors, Drug and Cosmetic colors, and External Drug and Cosmetic colors. The Service and Regulatory Announcement, FD and C No. 3, September 1940, listed colors that were approved at that time and the specification and regulations concerning manufacturing, certification, sale, etc. The Food and Drug Administration began testing colors in the early 1950s following an incident in which children became sick after eating candy and colored popcorn. Unfavorable findings resulted in the banning of FD and C Orange 1, FD and C Orange 2, and FD and C Red 32. The FDA's position was that the term harmlessness as defined in the 1938 Act meant safe regardless of the amount used. Later, the Supreme Court ruled that the Food and Drug Administration could not establish limits unless the certified color in any quantity caused harm. The Color Additives Amendment of 1960 (PL-86-618) required the following: existing colors could be used pending further testing; limits of use were established; all colors were to be included, not just the coal tar colors; the Secretary was to determine which colors were to be certified and which would be exempted; producers and consumers were to provide data to obtain permanent listings; and provisional listing referred to colors for which additional data were necessary to secure permanent listing.

Uses of Colors

Foods. Colors are added (1) to foods that have no color of their own (beverages, gelatin dessert, candies, ice cream); (2) where the natural color has been lost in processing or storage; (3) where color of the food varies with the season of the year (geographic origin, for example dairy products, oranges); (4) to make foods recognizable and attractive, enhancing their aesthetic value. The meat inspection stamp is also colored.

Drugs. Colors are added to drugs for purposes of identification, standardizing batches, to mask unsatisfactory natural colors, and for appeal (colorless products are not aesthetic).

Cosmetics. Cosmetics require the addition of colors for effectiveness. Colors may be added to enhance the aesthetic value, for example to after shave lotion and shampoo, or to serve a functional purpose, for example in eye brow pencil, nail polish, lipstick, etc. The amounts used in cosmetics is greater than is used in foods and drugs.

Acceptable Daily Intake (ADI)

The amount of the material that can be ingested without unreasonable risk of adverse health effects may be considered an acceptable daily intake. This refers primarily to food chemicals. To arrive at an acceptable daily intake, appropriate toxicological tests and safety factors are involved. ADIs have been established by the U.S. Food and Drug Administration, the World Health Organization, the Joint Expert Committee on Food Additives, and the European Economic Community.

Background of the Current Testing Program

The Food and Drug Administration determined that the provisional listing of colors was to be eliminated. Colors were to be either permanently listed or to be prohibited from use. Also, there was concern about colors that were permanently listed. The concern was not based on adverse health effects nor on the generation of a significant amount of toxicological data, but presumably on a teratology study of Aramanth (Red No. 2) that appeared in Russian literature. The findings were not confirmed when the study was redone by the Food and Drug Administration and by the Certified Colors Manufacturers Association. There was some concern that colors were not necessary since they are non-nutrive. This neglects the aesthetic value of foods. Colors were also re-evaluated, presumably because of the cyclic review and re-evaluation program at FDA. The industry was requested by FDA to re-test all FD and C and D and C colors. Specifically, the color manufacturers were requested to prove safety. If safety is defined as the absence of toxicity, then it can never be proved since one cannot prove a negative. If safety is defined as the very low probability that an adverse effect will occur under certain conditions of use, then appropriate studies can be designed and levels determined. Harmlessness must be defined under certain conditions of use. In order to respond to FDA's request, life-time studies were conducted in the mouse and the rat to establish safety (reasonable certainty that no harm will occur when the material is used under certain conditions).

Prior to initiating these studies, a thorough search of the literature was conducted and the extent of oral toxicity tests was determined. It was found that the colors have a very low order of acute oral toxicity. An experimental design was then developed. Potential reproductive toxicities were evaluated in multigeneration reproductive and teratological studies. No adverse effects were reported at any of the levels examined.

Experimental Design

The FD and C colors evaluated are listed in Table I. The chemical structures, molecular weights and chemical names appear in Table II. The suppliers of the colors are identified in Table III. Other experimental details are summarized in Tables IV through VII.

The chronic toxicity/carcinogenicity studies were designed as definitive studies to address the issue of safety. The experimental design involved in utero exposure of rats and the use of weanling mice. Only certified batches of color from the various suppliers were used. Two laboratories were selected following an extensive evaluation of the facilities available at that time.

The colors were analyzed on a regular basis to evaluate stability, and microbiological contamination. Feed analyses were conducted on a weekly basis for the first 13 weeks of the study, and then at monthly intervals thereafter by the contract laboratory and by independent laboratories. Good laboratory practices monitoring occurred at least monthly.

Results

The results of these studies are summarized in Tables VIII through XIII.

These data failed to identify any carcinogenic potential of the Food, Drug and Cosmetic colors. There were no consistent, biologically significant compound-related effects at any level in either species.

Future Studies

The genetic toxicological aspects of the colors are being evaluated. The data generated to date failed to demonstrate genotoxicity of the six F D and C colors evaluated. Comparative biotransformation and kinetic studies are essential and these are in progress.

Special studies are being considered including interactions, sensitization or allergies, and assessment of the value of color in human nutrition.

Summary and Conclusions

The Food, Drug and Cosmetic colors have been extensively evaluated (few food chemicals have been so extensively studied). The Food, Drug and Cosmetic colors do not pose a threat to human health at levels currently in use or at levels greater than those currently used. There is no biological evidence in animals or human that the Food, Drug and Cosmetic colors are unsafe or hazardous to human health.

Table I

FD AND C COLORS

Chronic Toxicity Studies
1977–1981

Chemical Class			Year approved by FDA/USDA
Triphenylmethane:	FD and C Blue No. 1	(Brilliant Blue FCF)	1929
	FC and C Green No. 3	(Fast Green FCF)	1927
Indigoid:	FD and C Blue No. 2	(Indigotine)	1907
Monoazo:	FD and C Yellow No. 6	(Sunset Yellow FCF)	1929
Pyrazolone:	FD and C Yellow No. 5	(Tartrazine)	1916
Xanthene:	FD and C Red No. 3	(Erythrosine) (Tetraiodo Fluorescein)	1907

Table II.   Chemical Structures, Names, and Molecular Weights
            of the FD&C Colors Evaluated

Color	Empirical Formula	Molecular Weight
FD&C Red No. 40 (Allura Red AC)	$C_{18}H_{14}O_8N_2S_2Na_2$	496.40
FD&C Red No. 3 (Erythrosine)	$C_{20}H_6I_4Na_2O_5$ or $C_{20}H_6I_4K_2O_5$	879.87 912.10
FD&C Yellow No. 5 (Tartrazine)	$C_{16}H_9N_4Na_3O_9S_2$	534.37
FD&C Yellow No. 6 (Sunset Yellow FCF)	$C_{16}H_{10}N_2Na_2O_7S_2$	452.37
FD&C Blue No. 2 (Indigotine)	$C_{16}H_8N_2Na_2O_8S_2$	466.36
FD&C Green No. 3 (Fast Green FCF)	$C_{37}H_{34}N_2Na_2O_{10}S_3$	808.86

Continued on next page

Table II.   Chemical Structures, Names, and Molecular Weights

Color	Dye Type	Structure
FD&C Red No. 40 (Allura Red AC)	Monoazo	
FD&C Red No. 3 (Erythrosine)	Xanthene	R = Na or K
FD&C Yellow No. 5 (Tartrazine)	Pyrazolone	
FD&C Yellow No. 6 (Sunset Yellow FCF)	Monoazo	
FD&C Blue No. 2 (Indigotine)	Indigoid	
FD&C Green No. 3 (Fast Green FCF)	Triphenylmethane	

of the FD&C Colors Evaluated -- Continued

Chemical Name	CFR Reference
Disodium salt of 6-hydroxy-5-[(2-methoxy-5-methyl-4-sulfophenyl)-azo]-2-napththalenesulfonic acid	21 CFR 74.340
Monohydrate of 9-(O-carboxy-phenyl)-6-hydroxy-2,4,5,7-tetraiodo-3H-xanthen-3-one, disodium or dipotassium salt, with similar amounts of lower iodinated fluoresceins	21 CFR 74.303
5-Oxo-1-(p-sulfophenyl)-4-[(p-sulfophenyl)azo]-2-pyrazoline-3-carboxylic acid, trisodium salt	21 CFR 74.705
Disodium salt of 1-p-sulfophenyl-azo-2-naphthol-6-sulfonic acid	21 CFR 82.706
Principally the disodium salt,of 5,5'-disulfo-3,3'-dioxo- $\Delta^{2,2'}$ - biindoline with smaller amounts of the isomeric disodium salt of 5,7'-disulfo-3,3'-dioxo-$\Delta^{2,2'}$-biindoline	21 CFR 74.1102
4-[(4-Ethyl-p-sulfobenzylamino)-phenyl]-(4-hydroxy-2-sulfoniumphenyl)-methylene}-[1-(N-ethyl-N-p-sulfobenzyl)-$\Delta^{2,5}$-cyclohexadienimine]	21 CFR 82.203

Table III

FD AND C COLORS

Chronic Toxicity Studies
1977–1981

SUPPLIERS OF COLORS

Color	Manufacturer
FD and C Blue No. 1	Hilton–Davis Chemical Co.
FD and C Green No. 3	Warner–Jenkinson Co.
FD and C Blue No. 2	Hilton–Davis Chemical Co.
FD and C Yellow No. 6	Stange Co. Hilton–Davis Chemical Co.
FD and C Yellow No. 5	Warner–Jenkinson Co.
FD and C Red No. 3	H. Kohnstamm

Table IV

FD AND C COLORS

Chronic Toxicity Studies
1977–1981

MATERIALS AND METHODS: ANIMALS

Laboratory	Species	Strain	Colony
Biodynamics	Rat Mouse	Charles River CD Rats Charles River CD-1 Mice	Wilmington, MA
International Research and Development Corp.	Rat Mouse	Charles River CD Rats Charles River CD-1 Mice	Portage, MI

MATERIALS AND METHODS: ANIMAL FEED

Laboratory	Species	Feed
Biodynamics	Rat and Mouse	Purina Rodent Laboratory Chow
International Research and Development Corp.	Rat and Mouse	Purina Rodent Laboratory Chow After 8/79: Purina Certified Laboratory Chow

Table V

FD AND C COLORS

Chronic Toxicity Studies
1977–1981

MATERIALS AND METHODS: MICE   (Charles River, CD-1)

Observation

General changes, moribundity,
  mortality (3 x daily)

Body Weight/Food Consumption
  (weekly: weeks 1–14;
  bi–weekly: weeks 16–26
  every 4 weeks thereafter)

Detailed Physical Examination
  (weekly: weeks 1–14;
  bi–weekly: weeks 16–16;
  every 4 weeks thereafter)

Pathology

Gross pathology on all animals

  DOS animals

  Terminal Sacrifice

Statistical Analysis

Appropriate tests

Test Diet Analysis

Independent analysis by contract
  lab and CCMA member company labs

Clinical Laboratory Tests

Hematology (3, 6, 12, 18 months;
  terminal)
Hemoglobin
Hematocrit
Total erythrocyte
Erythrocyte morphology
Total and differential leucocyte
  (10 M, 10 F from each group)

Histopathology

Adrenal (2)
Aorta (abdominal)
Bone and bone marrow (femur)
Blood smear
Brain (3 sections, including
  frontal cortex and basal
  ganglia, parietal cortex and
  thalamus; cerebellum and pons)
Esophagus
Eye (2-with optic nerve)
Gall bladder
Heart (with coronary vessels)
Intestine
  cecum
  colon
  duodenum
  ileum
Kidneys (2)
Liver (2)
Lung and mainstem bronchi
Lymph nodes
  (mesenteric, mediastinal)

Table V (Continued)

Histopathology

Mammary gland (inguinal)
Nerve (sciatic)
Ovaries
Pancreas
Pituitary
Prostate
Salivary gland (mandibular)
Seminal vesicles (2)
Skeletal muscle (biceps femoris)
Skin
Spinal cord (cervical)
Spleen
Stomach
Testes with epididymides
Thymus
Thyroid/parathyroid
Trachea
Urinary bladder
Uterus
Gross changes or uncertain nature
  (including a section of normal-
  appearing portion of same
  tissue)
Tissue masses or suspect tumors
  with regional lymph nodes

Table VI

FD AND C COLORS

Chronic Toxicity Studies
1977–1981

MATERIALS AND METHODS: RATS

In Utero Segment

Group	Male	Female	Min. No. Litters	Dosage Levels
1-A	60	60	70	Control
1-B	60	60	70	Control
2	60	60	35	Low
3	60	60	35	Mid
4	60	60	35	High

RANDOM SELECTION

Chronic Feeding Segment

Group	Male	Female	Dosage Levels
1-A	70	70	Control
1-B	70	70	Control
2	70	70	Low
3	70	70	Mid
4	70	70	High

Table VII

FD AND C COLORS

Chronic Toxicity Studies
1977-1981

MATERIALS AND METHODS: RATS (Charles River, CD-1)

Observation	Clinical Laboratory Tests

Observation

General changes, moribundity,)
  mortality (3 x daily)

Body Weight/Food Consumption
  (weekly: weeks 1-14;
  bi-weekly: weeks 16-26
  every 4 weeks thereafter)

Detailed Physical Examination
  (weekly: weeks 1-14;
  bi-weekly: weeks 16-16;
  every 4 weeks thereafter)

Clinical Laboratory Tests

Hematology (3, 6, 12, 18,
  24 months; terminal)
Hemoglobin
Hematocrit
Total erythrocyte
Erythrocyte morphology
Total and differential leucocyte
  (10 M, 10 F from each group)

Blood Chemistry (3, 6, 12,
  18, 24 months; terminal)
  Serum glutamic oxaloacetic
    transaminase
  Serum glutamic pyruvic
    transaminase
  Alkaline phosphatase
  Blood urea nitrogen
  Fasting glucose
  Total protein
  Creatinine

Pathology

Gross pathology on all animals
DOS animals
Interim Sacrifice
Terminal Sacrifice

Urinalysis (3, 6, 12, 18
  24 months; terminal)
  Gross appearance
  Specific gravity
  pH

Statistical Analysis

Appropriate tests

  Protein
  Glucose
  Ketones

Test Diet Analysis

Independent analysis by contract
  lab and CCMA member company la

  Bilirubin
  Occult blood
  Microscopic analysis

(Continued)

Table VII (Continued)

Histopathology	Ophthalmoscopic Examination
Adrenal (2)	3, 6, 12, 18, 24 months
Aorta (abdominal)	
Blood smear	
Bone and bone marrow (femur)	
Brain (3 sections, including frontal cortex and basal ganglia, parietal cortex and thalamus; cerebellum and pons)	
Esophagus	
Eye (2 – with optic nerve)	
Heart (with coronary vessels	
Intestine	
cecum	
colon	
duodenum	
ileum	
Kidneys (2)	
Liver (2)	
Lung and mainstem bronchi	
Lymph nodes (mesenteric, mediastinal)	
Mammary gland (inguinal)	
Nerve (sciatic)	
Ovaries	
Pancreas	
Pituitary	
Prostate	
Salivary gland (mandibular)	
Seminal vesicles (2)	
Skeletal muscle (biceps femoris)	
Skin	
Spinal cord (cervical)	
Spleen	
Stomach	
Testes with epididymides	
Thymus	
Thyroid/parathyroid	
Trachea	
Urinary bladder	
Uterus	
Gross changes of uncertain nature (including a section of normal-appearing portion of same tissue)	
Tissue masses or suspect tumors with regional lymph nodes	

Table VIII   FD AND C BLUE NO. 1

International Research and Development Corporation

Species	Number/Group Dose Levels	Initiation Termination	Effects
Rat	70/Sex/Group	Initiation:	No consistent biologically significant compound related adverse effects
	0.1% (50 mg/kg/day)	11 October 1977	
	1.0% (500 mg/kg/day)		
	2.0% (1000 mg/kg/day)	Termination:	
		Males – 28 December 1979	
	2 Concurrent Controls	Females – 15 November 1979	
Mouse	60/Sex/Group	Initiation:	No consistent biologically significant compound related adverse effects
	0.5% (750 mg/kg/day)	26 April 1978	
	1.5% (2250 mg/kg/day)		
	5.0% (7500 mg/kg/day)	Termination:	
		Males – 28–30 April 1978	
	2 Concurrent Controls	Females – 28–30 April 1980	

Table IX   FD AND C GREEN NO. 3 Bio/Dynamics, Inc.

Species	Number/Group Dose Levels	Initiation Termination	Effects
Rat	70/Sex/Group	Initiation:	Statistically significant increase in hyperplasia and tumors in urinary bladders of high-dose male rats.
	1.25% (625 mg/kg/day)	12 October 1977	
	2.5% (1250 mg/kg/day)		
	5.0% (2500 mg/kg/day)	Termination:	
		Males – 4 March 1980	
	2 Concurrent Controls	Females – 18 April 1980	
Mouse	60/Sex/Group	Initiation:	No consistent biologically significant compound related adverse effects
	0.5% (750 mg/kg/day)	11 May 1978	
	1.5% (2250 mg/kg/day)		
	5.0% (7500 mg/kg/day)	Termination:	
		16 May 1980	
	2 Concurrent Controls		

Table X

FD AND C BLUE NO. 2

Bio/Dynamics, Inc.

Species	Number/Group Dose Levels	Initiation Termination	Effects
Rat	70/Sex/Group	Initiation:	Brain Gliomas and Granular Cell Tumors (Males)*
	0.5% (250 mg/kg/day)	18 October 1977	
	1.0% (500 mg/kg/day)		
	2.0% (1000 mg/kg/day)	Termination:	Bladder Tumors (Males)*
		Males – 18-19 February 1980	Mammary Tumors (Males)*
	2 Concurrent Controls	Females – 3-4 April 1980	*Not biologically significant
Mouse	60/Sex/Group	Initiation:	No consistent biologically significant compound related adverse effects
	0.5% (750 mg/kg/day)	16 May 1978	
	1.5% (2250 mg/kg/day)		
	5.0% (7500 mg/kg/day)	Termination:	
		Males – 21-22 February 1980	
	2 Concurrent Controls	Females – 14-15 April 1980	

*Statistically significant with high dose males only.

Table XI

FD AND C YELLOW NO. 6

Bio/Dynamics, Inc.

Species	Number/Group Dose Levels	Initiation Termination	Effects
Rat	70/Sex/Group	Initiation:	
	0.75% (375 mg/kg/day)	3 November 1977	No consistent biologically significant compound related adverse effects
	1.5% (750 mg/kg/day)	5.0% – 26 February 1979	
	3.0% (1500 mg/kg/day)	Termination:	
	5.0% (2500 mg/kg/day)	Males – 22 April 1980	
	2 Concurrent Controls	Females – 7 March 1980	
		5.0% – March 1981	
Mouse	60/Sex/Group	Initiation:	
	0.5% (750 mg/kg/day)	16 May 1978	No consistent biologically significant compound related adverse effects
	1.5% (2250 mg/kg/day)	Termination:	
	5.0% (7500 mg/kg/day)	Males – 29 December 1979	
	2 Concurrent Controls	Females – 30 March 1980	

Table XII FD AND C YELLOW NO. 5
International Research and Development Corporation

Species	Number/Group Dose Levels	Initiation Termination	Effects
Rat	70/Sex/Group	Initiation:	
	0.1% (50 mg/kg/day)	25 October 1977	No consistent
	1.0% (500 mg/kg/day)	5.0% – 9 October 1978	biologically significant
	2.0% (1000 mg/kg/day)	Termination:	compound related adverse effects
		31 December 1980	
	2 Concurrent Controls	5.0% – 24 February 1981	
Mouse	60/Sex/Group	Initiation:	
	0.5% (750 mg/kg/day)	3 May 1978	No consistent
	1.5% (2250 mg/kg/day)		biologically significant
	5.0% (7500 mg/kg/day)	Termination:	compound related adverse effects
		2 May 1980	
	2 Concurrent Controls		

Table XIII   FD AND C RED NO. 3

International Research and Development Corporation

Species	Number/Group Dose Levels	Initiation Termination	Effects
Rat	70/Sex/Group	Initiation:	No consistent biologically significant compound related adverse effects
	0.1% (50 mg/kg/day) 0.5% (250 mg/kg/day) 1.0% (500 mg/kg/day) 4.0% (2000 mg/kg/day)	18 October 1977 4% – 4 October 1978	
	2 Concurrent Controls	Termination:	
		27 March 1980 4% – 24 February 1981	
Mouse	60/Sex/Group	Initiation:	No consistent biologically significant compound related adverse effects
	0.3% (500 mg/kg/day)	25 April 1978	
	1.0% (1500 mg/kg/day) 3.0% (4500 mg/kg/day)	Termination:	
		23 April 1980	
	2 Concurrent Controls		

Analysis of Carrot Constituents: Myristicin, Falcarinol, and Falcarindiol

S. G. YATES, R. E. ENGLAND, and W. F. KWOLEK

Northern Regional Research Center, Agricultural Research Service, U.S. Department of Agriculture, Peoria, IL 61604

P. W. SIMON

Department of Horticulture, University of Wisconsin, Madison, WI 53706

Falcarinol, falcarindiol, and myristicin contents of carrots, Daucus carota L., were determined by a sequence of dichloromethane extraction, column chromatographic purification, and gas-liquid chromatographic analysis. High Color 9, Long Imperator 58, Danvers 126, and Spartan Bonus varieties were grown in Wisconsin (1979-1982), Florida (1980-1982), California (1980-1982), Arizona (1981), and Illinois (1981-1982). Gold Pak, Nantes Half Long, Red Cored Chantenay, and Royal Chantenay varieties were grown in Illinois (1980). The overall mean of falcarinol for 510 observations of these eight commercial varieties was 24.1 mg/kg; that of falcarindiol for 389 observations was 65.1 mg/kg. The standard error of a mean based on 2 samples of 4 carrots, with 2 aliquots per sample, was 2.8 for falcarinol and 4.8 for falcarindiol. Varietal means ranged from 11.3 to 28.2 for falcarinol and 53.3 to 106.9 for falcarindiol. Myristicin was detected in only one variety of carrots (Spartan Bonus) harvested in Wisconsin in 1981; the mean of 12 observations, 2 samples, was 1.4 mg/kg with a range of 1.3 to 1.5 mg/kg.

        Crosby and Aharonson (1), in the course of their
investigation of naturally occurring toxicants in foods,
discovered that an acetone extract of carrots was toxic to the
organism Daphnia magna Straus. The purified toxin had an LD_{50}
in mice of 100 mg/kg. They gave this substance the trivial
name "carotatoxin" and published a tentative structure. Bentley
and Thaller (2) published a corrected structure and gave proof
that the compound Crosby and Aharonson isolated was falcarinol,
a polyacetylenic alcohol (I) (Figure 1) first isolated by
Bohlmann et al. (3), from Falcaria vulgaris Bernh. Other such
compounds have since been isolated from carrots (falcarindiol II,
acetylfalcarindiol III, and falcarinolone IV) (4). Recently,
the function of falcarindiol as an antifungal agent in the
disease response mechanism of carrots was recognized (5-7).
The LD_{50}, ip, in mice of falcarindiol was found to be 133 mg/kg
(8).
        Myristicin V, a phenylpropenoid, is frequently found in
carrots (9). It is known to stimulate central nervous system
activity (10) and to enhance the activity of certain insecticides
(11), and it is suspected of being involved in the disease
response mechanism of carrots (12).
        Carrots were analyzed for falcarinol, falcarindiol, and
myristicin to determine if concentrations varied with respect
to genetic (variety) and/or environmental changes (location and
year). The data generated define the level of those toxicants
normally present in carrots grown for processing (Danvers 126,
Spartan Bonus, Royal Chantenay, Red-Cored Chantenay, and Nantes
Half Long), for fresh market (Long Imperator 58, High Color 9,
and Gold Pak), and for genetic studies (B10138, B9304, B0493,
B3615, and B10720).

Experimental Section

Plant Materials. Carrot roots, Daucus carota L., were grown at
NRRC or at the following locations as directed by the Department
of Horticulture, University of Wisconsin, Madison: Wisconsin,
Florida, California, and Arizona.
        Carrots were harvested by hand and shipped unwashed to
NRRC in plastic bags. Analysis of the four varieties was
completed 1 to 2 weeks after each harvest sample was received.
Carrots grown in Illinois (NRRC) were harvested by hand and
analyzed immediately.

Chromatography Equipment and Conditions. Gas-liquid
chromatography was performed with a Bendix 2600 instrument
(flame ionization detectors); injector temperature was 250°C
and detector temperature was 270°C, with helium carrier gas at
10-20 ml/min, air at 500-600 ml/min, and hydrogen at 50 ml/min.
Columns were programmed from 80 to 250°C at 4°C/min with a

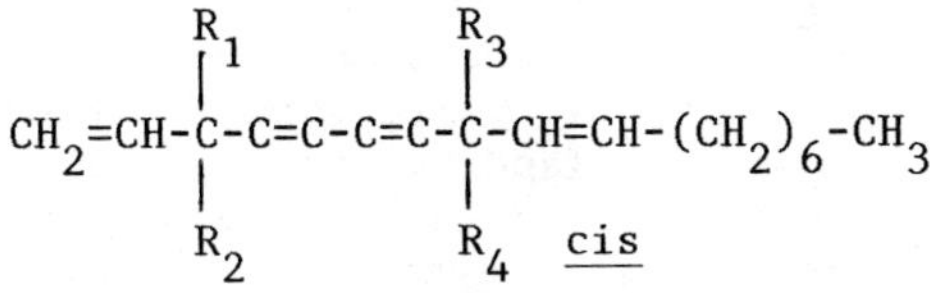
R1
R3
CH2=CH-C-C=C-C=C-C-CH=CH-(CH2)6-CH3
R2
R4
cis

		R_1, R_2	R_3, R_4
I	Falcarinol	(OH, H)	(H, H)
II	Falcarindiol	(OH, H)	(OH, H)
III	Acetylfalcarindiol	(OAc, H)	(OH, H)
IV	Falcarinolone	(=O)	(OH, H)

V Myristicin

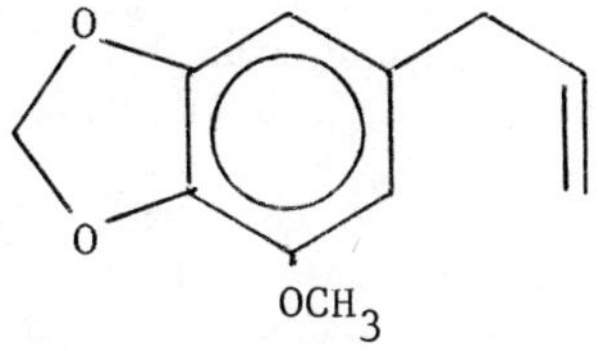
O
O
OCH3

Figure 1. Structures of carrot constituents.

5-min final hold. Glass columns 6 ft by 1/8 in. were used, one packed with 3% SE-52 (Applied Science Laboratories, Inc.) on 80-100 mesh Gas-Chrom Q (nonpolar), and one packed with 3% OV-17 (Supelco Inc.) on 100-120 mesh Chromosorb W HP (intermediate polarity).

Dichloromethane Extraction, Column Chromatographic Purification and Gas-Liquid Chromatographic (DE-CCP-GLC)

Analysis of Carrots. A longitudinal quarter was removed from each carrot included in the sample. Each quarter was cut into 2-mm cross sections, and these were immediately placed in a 2 ℓ stainless steel blending container. Antioxidant (Antioxidant 330, Ethyl Corp. or Ionox 330, Shell Chemicals) (2 mg/5 g carrot fresh weight) and dichloromethane (10 ml/5 g carrot) were added quickly, and the constituents were blended in a commercial Waring Blendor at moderate speeds for a total of 12 min. Alternate cycles of blending and cooling (4 min each) reduce evaporation of dichloromethane. Any solvent losses were corrected for by weighing the capped blender and contents before and after blending and then replacing the lost solvent. Maximum blending efficiency was obtained with 300- to 500-g of carrots. Teflon seals were inserted in the blender cup blade assembly to replace the standard seals. After dichloromethane lost by evaporation was replaced, the mixture was blended for an additional 30 s and aliquots transferred to 250-ml centrifuge bottles capped with a screw cap or Saran Wrap. The mixture was centrifuged for 15 min at 1500 g, and then 50 ml of the clear extract was removed with a large syringe fitted with a long 17-gauge needle passed through the pulp. One mg of methyl palmitate as internal standard was added to each of two 50-ml aliquots of centrifuged extract. These aliquots were concentrated under vacuum on a rotating evaporator at 25°C to about 3 ml; 7 ml of hexane was added and the solution was reconcentrated to 3 ml; 4 ml of hexane was added and the solution was reconcentrated to 1 ml. The resulting hexane solution was chromatographed on 2 g of Silica gel (70-325 mesh; EM Reagents). Glass columns 6 X 140 mm, fitted with 50-ml reservoirs, were constructed from 8 mm o.d. glass tubing and 25 X 140 mm test tubes. Yellow pigments were eluted with hexane until the hexane eluate was colorless (40 to 60 ml). The fraction of interest was eluted with 20 ml of ether-hexane (45:55). The eluate was concentrated to about 0.75 ml and transferred to a ½ dram vial with teflon-lined cap. Analysis by GLC (3-6 μl injection) gave symmetrical peaks, which were integrated electronically.

Quantities of individual toxicants were calculated by using the formula

$$\frac{\text{mg of toxicant}}{\text{kg of sample}} = F_t \frac{A_t \ W_p \ V_a}{A_p \ W_c \ V_r} \times 10^3$$

where F_t is the response factor of the toxicant in relation to methyl palmitate, A_t and A_p are the areas of the toxicant and methyl palmitate gas chromatographic peaks, respectively, W_p is the quantity of methyl palmitate added in milligrams, W_c is the initial weight of carrots used, V_a is the initial volume of solvent used for extraction, and V_r is the volume of solvent taken after centrifuging as the analysis aliquot. Response factors were determined by chromatographing a mixture of known weights of the toxicants myristicin, falcarinol, and falcarindiol, with a known weight of methyl palmitate (13).

Results and Discussion

Carrots (Daucus carota L.) make a significant contribution to the American diet by providing fiber, minerals, and vitamins (14). These essential nutrients must be maintained at present levels or improved as the plant breeder attempts to develop carrots of better culinary quality. Other components of carrots, those that contribute to the plant's defense against damage, disease, and insects, must be monitored to ensure that they do not increase or decrease to a troublesome level. Therefore, today more than ever, the plant breeder and chemist need to cooperate in developing new varieties.

Most of the carrots grown in the USA (80%) are for fresh market, the remainder are grown for processing (15). An unestimated, but significant, carrot crop also is produced in the home garden. The main thrust of this study involved four commercial varieties (for fresh markets, Long Imperator 58 and High Color 9; for processing, Danvers 126 and Spartan Bonus) grown in Wisconsin, Florida, California, Arizona, and Illinois during 1979-1982. Other varieties commonly grown in home gardens also were examined (Royal Chantenay, Red Cored Chantenay, Gold Pak, Nantes Half Long) as well as experimental genetic material from the USDA Carrot Improvement Program (low volatile inbreds B10138 and B9304, high volatile inbreds B0493 and B3615, and white carrot B10720).

During the early stages of the study (1979-1980), only falcarinol was measured; later measurements (1980-1982) included falcarindiol and myristicin. Identification of peaks in the chromatographic record was based on elution times relative to methyl palmitate (internal standard) in nonpolar (3% SE-52) and intermediate polarity (3% OV-17) packed columns. Identification of myristicin, a small peak, was generally confirmed by GC/MS.

The data acquired were divided into three main groups, depending on sampling and analysis protocol, for further evaluation: (a) Type 1: 22 selections, with four samples each; sample weight was 50 g, with 4 carrots per sample. Aliquots of each sample were analyzed. (b) Type 2: 5 selections, with 5 to 18 carrots per sample. Carrots were quartered, and aliquots of two quarters each were analyzed in duplicate. (c) Type 3: 28 selections with two samples each; sample weight was 300 to 500 g, with 10 to 30 carrots per sample. Aliquots of each sample were analyzed in duplicate. Although sampling procedures differed, there were 8 observations of each toxicant for each carrot selection. Analysis of variance was computed for each group; the least significant difference (LSD, 0.05 level) is reported where appropriate (16).

The largest sources of variation in the analysis are due to sampling and lack of agreement between GC columns. Larger composite samples (Type 3) gave less variation for falcarindiol; falcarinol generally gave good agreement with all sampling types. Agreement between GC columns also was much better for falcarinol than for falcarindiol. One probable explanation for these results is that the elution time for falcarinol is very close to that of methyl palmitate, whereas elution time for falcarindiol was somewhat later. Also, in the OV-17 column, establishment of a base line at the falcarindiol peak was complicated because of minor peaks that were not completely resolved from falcarindiol. Minor constituents may have coeluted with falcarindiol.

Myristicin was detected in only one variety of carrots (Spartan Bonus) harvested in Wisconsin in 1981; the mean of 12 observations, 2 samples, was 1.4 mg/kg with a range of 1.3 to 1.5 mg/kg. Wulf et al. (9) also report myristicin in carrots. They show 15 mg/kg for the variety Imperator, with lesser amounts for other varieties. The polyacetylenes, on the other hand, were found in all varieties (Table I).

The overall mean of falcarinol for 510 observations of all commercial varieties was 24.1 mg/kg; that of falcarindiol for 389 observations was 65.1 mg/kg. Previous reports on toxicant levels, except for those relating to disease response, tended to overlook the falcarindiol content. The mean of the falcarindiol/falcarinol ratio was 4.4, reflecting the higher concentration of falcarindiol.

The standard error of a mean based on 2 samples (4 carrots per sample), 2 aliquots per sample, and 2 runs per sample, or 8 observations, was 2.8 for falcarinol and 4.8 for falcarindiol. For single observations, the respective standard deviations were 15.2 and 24.8. About 70% of the variation for falcarinol was associated with sample, but only about 25% for falcarindiol. For falcarindiol, variation associated with the assay differences contributed most of the variation. Precision for both toxicants

Table I. Summary of Means of Falcarinol and Falcarindiol for Thirteen Carrot Varieties[1]

		Falcarinol		Falcarindiol	Mean ratio falcarindiol/
Variety	N[2]	mg per kg	N	mg per kg	falcarinol
High Color 9	104	11.3	72	54.5	9.0
Long Imperator 58	114	28.1	85	69.0	2.8
Danvers 126	124	28.2	92	59.3	2.7
Spartan Bonus	118	28.1	90	74.4	4.2
Mean	460	24.3	339	64.7	4.4
Gold Pak	10	13.4	10	106.9	8.0
Nantes Half Long	8	22.2	8	59.9	2.7
Red Cored Chantenay	8	22.6	8	67.8	3.1
Royal Chantenay	24	25.6	24	53.3	2.6
Mean	50	22.1	50	67.4	3.8
Overall mean[3]	510	24.1	389	65.1	4.4
Low volatiles B10138	8	10.5	8	78.0	7.6
Low volatiles B9304	8	12.3	8	38.0	3.1
High volatiles B0493	8	6.1	8	58.9	9.8
High volatiles B3615	12	9.2	12	284.6	52.4
White carrot B10720	8	9.4	8	129.1	14.2
Mean	44	9.5	44	132.9	20.6
Overall means[3]	564	22.7	433	76.8	7.1
Minimum single value		0.4		16.7	0.8
Maximum single value		53.5		384.2	82.9

[1] High Color 9, Long Imperator 58, Danvers 126, and Spartan Bonus varieties were grown in Wisconsin (1979-1982), Florida (1980-1982), California (1980-1982), Arizona (1981), and Illinois (1981-1982). Gold Pak, Nantes Half Long, Red Cored Chantenay, and Royal Chantenay varieties were grown in Illinois (1980), and the experimental genetic materials were grown in Wisconsin (1980-1981).

[2] N Number of analyses ignoring sampling design.

[3] Means of all varieties listed above.

Table II. Falcarinol and Falcarindiol Means by
Location, Year, and Variety

	Falcarinol	Falcarindiol
	mg/kg	mg/kg
Location		
Illinois (NRRC)	15.6[1]	75.1
Wisconsin	15.1	52.4
Florida	33.5	62.8
California	25.2	56.2
LSD[2]	5.0	8.8
Year		
1980	22.5	--
1981	25.9	65.8
1982	25.4	57.6
LSD	5.0	6.2
Variety		
High Color 9	12.1	46.9
Long Imperator 58	28.8	65.2
Danvers 126	27.9	57.4
Spartan Bonus	29.6	70.2
LSD	5.8	8.8

[1] Based on 1981 and 1982 only.

[2] Least significant difference (0.05 level)
between two means.

Table III. Falcarinol and Falcarindiol
Means Associated with the Interaction of
Location and Year[1]

Location	Year		
	1980	1981	1982
	Falcarinol mg/kg		
Wisconsin	18.0	27.2	21.9
Florida	13.4	40.5	23.7
California	13.8	32.8	29.6
LSD[2]= 8.6			
	Falcarindiol mg/kg		
Illinois	--	95.3	54.9
Wisconsin	--	56.8	48.1
Florida	--	56.9	68.8
California	--	54.0	58.4
LSD = 12.4			

[1] Each mean is for High Color 9, Long
Imperator 58, Danvers 126, and Spartan
Bonus varieties.

[2] Least significant difference (0.05 level)
between two means.

Table IV. Falcarinol and Falcarindiol Means by Variety and Location

Variety	Illinois	Wisconsin	Florida	California
		Falcarinol mg/kg[1]		
High Color 9	--	6.2	14.9	13.2
Long Imperator 58	--	22.3	37.1	29.8
Danvers 126	--	18.6	40.5	22.5
Spartan Bonus	--	13.3	41.5	34.8
LSD = 10.0				
		Falcarindiol mg/kg[2]		
High Color 9	49.6	69.6	56.8	48.8
Long Imperator 58	60.4	67.6	71.2	51.6
Danvers 126	81.6	90.0	74.8	54.0
Spartan Bonus	48.8	59.2	68.4	33.2
LSD = 16.8				

[1] 1980, 1981, 1982.

[2] 1981, 1982.

was improved by a factor of 2 when sample size was increased
from 4 to 18 carrots.

The means by location, year, and variety for four selected
commercial varieties are shown in Table II. The combination of
data for all years and varieties shows that the Florida location
produced the highest concentration of falcarinol. However,
location differences are dependent on year; the high value of
falcarinol occurred at a different location each year (Table III).
Table II also shows that falcarindiol concentration is highest
in those carrots grown in Illinois; however, Table III again
shows that the high toxicant level is in a different location
each year. Therefore, the significant effects of location in
Table II must be judged in the light of a significant
year-location interaction.

Tables II and III indicate that the levels of both toxicants
were highest in 1981. Perhaps these results account for variation
in resistance to rot that is observed in carrots from year to
year (6). The interaction of varieties with year was not
significant, suggesting that varietal differences tended to
remain the same from year to year.

An interaction of variety and location was observed for
falcarinol (Table IV). Long Imperator 58, Danvers 126, and
Spartan Bonus show considerable variation among locations, but
High Color 9 has the lowest values at all three locations.
High Color 9 has low levels of falcarindiol, whereas Danvers 126
consistently had high levels.

Sensory scores on a scale of 1 to 3 were tabulated by one
of the authors with a limited number of carrots for four sensory
evaluations: sweetness, harsh aftertaste, crispness, and
overall preference. There was no indication of association
between toxicant levels and sensory evaluations in a plot of
toxicants versus sensory evaluation. Therefore, it seems
highly probable that culinary quality can be improved without
increasing toxicant levels.

Literature Cited
1.   Crosby, D. G.; Aharonson, N. Tetrahedron 1967, 23, 465-472.
2.   Bentley, R. K.; Thaller, V. Chem. Commun. 1967, 439-440.
3.   Bohlmann, F.; Niedballa, V.; Rode, K. M. Chem. Ber. 1966,
      99, 3552-3558.
4.   Bentley, R. K.; Bahattacharjee, D.; Jones, E. R. H.;
      Thaller, V. J. Chem. Soc. C 1969, 685-688.
5.   Garrod, B.; Lewis, B. G. Trans. Br. Mycol. Soc. 1980, 75,
      166-169.
6.   Harding, V. K.; Heale, J. B. Ann. Appl. Biol. 1981, 99,
      375-383.
7.   Garrod, B.; Lewis, B. G.; Brittain, M. J.; Davies, W. P.
      New Phytol. 1982, 90, 99-108.

8.   Ho, A. K. S. Dept. Basic Sciences, University of Illinois
     College of Medicine, Peoria School of Medicine, Peoria,
     Illinois 61656, unpublished data, 1982.
9.   Wulf, L. W.; Nagel, C. W.; Branen, A. L. J. Agric. Food
     Chem. 1978, 26, 1390-1393.
10. Forrest, J. E.; Heacock, R. A. Lloydia 1972, 35, 440-449.
11. Fuhremann, T. W.; Lichtenstein, E. P. J. Agric. Food Chem.
     1979, 27, 87-91.
12. Surak, J. G. Proc. Fla. State Hort. Soc. 1978, 91, 256-258.
13. Yates, S. G.; England, R. E. J. Agric. Food Chem. 1982,
     30, 317-320.
14. Senti, F. R.; Rizek, R. L. Crop Soc. Am. Spec. Publ.,
     No. 5, 1974, 7-20.
15. Simon, P. W.; Peterson, C. E.; Lindsay, R. C. "Quality of
     Selected Fruits and Vegetables of North America"; Teranishi,
     R.; Barrera-Benitez, H., Eds.; ACS SYMPOSIUM SERIES,
     No. 170, ACS: Washington, D.C., 1981; p. 109-118.
16. Steel, R. G. D.; Torrie, J. H. "Principles and Procedures
     of Statistics," 2nd ed., McGraw-Hill Book Co., NY, 1980.

RECEIVED July 6, 1983

Ingestion of Pyrrolizidine Alkaloids: A Health Hazard of Global Proportions

JAMES N. ROITMAN

Natural Products Chemistry Research, Western Regional Research Center, Agricultural Research Service, U.S. Department of Agriculture, Berkeley, CA 94710

Pyrrolizidine alkaloids, about 200 of which have been identified, occur in a number of unrelated plant families distributed throughout the world. These alkaloids have been shown to be responsible for the long known hepatotoxicity in humans and animals associated with ingestion of certain plants. Because the onset of symptoms often occurs only after considerable time has elapsed (up to several years), it is likely that many, if not most, cases of pyrrolizidine alkaloid-caused liver damage are ascribed to other causes. The diverse physiological effects as well as the underlying mode of toxicity are presented. The chemical properties and analytical methods employed are summarized and the manner in which pyrrolizidine alkaloids enter the human food chain via contaminated foodstuff and the use of herbs is discussed as well as the nature of the problem in the U.S. today. Reasons for increasing consumption of herbal teas are suggested.

It was eighty years ago that Gilruth demonstrated by feeding experiments that tansy ragwort (Senecio jacobaea) was responsible for a disease of horses and cattle in New Zealand called Winton disease (1). Other feeding experiments established that certain species of Senecio (Compositae) were responsible for Pictou disease of cattle (Canada, 1906) (2), Molteno disease (Cape Colony, South Africa, 1904) (3), "dunsiekte" disease of horses (South Africa, 1918) (4), and "walking disease" of horses (northwestern Nebraska, 1929) (5). Feeding experiments with various species of Crotalaria (Leguminosae) established the etiology of several diseases of horses exhibiting symptoms similar to those caused by Senecio although the genera are unrelated botanically. Diseases known as "jaagsiekte" in S. Africa and "walkabout" in Australia were reproduced by feeding horses Crotalaria dura and C. retusa respectively (6,7). A number of plants in the family Boraginaceae were also demonstrated to cause assorted related diseases: Heliotropium species were responsible for liver dystrophy prevalent in central Asia during the period 1931-45 in man and domestic animals (8-12) as well as sheep poisoning in Australia (13); Trichodesma incanum was responsible for an Asian disease of horses and cattle, called "suiljuk" (14), Echium lycopsis caused sheep poisoning in Australia (13,15), and Amsinckia intermedia produced cirrhosis in horses and "hard liver disease" in cattle and pigs in the Pacific Northwest of the U.S. (16). Although the plants associated with these various, often lethal, diseases occur in three unrelated plant families, a common feature of all is their production of pyrrolizidine alkaloids. These have been shown to be capable of causing the physiological changes characteristic of the above-mentioned diseases although other plant constituents may play a role in exacerbating or mediating the effects of the alkaloids and may in part explain some of the inconsistencies observed in animal feeding experiments.

Chemistry of Pyrrolizidine Alkaloids

There are currently about 200 pyrrolizidine alkaloids known, most of which are mono- and di-esters of the saturated and 1,2-unsaturated amino-alcohols (commonly known as necines or necine bases) shown in Figure 1 (17a). Numerous toxicological studies on small laboratory animals have shown that acute and chronic toxicity are caused only by esterified 1,2-unsaturated necines although an unrelated per-acute syndrome, manifested by rapid mortality, can be induced by very large doses of saturated necine esters (17b,18). The structures of some representative pyrrolizidine alkaloids are shown in Figures 2 thru 4. The esterifying acids are highly branched and infrequently found elsewhere in nature. Although the structures are not especially complex, the number of asymmetric centers renders unequivocal structure determination difficult. Furthermore, mixtures of diastereomers and geometric isomers often coexist in plant extracts, and separation of these is laborious and involves special techniques. These problems confounded a number of the early chemical investigations especially since mixtures of the alkaloids often crystallize as if they were single substances.

An additional feature of pyrrolizidine alkaloids is that they often occur admixed with their N-oxides. The latter are highly water soluble and consequently are not extracted from aqueous solutions by the normal extraction procedures employed to isolate alkaloids. However total plant alkaloids may be 90% in the form of N-oxides, rendering meaningless any estimates of alkaloid content determined by normal extraction techniques. Chemical reducing agents added during isolation procedures rapidly convert N-oxides to the corresponding alkaloid bases allowing isolation from aqueous alkaline solution by solvent extraction (17c).

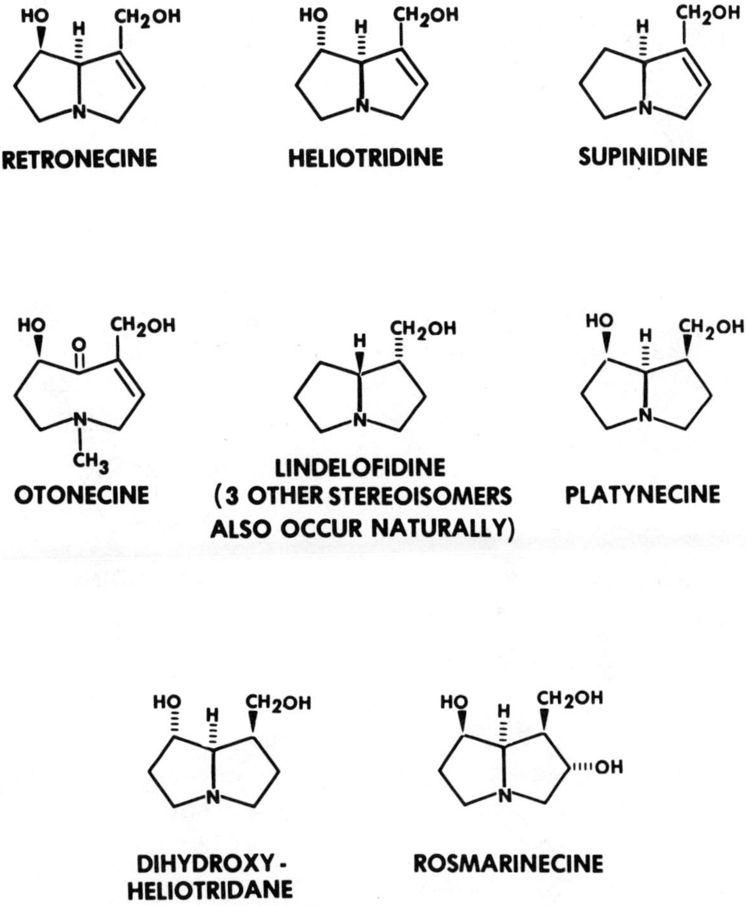

Figure 1. *Structures of necine bases, esters of which are hepatotoxic (retronecine, heliotridine, supinidine, otonecine) or nonhepatotoxic (platynecine, dihydroxyheliotridane, rosmarinecine, lindelofidine) pyrrolizidine alkaloids.*

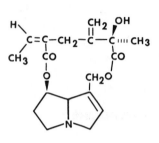

SENECIONINE

SENECIPHYLLINE

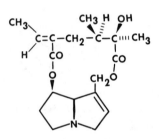

INTEGERRIMINE

SPARTIOIDINE

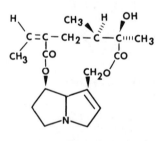

PLATYPHYLLINE

NEOPLATYPHYLLINE

Figure 2. Macrocyclic diester pyrrolizidine alkaloids.

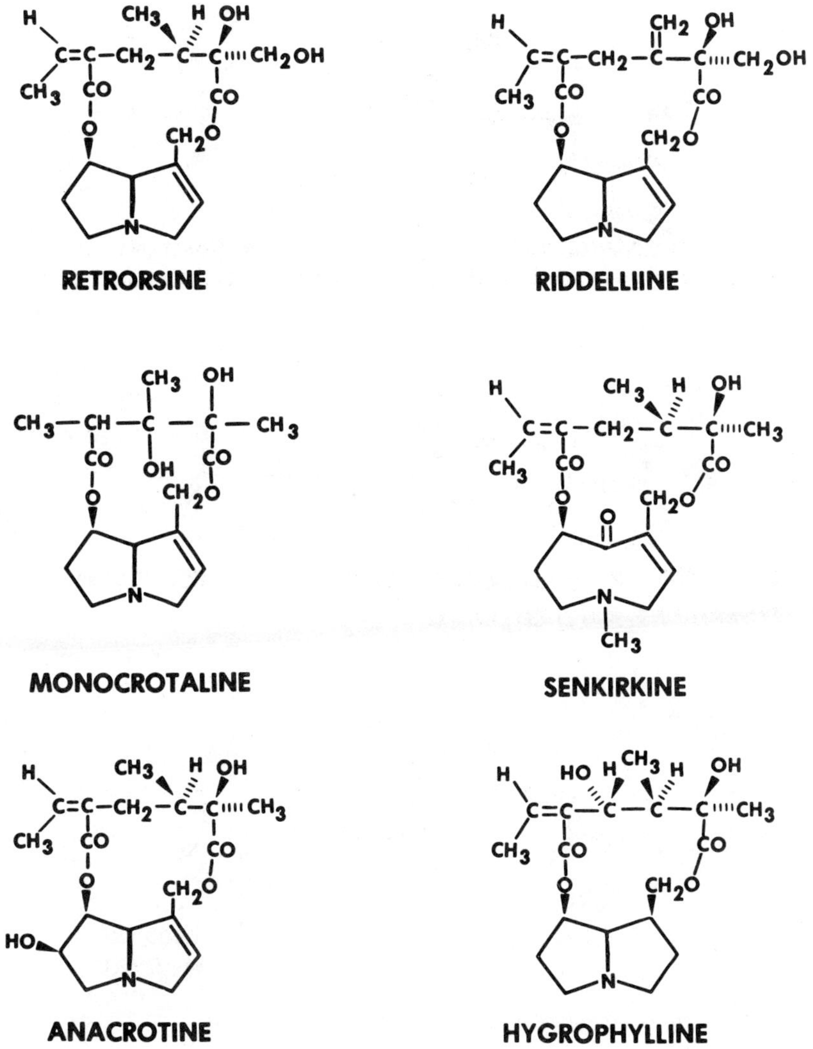

Figure 3. Macrocyclic diester pyrrolizidine alkaloids.

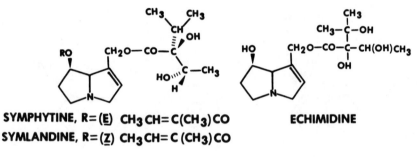

LYCOPSAMINE, R=H

7-ACETYL-LYCOPSAMINE, R=CH₃CO

INTERMEDINE, R=H

7-ACETYL-INTERMEDINE, R=CH₃CO

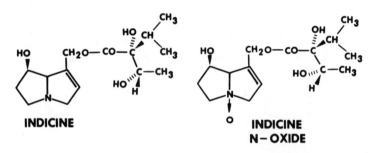

SYMPHYTINE, R=(E) CH₃CH=C(CH₃)CO

SYMLANDINE, R=(Z) CH₃CH=C(CH₃)CO

ECHIMIDINE

INDICINE

INDICINE
N-OXIDE

Figure 4. *Mono- and diester pyrrolizidine alkaloids and a pyrrolizidine N-oxide.*

The chemical stability of the pyrrolizidine alkaloids varies considerably with structural type and purity. The macrocyclic alkaloids such as senecionine, monocrotaline, and senkirkine are more stable than mono- and di-ester alkaloids such as lycopsamine and echimidine under normal storage conditions. This may be a result of steric inhibition of decomposition processes or the lack of crystallinity often characteristic of non-macrocyclic alkaloids; we have noticed that their decomposition seems to be enhanced and catalyzed by the presence of impurities. In some cases alkaloid levels in dried plant material are considerably lower than in fresh plant, an important factor to be considered when attempting to reproduce livestock poisoning experimentally by feeding dried plant material. Losses of up to 80% of the alkaloids upon drying of plant material have been reported, but this phenomenon varies greatly with the particular species and is probably caused by enzymes liberated during wilting (17c). Unless evidence to the contrary is available, crude alkaloid extracts, mixtures, and even pure non-crystalline alkaloids ought to be considered as having limited stability and stored at low temperature in the absence of air. Failure to appreciate possible alkaloid loss via decomposition during the course of a long term toxicological study could certainly lead to spurious results.

Analysis of Pyrrolizidine Alkaloids

Although gravimetric and titrimetric procedures have been used extensively to measure levels of pyrrolizidine alkaloids, these methods are subject to increasingly great errors when alkaloid levels are low. A much more specific analytical method based on formation of a characteristic purple color, which can be readily measured by ultraviolet spectroscopy, has been widely used (19,20). The color is formed by acid-catalyzed condensation of 4-(N,N-dimethylamino)-benzaldehyde (Ehrlich's reagent) with the pyrrole ring formed from the pyrrolizidine alkaloid by N-oxidation, acetylation, and subsequent Polonovski rearrangement (Scheme 1). The reaction sequence requires 1,2-unsaturation, and thus alkaloids lacking this double bond are not detected. But 1,2-unsaturation is also a structural prerequisite for hepatotoxicity; the colorimetric procedure therefore automatically excludes the non-toxic saturated alkaloids. Unfortunately it also gives negative results with seco alkaloids, such as senkirkine and other otonecine based alkaloids, whose physiological properties are largely unknown.

Tlc. We have used a modification of the colorimetric method to detect pyrrolizidine alkaloids on thin layer chromatograms. Alkaloid spots when sprayed with o-chloranil are converted directly to the pyrrole derivatives which then can be detected by spraying with Ehrlich's reagent (21). As expected, seco and saturated alkaloids give negative results.

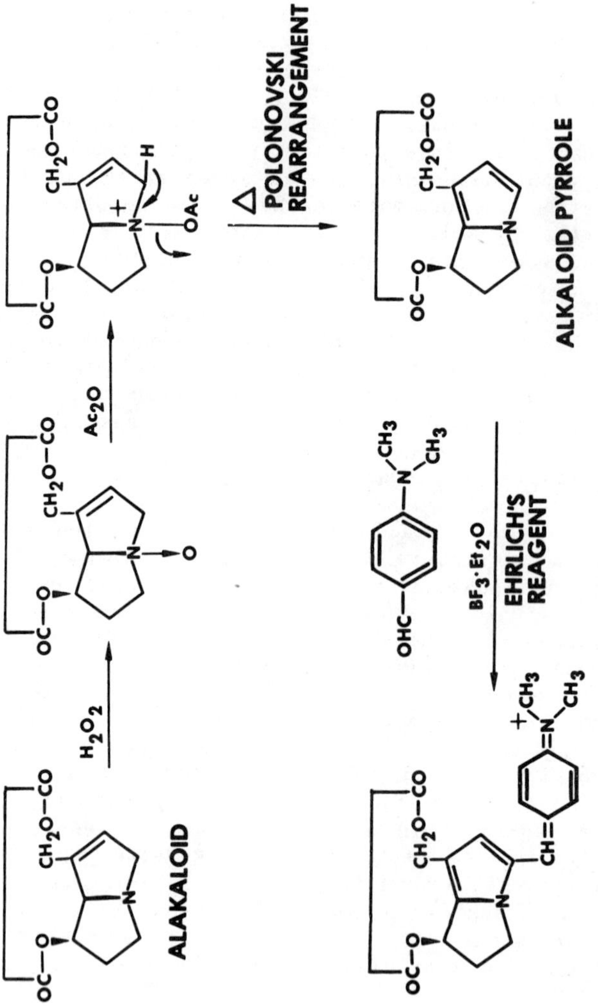

Scheme 1. Colorimetric determination of pyrrolizidine alkaloids.

Pmr. Proton magnetic resonance (pmr) spectroscopy provides a reliable analysis of pyrrolizidine alkaloids if sufficient quantities of alkaloid ($>$ 1 mg) are present. The amount of total alkaloid is estimated by comparison of the area of the vinyl proton (H2) signal (present in all 1,2-unsaturated and seco alkaloids) with that of an added internal standard (p-dinitrobenzene) (22). In certain fortuitous instances the relative amounts of individual alkaloids may be simultaneously determined by integration of other diagnostic signals.

Hplc. High pressure liquid chromatography (hplc), particularly with reverse-phase columns, is very useful in the analysis of pyrrolizidine alkaloid mixtures and can be used to isolate pure alkaloids on a preparative scale (23-27). However, because ultraviolet detection is used and the alkaloids have an absorption maximum near 220 nm, choice of solvents is limited and small amounts of impurities with large extinction coefficients can give very misleading profiles. With current hplc instrumentation, detection of microgram quantities of pyrrolizidine alkaloids is practical. Furthermore separations of alkaloids differing in two hydrogen atoms at C13 (e.g., senecionine vs. seneciphylline or retrorsine vs. riddelliine, Figure 2) are readily achieved; such separations have been very difficult in the past necessitating countercurrent distribution or specialized partition chromatography (27). It has been impossible, however, to separate the C15-C20 double bond isomers which often co-occur naturally (e.g., senecionine vs. integerrimine or seneciphylline vs. spartioidine, Figure 2). Nor have any reports of separation of diastereomeric pyrrolizidines by hplc appeared, although they, too, frequently occur as mixtures in plant extracts. We have tried unsuccessfully to separate the diastereomeric alkaloids lycopsamine and intermedine (Figure 4) by reverse phase hplc.

Gc. Gas chromatography (gc) has been used for pyrrolizidine alkaloid analysis although most of the work has been qualitative in nature. Thermal instability coupled with low volatility and high polarity make special precautions such as all glass systems necessary (28). Because char was reported at the front of the columns, necessitating frequent replacement of some of the packing material, it is clear that a considerable portion of the injected sample never reached the detector. The technique is capable of resolving E and Z isomers of macrocyclic diester alkaloids but is less successful with mixtures of diastereomers such as lycopsamine and intermedine (Figure 4). A sensitive method for total alkaloid analysis, based on electron capture gc of fluorinated esters of retronecine, has been reported (29). Alkaloid mixtures are hydrolyzed; then the basic amino-alcohol portion (necine) is acylated with a fluorinated acid derivative. The disadvantage of this technique is that no information regarding the individual alkaloids can be obtained and further that it may not be applicable to <u>seco</u> alkaloids, since otonecine is substantially destroyed by the alkaline hydrolytic conditions (<u>30</u>).

We have recently explored the application of glass capillary gc to trimethylsilyl (tms) ether derivatives of pyrrolizidine alkaloids. The high resolution capabilities of capillary columns offered promise in separating the complex and closely related alkaloid mixtures often encountered in plant extracts. The gc trace shown in Figure 5 illustrates the application of a capillary system to a mixture of tms-ethers of the 12 pure macrocyclic di-ester alkaloids shown in Figures 2 and 3.

The compounds were eluted from the non-polar column with good peak shape and resolution, and when checked by a combined gc-mass spectroscopy (gc-ms) experiment gave molecular ions corresponding to the expected per-silylated ethers. Both flame ionization (FI) and nitrogen-phosphorus (NP) detectors permit facile detection of alkaloids down to levels of 1 ng or less; the selective NP detector has as its major advantages over FI increased sensitivity (5-10 times) and the ability to suppress peaks of non-nitrogenous impurities which hamper analyses at high sensitivity. Separation of closely related compounds was successful, but some problems were encountered with several alkaloids, notably jaconine and jacobine (Figure 6) each of which gave several signals but not reproducibly. The chlorohydrin moiety of jaconine and the epoxide of jacobine are chemically labile and apparently undergo various transformations during preparation of the tms ethers.

We have since applied this technique to mixtures of alkaloids isolated from herbal teas. A gc trace of comfrey root alkaloids is shown in Figure 7. The alkaloids were identified after comparing a gc-ms run with the reported alkaloid contents of comfrey (<u>31</u>). Although the geometric isomers symphytine and symlandine (Figure 4) were incompletely resolved, the epimers lycopsamine and intermedine and their 7-acetates were clearly separated. As a further illustration of the resolution of capillary gc we prepared a tms derivative of indicine (another epimer of lycopsamine (Figure 4)), and showed by co-injection with lycopsamine and intermedine tms ethers that all three diastereomers were cleanly separated.

<u>Ms</u>. Mass spectroscopy has been used to characterize pyrrolizidine alkaloids since the mid 1960's and the major fragmentation patterns have been determined (<u>32-34</u>). We have found that the rather low-intensity molecular ions observed in electron impact (EI) spectra can be dramatically enhanced by use of chemical ionization (isobutane) where intense ions corresponding to the molecular ion plus hydrogen are observed. The EI and CI spectra of lycopsamine shown in Figure 8 illustrate this phenomenon.

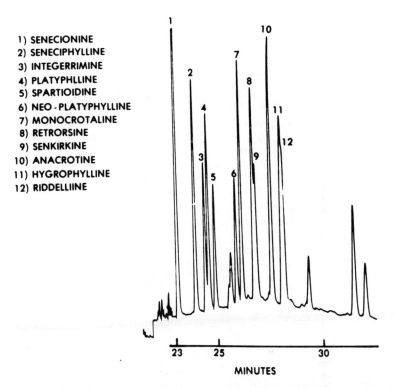

1) SENECIONINE
2) SENECIPHYLLINE
3) INTEGERRIMINE
4) PLATYPHLLINE
5) SPARTIOIDINE
6) NEO - PLATYPHYLLINE
7) MONOCROTALINE
8) RETRORSINE
9) SENKIRKINE
10) ANACROTINE
11) HYGROPHYLLINE
12) RIDDELLIINE

Figure 5. Gas chromatogram of 12 pyrrolizidine alkaloid TMS ethers. Conditions: 0.32 mm × 25 mm, wall-coated (SE52) open tubular glass capillary; flame ionization detector; carrier gas: helium, flow 28 cm/s; temperature program: 60– 180 °C at 30 °C/min; 180–325 °C at 5 °C/min.

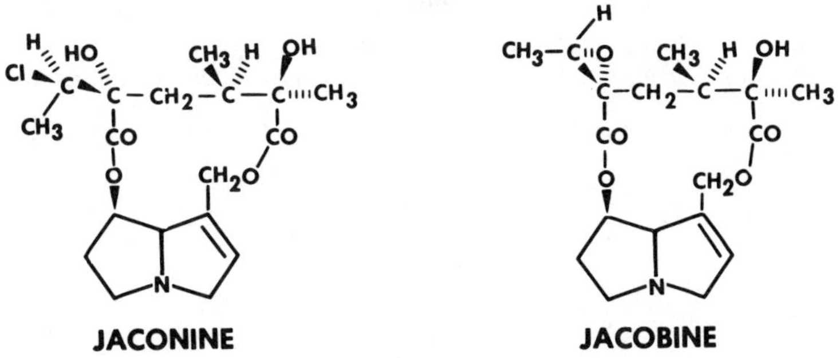

JACONINE

JACOBINE

Figure 6. Structures of jaconine and jacobine.

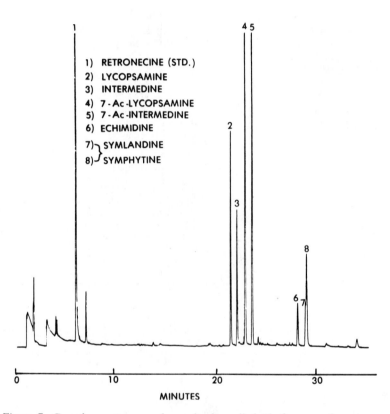

1) RETRONECINE (STD.)
2) LYCOPSAMINE
3) INTERMEDINE
4) 7-Ac-LYCOPSAMINE
5) 7-Ac-INTERMEDINE
6) ECHIMIDINE
7) ⌐ SYMLANDINE
8) ⌙ SYMPHYTINE

MINUTES

Figure 7. Gas chromatogram of pyrrolizidine alkaloids from comfrey root tea. Nitrogen–phosphorus selective detector; all other conditions identical to those listed in Figure 5.

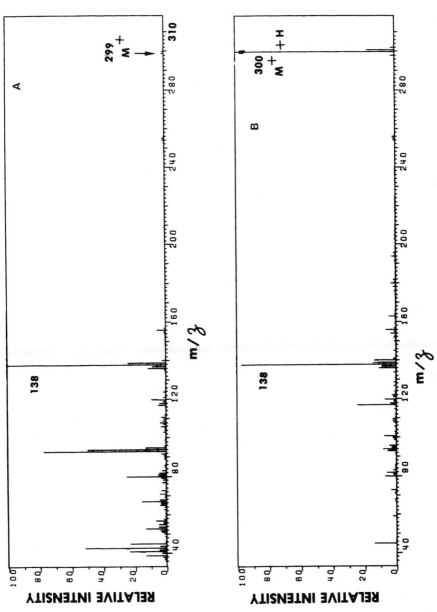

Figure 8. Mass spectra of lycopsamine; electron impact (a); chemical ionization (isobutane) (b).

Toxic Actions of Pyrrolizidine Alkaloids

Many studies have been undertaken to elaborate the toxic effects of pyrrolizidine alkaloids by feeding the alkaloids, or plants which contain them, to a variety of animals; several extensive reviews have appeared (17,18,35). In Table I are listed the affected organs and the animal species in which the observations

Table I. Animal Species and Organs Affected by Pyrrolizidine Alkaloids

Species	Liver	Lung	Kidney	Heart	Pancreas	Gastric mucosa	Muscle
man	+						
monkey	+	+	+	+			
horse	+	+	+				
pig	+	+	+		+	+	
sheep	+	+	+				
goat	+	+					
cattle	+	+					
dog	+						
mouse	+		+				
rat	+	+		+		+	
chicken	+	+	+				+
turkey	+	+					+

have been made. The sensitivity to alkaloid toxicity varies greatly among the various species as do the primary sites of damage. Furthermore even within a single species the nature of the toxic effect as well as the organ affected can be altered by changing the dose rate and span.

The comparative susceptibilities of various animal species to chronic pyrrolizidine alkaloid poisoning as determined by plant feeding experiments are shown in Table II. The relative insensi-

Table II. Susceptibility of Animals to Pyrrolizidine Alkaloid Toxicity.*

Animal	Relative Amount of Plant Necessary to Cause Chronic Poisoning	Tolerance to Poisoning
sheep (goat)	200	high
mouse	150	
rat	50	
cattle (horse)	14	
chicken	5	
pig	1	low

* Data were drawn from reference 36.

tivity of sheep and goats probably lies in their ability (via ruminal micro-organisms) to convert the alkaloids to nontoxic metabolites (17d,37). Where man might lie in such a ranking is presently unknown although, based on reported human poisoning incidents, it may be inferred that he would appear in the lower part of Table II.

As can be seen from Table I, the most commonly affected organ is the liver followed closely by the lungs. The effects on other organs have been less frequently observed and appear to be more species specific. The possibility that plant constituents other than alkaloids influence the course of toxic effects cannot be overlooked, especially when attempts to evaluate the significance of diverse feeding experiments are made.

Liver Toxicity. Three major effects of pyrrolizidine alkaloids on the liver are commonly observed in many animals: 1) acute necrosis (death of liver cells), 2) megalocytosis (formation of greatly enlarged cells), and 3) veno-occlusive disease (blockage of hepatic veins) (17,18,35,36). The first of these is the result of relatively large doses of alkaloids and is manifested by extensive death of liver parenchymal cells, which occurs rapidly and results in hemorrhage of the liver and death. Animals surviving acute necrosis go on to develop veno-occlusive disease, a vascular lesion marked by progressive formation of fibrous connective tissue in the hepatic veins, culminating in their occlusion. The resulting blockage of blood flow out of the liver results in portal hypertension, ascites, and engorgement of the liver (18). When low doses of alkaloids are administered over long periods of time the livers of numerous animals exhibit many greatly enlarged cells (megalocytes). These are thought to be a result of the cells' inability to divide while DNA synthesis continues. Ultimately the number of these abnormal cells becomes so great that liver failure results; these megalocytes are incapable of performing normal liver functions (17,18).

Lung Toxicity. The changes which occur in the lungs of rats and monkeys parallel those of veno-occlusive disease in the liver: attack on endothelial cells resulting in destruction of the capillary bed and consequent pulmonary vascular failure often accompanied by subsequent hypertrophy of the right heart (18,38, 39). Although lung damage is usually accompanied by liver damage some experiments with rats have produced the lung-heart lesions with no discernable liver damage (38). The deleterious effects seen in the lungs of livestock are quite different from the vascular lesions observed in rats and monkeys and are characterized by interstitial pneumonia resulting from edema, fibrosis, epithelialization, and emphysema (40).

Carcinogenicity. The carcinogenicity of pyrrolizidine alkaloids has been debated since it was first reported, in part because of

disagreements in characterization of the lesions (17,18,41). Many
of the earlier experiments were marred by high death rates of the
test animals due to liver failure as well as the possible contamination of the plant material with carcinogenic mycotoxins (41).
It has since become clear that low dose rates are necessary and
that a long period of latency exists. Relatively few pyrrolizidine alkaloids have been tested for carcinogenicity, but all the
hepatotoxic ones thus far examined have also been shown to be
carcinogenic; from the limited data available it seems that the
carcinogenic activity of the individual alkaloids parallels their
mutagenic behavior but not their relative hepatotoxicities (41).
It is presently believed that pyrrolizidine alkaloids capable of
exhibiting hepatotoxicity should also be considered carcinogenic
but that carcinogenicity overall is weak (41). This latter feature is supported, albeit in a negative way, by the failure to
find abnormal rates of liver cancer in human populations exposed
to pyrrolizidine alkaloids in food or herb teas although the
characteristic signs of liver toxicity associated with pyrrolizidine alkaloids have been observed. Carcinogenicity has not been
observed in livestock either, although this may be related to the
rather young age at which the animals are slaughtered relative to
their lifespans.

Other Effects. Additional effects of pyrrolizidine alkaloids have
also been reported; they can act as teratogens and abortifacients
(42, 49), mutagens (17e,18) and cause chromosome damage (17f,18,
50). Chromosome damage has been observed in the blood of humans
suffering from pyrrolizidine-alkaloid-induced veno-occlusive disease (51). The alkaloids also show anti-tumor properties, doubtless related to their antimitotic effects (52,53). Clinical
testing of the N-oxide of indicine (Figure 4) is currently underway in the United States, and although significant remissions
have been achieved with leukemia patients, the problem of concom-
mitant liver damage makes its future use unlikely (54,55).

Mechanism of Pyrrolizidine Toxicity

It was first suggested that the toxic effects of pyrrolizidine alkaloids may be due to the ability of the allylic esters to
undergo nucleophilic attack by cell constituents thereby alkylating them (56). However the alkaloids are not readily alkylated
in vitro and are no longer considered to be the actual active
toxins. But oxidation of 1,2-unsaturated pyrrolizidine alkaloids to form pyrroles has been demonstrated by incubation of
pyrrolizidine alkaloids in vitro with liver microsomal enzymes
from numerous animal species (57,58). Furthermore the presence
of these pyrroles can be detected in vivo in rat livers, and the
amounts present one hour after administration of alkaloid corre-
late well with the relative toxicities of a number of individual
alkaloids (58). Studies with the pyrrolic alkaloids have shown

them to be not only very reactive alkylating agents but also capable of alkylation at both ester groups (59,60). The ability to
act as bifunctional alkylating agents suggests that crosslinking
of nucleic acids may account for some of the toxic effects, especially antimitosis (18).

Additional studies have shown that the oxidation of alkaloid
to its N-oxide occurs and competes with pyrrole formation.   N-
oxides when administered intravenously to rats or when treated
with liver microsomal enzymes are not converted to pyrroles. Hence
they are non-toxic in the liver, and, by their highly hydrophilic
nature, provide a pathway for detoxification. When administered
orally to rats and sheep however, N-oxides are converted in the
rumen (sheep) or gut (rats) to the parent alkaloids which are
then metabolized in the liver causing the normal toxic sequelae.
The toxicity (or lack thereof) of the pyrrolizidine N-oxides depends on whether or not they are reduced in vivo before reaching
the liver (61).   After intravenous administration of indicine
N-oxide to human cancer patients, free alkaloid has been detected
in the blood and subsequent liver damage has been observed (55).

Another important process occurring concommitantly with pyrrole formation and N-oxidation is hydrolysis of the ester groups.
If this occurs before pyrrole formation, the necine formed, being
highly water soluble is likely to be rapidly excreted.   And unlike the parent alkaloids, unesterified necine bases do not form
pyrroles when treated in vitro with liver microsomal enzymes nor
are they metabolized to pyrroles in vivo (58,62).   On the other
hand, if ester hydrolysis occurs after the alkaloid has been converted to its pyrrolic metabolite the resulting necine pyrrole is
still capable of producing toxicity.   These findings are summarized in Scheme 2.   That hydrolysis prior to oxidation results in
detoxification is supported by experiments in which esterase-
activating drugs administered prior to alkaloid dosing reduced
toxicity dramatically while esterase inhibitors increased the
toxic effects (62).   Analogous experiments aimed at the liver
microsomal enzyme system have also been performed, but the results
are not completely consistent and seem to depend very much on the
particular alkaloid employed.

Other significant experiments have corroborated the metabolic
pyrrole hypothesis. When cells other than those capable of microsomal oxidation (i.e., cells other than liver) were incubated with
pyrrolizidine alkaloids toxicity was not observed. However when
these cells were exposed to synthetically prepared necine pyrroles, severe mitotic inhibition was observed.   The chemical
stability of the pyrrolic alkaloids is much less than that of the
corresponding necine pyrroles and the former have not been detected in vivo.   However when synthetic monocrotaline pyrrole was
injected into the mesenteric vein of rats it produced the lesions
typical of pyrrolizidine alkaloid poisoning: portal vascular
degeneration, hepatic necrosis, and inhibition of hepatocyte
mitosis (63,64).   Injected into the jugular veins of rats and dogs

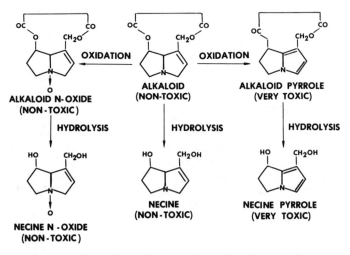

Scheme 2. Metabolism of pyrrolizidine alkaloids in the liver.

the same substance caused severe vascular lesions in the lung similar to the effects seen when monocrotaline itself was administered (64,65).

Because of its increased chemical stability, retronecine pyrrole has been detected in the liver, blood, and urine of rats treated with monocrotaline (66). When synthetic retronecine pyrrole was injected subcutaneously into rats, ulceration and hemorrhage of the stomach wall was observed as well as inhibition of liver parenchymal cell mitosis; furthermore the production of cancerous lesions at the site of injection was high (67-69).

Structure Activity Relationship. Attempts to relate alkaloid structure to toxicity have been based on studies with rats in which single doses of alkaloids were administered via intraperitoneal or intravenous injection. The objective of the early studies was establishment of median lethal doses (LD_{50}) based on 3-day or 7-day survival times (17g). This procedure was expanded to include the determination of the minimum dose of many alkaloids necessary to cause: 1) acute toxicity, 2) chronic megalocytosis and 3) lung lesions (70). Another approach has employed the measurement of pyrrole levels in the liver two hours after administration of alkaloids, semisynthetic alkaloids, and synthetic analogs (58,62).

The results may be summarized as follows: Necine bases and alkaloids of saturated necine bases are non-toxic; esters of the monohydroxy-necine, supinidine, are only slightly toxic; monoesters of dihydroxy-necines are slightly more toxic and diesters are considerably more so; macrocyclic diester alkaloids are the most toxic. Necine bases esterified synthetically with n-aliphatic acids are non-toxic indicating that branching of the acid side chain is required for toxicity (58,62,70). Relative toxicities also appear to be inversely related to water solubilities of the alkaloids.

These observations can be accommodated by the pyrrole hypothesis (Scheme 2). Necines are not converted to pyrroles and hence are non-toxic; the esters of supinidine can form pyrroles but these are not bifunctional alkylating agents. Monoesters of diol necines form pyrroles which are weak bifunctional alkylating agents whereas diesters form highly reactive ones. Macrocyclic diesters have fairly rigid conformations which may hinder their hydrolysis but not their conversion to pyrroles. The requirement for branched side chains can also be explained by retardation of hydrolysis. High water solubility considerably lowers the amount of alkaloid reaching the necessary (lipophilic) enzyme sites for pyrrole conversion.

It must however be kept in mind that the above generalizations are based on only one species of test animal (rat), single rather than multiple doses, and intraperitoneal and intravenous rather than oral administration. Extrapolation to other species receiving multiple doses orally may be highly misleading. And

there are many gaps in the data because of the lack of pure alkaloids for testing. The role of the seco alkaloids is largely
unknown; although their carcinogenicity has been demonstrated,
liver or other organ toxicity has seldom been reported (41,71).

Because pyrrolizidine alkaloids require metabolic activation
to exhibit their toxic effects, characterization of the problem
is extremely complex and the observed effects may depend on many
factors such as: 1) the species of animal, 2) the status of the
individual animal's metabolizing enzymes, 3) synergistic or antag-
onistic influences of other foods taken, 4) structure of individual alkaloids, 5) dose-time relationships. One of the most
vexing problems is that visible evidence of organ damage is often
absent for very long periods and finally appears only months after
administration of alkaloid has ceased. If the toxicity is in
fact caused by pyrrole derivatives and they are highly reactive
as had been observed, one would expect the toxic effects to be
readily expressed. At present there is no explanation for this
long delay period.

Human Poisoning by Pyrrolizidine Alkaloids

Humans have been poisoned by pyrrolizidine alkaloids in many
areas of the world, sometimes massively; furthermore it is likely
that the reports in the literature are but a fraction of those
which have occurred. The problem was first recognized in South
Africa in 1920 and was traced to bread contaminated with seed of a
Senecio species (72). Subsequently a large number of cases were
seen in Jamaica and associated with consumption of so-called "bush
teas" consumed regularly by adults and given medicinally to children (73,74). Further study in Jamaica resulted in a complete
clinical description including collagenous occlusion of small
branches of the hepatic venous system; the disease was named
veno-occlusive disease (75,76). Of the patients affected 50%
recovered from the acute stages, 20% died, and the remainder prog-
ressed to a chronic form of the disease; one third of these
patients subsequently died of cirrhotic liver failure and the
other two thirds recovered (77). The cirrhosis was atypical and
recognizable to pathologists because it was largely non-portal;
this type of cirrhosis was present in one third of the total
cirrhotic livers seen in Jamaica at autopsy in 1961 (78). Crotalaria species were implicated in the Jamaican poisonings.

Other cases of poisoning, reported in Central Asia in 1952
and 1965, have been attributed to species of Heliotropium;
victims suffered ascites and hepatosplenomegaly one year after
acute intoxication (10,11). A more recent outbreak occurred in
central India caused by cereal grain contaminated with Crotalaria
seeds; of the 67 cases seen in the four affected villages, 42%
were fatal (79). Finally a massive outbreak of the disease was
observed in Afghanistan in the early 1970's (80). A severe
drought in 1970-72 caused a serious food shortage in an area of

35000 inhabitants; by 1974 cases of ascites began to appear with fatality 3-9 months later being normal. Examination of 7200 residents in 1976 showed one quarter to have evidence of liver disease, eventually traced to bread made from flour contaminated with Heliotropium seeds (80).

A few other cases of pyrrolizidine alkaloid poisoning have been traced to consumption of herbal teas. A woman in Britain suffering from severe veno-occlusive disease, traced to a locally purchased herb tea, died of liver failure although surgery to alleviate the condition had been performed; the identity of the tea could not be determined but it was shown to contain pyrrolizidine alkaloids (81). An Ecuadorian woman upon seeking advice from a local herbalist was given 7 herbal teas, one of which was later identified as Crotalaria juncea. Several months later she suffered abdominal distension and was diagnosed as having portal hypertension due to cirrhosis; subsequent diagnosis in the United States, including liver biopsies, revealed veno-occlusive disease, and after a successful portocaval shunt operation she recovered completely (82). Two additional cases of veno-occlusive disease, one of which was fatal, were observed in young children from the Mexican-American population of Arizona (83,84). They resulted from administration of a medicinal tea known as "gordolobo yerba" shown to be Senecio longilobus, a range plant well known for its toxicity to livestock.

The effects of pyrrolizidine alkaloid poisoning on humans are similar to the acute toxicity observed in rats and other animals, namely ascites, liver cell necrosis, and fibrotic occlusion of the hepatic venous system. However the effects of chronic poisoning are unclear. The available evidence suggests that a type of cirrhosis results; the commonly observed chronic effect in many animals, megalocytosis, has never been observed in human victims. The effects of repeated exposure to small doses have never been reported, but this does not mean that there are none. There are a number of reasons for lack of information on this important subject which are related to the time necessary to develop symptoms. In order to be reported, the association between the etiological factor and the symptoms must be established; this is possible when symptoms appear rapidly, but much less likely after considerable time has elapsed. Thus even the acute poisonings with pyrrolizidine alkaloids have been observed only because outbreaks were large or astute medical observation detected the unusual effects. Furthermore in many non-industrialized areas of the world medical care is inadequate, contaminated food supplies, disease, and malnutrition are prevalent, and use of herbal medicine is widespread. Chronic pyrrolizidine poisoning is likely to escape detection under such circumstances and will doubtless continue to be a problem in Third World countries.

Sources of Pyrrolizidine Alkaloid Poisoning in the United States.

The methods by which pyrrolizidine alkaloid ingestion may occur in the United States are, as in the rest of the world, basically of two types, one involving contaminated foodstuffs, the other by consumption of herbal teas. Contamination of food may occur if seeds of pyrrolizidine-bearing plants are accidentally included in grain crops. Thus far no reports of contaminated grain have appeared in the U.S., but grain crops are grown in areas where pyrrolizidine-containing weeds grow at the edges of and invade the fields. Thorough grain inspections in suspect areas could better define the potential extent of the hazard. Screening procedures and weed control measures could then be used to eliminate the problem. For example, producers are now penalized if Crotalaria seeds are found in their soybean crop (85).

The other major route of food contamination is by means of intermediary animals. When bees forage on plants containing pyrrolizidine alkaloids they transmit the alkaloids to their honey (86-88). Honey from bees foraging on Senecio jacobaea in Oregon was found to contain from 1-4 ppm of pyrrolizidine alkaloids (86,87). Perhaps more disturbing is the finding that cows and goats feeding on Senecio jacobaea transfer alkaloids into their milk (89,90). The current practice of pooling milk from a number of different areas doubtless reduces the hazard, but in those cases where milk is not blended (e.g., individuals producing milk for their own consumption) the risk is substantially greater. Unfortunately, little is known about what proportion of the alkaloids ingested by a grazing animal passes into its milk, what role structural differences of the alkaloids play in that distribution, and whether or not as yet undetected toxic metabolites may be present as well.

The possibility that pyrrolizidine alkaloids or some toxic metabolites may be present in muscle and organ meats has also been raised. The likelihood of finding intact alkaloids is negligible, although some sort of bound metabolite may certainly occur.

Assessment of risks due to food contamination by pyrrolizidine alkaloids is made difficult not only by the many complex toxicological effects as yet unexplained, but also lack of information about the plant sources of the pyrrolizidine alkaloids. Although pyrrolizidine alkaloids have been found in 11 plant families and are wider spread botanically than was previously thought, they have been found most often in three families: Leguminosae (genus Crotalaria), Boraginaceae (all members thus far examined) and Compositae (tribes Eupatoriae and Senecionae) (17, 91). The potential number of pyrrolizidine-alkaloid-bearing plants has been estimated at 6000 (about 3% of the world's flowering plants) (91). Of these the genus Senecio alone accounts for an estimated 1200 species worldwide over 100 of which can be found in the U.S. (92). The genus Crotalaria is found in many tropical areas of the world, but grows well in temperate regions,

including the southern U.S. where a number of species were introduced as nitrogen-fixing crops before it was known that they
contained pyrrolizidine alkaloids. There are many species of
the Boraginaceae which grow in the U.S., more than 150 in California alone (93). Of the potential plant species from which
pyrrolizidines may be expected only ca. 350 (5%) have been
investigated chemically. In the past chemical investigations
were initiated only after outbreaks of human or animal poisonings; prior knowledge of the chemical composition of suspect
plants would aid in preventing poisonings in the future.

Although botanic information on any of the known or suspect
species is available, it is often limited to morphological description and the geographical limits wherein the plant may be
found. The density of the plant within the geographic boundaries
is usually unrecorded or unknown as are changes in geographic
boundaries. It would certainly be prudent to conduct botanic
inventories in areas of grain, milk, and honey production to identify plants known or suspect of containing pyrrolizidine alkaloids. The U.S. Department of Agriculture in cooperation with the
U.S. Food and Drug Administration has begun efforts in this direction. The amounts of pyrrolizidine alkaloids in a number of
species (including Senecio, Crotalaria and Amsinckia) are being
determined monthly for several years at different locations in
order to determine the effects of climate, soil, weather patterns, and stage of growth. Although the study is not yet completed, some striking variations have been observed, including a
great variability in alkaloid content for the species Senecio
riddellii, a plant common in the arid rangeland of the American
southwest (94). Examination of food samples collected in areas
having high densities of pyrrolizidine containing plants has
recently begun.

Herbal Teas and Medicines

Because of the broad botanic and geographical distribution of
pyrrolizidine alkaloid-containing plants quite a number of them
have found use as herbal remedies. Their botanic distribution
suggests that herbs in the families Boraginaceae, Compositae
(tribes Eupatoriae and Senecionae) or Leguminosae (genus Crotalaria) are apt to contain pyrrolizidine alkaloids. A number of
herbs currently sold in U.S. fall into these suspect groups;
they are listed in Table III with their common names, Latin
binomials, and whether or not pyrrolizidine alkaloids have been
reported. This list is certainly incomplete since no attempt to
include the special plants used by various close-knit ethnic
groups was made. (An exception is "gordolobo yerba" used in the
American southwest by the Mexican-American population and included
because its use has resulted in known human poisoning incidents
(83,84).)

Table III. Herbal Teas Available in the U.S. in which the
Presence of Pyrrolizidine Alkaloids is Suspected or Proven.

Common Name	Latin Binomial	Alkaloids	Literature
	Boraginaceae:		
Borage	Borago officinalis	+	95
Lungwort	Pulmonaria spp.	+	95
Comfrey	Symphytum officinale	+	95–101
Comfrey	S. asperum	+	96,99,102,103
Russian Comfrey	S. X uplandicum	+	31,96,104
	Compositae: (Senecionae)		
Coltsfoot	Tussilago farfara	+	105,106
Fireweed	Erechtites hieracifolia	+	107,108
Gordolobo Yerba	Senecio longilobus	+	109–113
Life Root Plant	S. aureus	+	110,114
	(Eupatoriae)		
Gravel Plant	Eupatorium purpureum	+	115
Boneset	E. perfoliatum	?	--

Life Root Plant. Life root plant (Senecio aureus), also known
under the common names golden groundsel, squaw weed, and golden
senecio, was used originally by Catawba Indian women to reduce
the pains of childbirth and hasten labor (116). According to
another source, it is a "most useful plant..... employed for em-
menogogue, diuretic, pectoral and astringent qualities and as
treatment for the first stages of consumption" (117a). The plant
is reported to contain senecionine as a result of investigations
by Manske in the infancy of chemical studies on pyrrolizidine
alkaloids in the 1930's and has not been investigated since for
alkaloids (110,114).
     We have recently examined a sample of life root plant pur-
chased in San Francisco and found, rather than senecionine, its
C15–C20 double bond isomer, integerrimine, (Figure 2) in small
amount. However the major alkaloids were a series of seco alkaloids, doronine, florosenine, floridanine and otosenine, which,
with the exception of otosenine, have been rarely observed previously (91). All were isolated as single substances by chromatography and characterized by nmr and ms. The structures of the
alkaloids are shown in Figure 9. The toxicological properties
of the seco-alkaloids are largely unknown because their rarity
has precluded much biological evaluation. Although thus far
hepatotoxicity has been demonstrated in very young rats only,
carcinogenicity has been shown and in vitro incubation of liver
enzymes with seco-alkaloids leads to pyrrole formation presumably
via N-demethylation followed by ring closure and oxidation (or
elimination) (41,71,118–121).

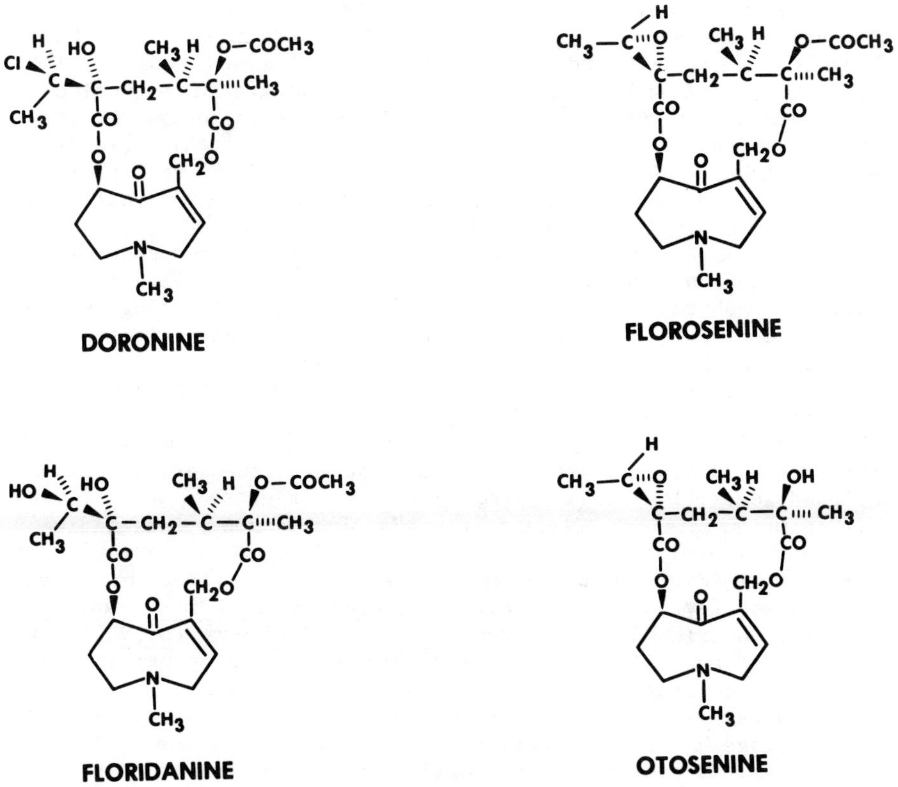

Figure 9. *Secopyrrolizidine alkaloids isolated from life root plant* (Senecio aureus).

Comfrey. Comfrey (Symphytum spp.) has been used since the time
of the Greeks for a great number of medicinal purposes (117b,
122a). One of the most prominent uses has been to promote healing
of broken bones and reduce swelling; this effect has been documented and is apparently caused by the allantoin present. The
action of allantoin may also explain the popularity of comfrey
as a treatment for bleeding of many sorts, both external and
internal (stomach, lungs, bowels). Because it contains a large
amount of mucilage, it has been used often for intestinal problems
(diarrhea, dysentery) as an emollient. Additional uses have
been as a demulcent and expectorant for colds and coughs. The
herb, both root and leaf, remain popular and are often included
as components of the numerous herbal mixtures sold today. Comfrey
appears to have assumed the attributes of a panacea. A single
modern herbal book (123), sold commonly in health food stores,
recommends the use of comfrey to alleviate some 47 ailments
(including allergies, anemia, emphysema, and diabetes) and affected body organs (including bladder, lungs, kidneys, and pancreas).
     A number of recent studies of the pyrrolizidine alkaloids in
various Symphytum species have succeeded in characterizing twelve
mono- and di-ester alkaloids of retronecine and heliotridine (31,
95-104). We have examined twelve samples each of comfrey root and
leaf sold as herbs in the U.S. As determined by nmr, the total
alkaloid content of the leaf samples was < 0.005%; the roots, on
the other hand, contained from 0.14-0.42% (130). Examination of
the root alkaloid mixture by capillary gc–ms after derivatization
allowed identification of seven alkaloids (Figures 4 and 7); in
all of the samples the first four peaks, lycopsamine, intermedine,
and their 7-acetyl derivatives, accounted for 75% or more of the
total alkaloids. The same seven alkaloids have been found in
Russian comfrey, a cross between Symphytum officinale and S.
asperum, sometimes called Symphytum X uplandicum (31,96,104).
     An aqueous infusion of one of the comfrey root samples was
prepared according to the package's directions and the aqueous
solution was analyzed for alkaloid by nmr after separation from
the mucilage by centrifugation, and extractive workup. Of the
total alkaloid content of the particular sample, one third (8 mg)
was in the supernatant liquid, while the remainder (17 mg) stayed
in the mucilage. However in actual practice the entire sample
would probably be consumed in order to benefit from the therapeutic properties of the mucilage. In this case the alkaloids consumed per cup of tea would range between 12 mg and 36 mg depending on the amount of alkaloid in the particular root sample (130).

Coltsfoot. Coltsfoot (Tussilago farfara), known since Roman
times, has been used widely for treatment of assorted lung and
breathing ailments including asthma, bronchitis, and coughing
(117c,122b). More recently an examination of this herb for alkaloids was made and the seco pyrrolizidine, senkirkine (figure 3),
was found (105,106). We have examined several samples obtained
locally and also found small amounts of senkirkine (ca. 0.004%).

Borage. Borage (Borago officinalis), another herb with a history
of use dating back to ancient times, has been used more recently
as a demulcent in the treatment of various pulmonary complaints
and as a diuretic (117d,122c). We have made a preliminary examination of a locally-purchased sample of borage tea and showed the
presence of pyrrolizidine alkaloids by tlc although in very small
amounts. Examination of the crude alkaloids by capillary gc after
derivatization showed only two major peaks which had retention
times identical to two peaks found in comfrey root, namely lycopsamine and 7-acetyl-lycopsamine, and suggests that these are the
major alkaloids of borage.

The foregoing examples make it clear that some herbs sold in
the U.S. do contain pyrrolizidine alkaloids; others will doubtless
be found especially if the herbals of various ethnic groups are
examined.

Why is the Use of Herbal Teas Increasing in the U.S.?

For a variety of reasons the use of herbal teas as medicine
is increasing in the U.S. at the same time that traditional medical practice has abandoned them. It is perhaps surprising that
much of the increase has come not from those close-knit ethnic
communities of recent immigrants where traditional use of herbs
is well established, but largely from the mainstream of society.
With the exception of the ethnic "gordolobo yerba", the herbs
listed in Table III are generally available throughout the country; they are to be found at most health food establishments as
well as special herb shops. These establishments are finding
increasing acceptibility and are as likely to be found in sub-
urban shopping centers as anywhere else. What accounts for
this new popularity of herbal medicine among segments of the
population who themselves had no history or tradition of herbal
medicine?   The explanations which follow are my own and are merely speculative.

During the last decade or two the word "chemical" has acquired a perjorative mantle and in the minds of many people is
equated with "toxic", "unhealthy", and "unnatural". On the contrary "nature" is perceived as "safe", "wholesome", and "natural".
Plants as part of "nature" of course possess its beneficial attributes; and pharmaceutical drugs, since they are "chemicals", are
"bad for you."

Second, herbal medicine has a very long history and tradition. It was, after all, the only form of medicine available
until rather recently, and although its use has all but disappeared from modern medical practice it remains an important source of
therapy in many areas of the world where the benefits of modern
medicine are simply unavailable or unaffordable. The use of
herbal medicine has a weighty and lengthy tradition and is seen

by some as the "Wisdom of the Ages"; in fact the origins of most
folk remedies lie as much in sorcery, magic, and other irrational-
ities as in keen empirical observation.

A third reason to use herbal medicine is cost; visits to
physicians, including tests, possible hospitalization and medica-
tion are expensive, whereas self-diagnosis followed by herbal medicine costs almost nothing. Diagnosis and treatment are readily
accomplished by purchase of any of a number of books stocked by
stores selling herb teas. These range from extensive historical
treatments to lists of ailments and the herbs to take for them
accompanied by enthusiastic endorsements which often border on
fanaticism (117,122,123,131).

Fourth there are those individuals who have availed themselves of modern medicine, have been informed that no effective
cure exists and then turn to unconventional methods of which
herbal medicine is only one facet. Finally the fact that herbal
medicine is, medically speaking, decidedly anti-establishment
may provide an irresistible attraction to many counterculture
enthusiasts.

The U.S. Government has established stringent requirements
to ensure the safety of food and drugs consumed in the U.S. However because of peculiarities in the regulations, herbs are not
considered as food or drugs and need not be proven safe or effective. The fact that herbs may contain toxic substances such as
pyrrolizidine alkaloids has caused concern about the effects on
an everwidening group of users. Because the effects of small
repeated doses of pyrrolizidine alkaloids in humans are presently
unknown, it would seem wise to discourage the use of herbs in
which they occur until they can be demonstrated to be safe. At
the very least warning labels outlining the risks ought to accom-
pany the herbs sold in retail establishments.

Conclusions

Because the pyrrolizidine alkaloids are distributed in plants
growing throughout the world and their toxic effects on livestock
and man have been documented since the turn of the 20th century,
many scientists worldwide have studied them. Through considerable
effort, both chemical and biological, the basic features of the
toxic action have been determined. There remain however many
unanswered questions. The relative sensitivity to and pathological effects of the pyrrolizidines are very much dependent on the
animal species involved. Even within a single species such as
the rat (the animal most studied) the physiological response is
very dose and time dependent. No satisfactory explanation has
been advanced to account for the observation of hepatic veno-
occlusion in certain instances, hepatic megalocytosis in others,
and endothelial lung lesions with (or without) liver damage in
yet others. The considerable delay between cessation of alkaloid
administration and the onset of pathologically observable effects

when small amounts of alkaloids are involved remains a baffling puzzle.

The role played by alkaloid N-oxides when ingested is unknown except in rats (where they pass into the gut, are reduced therein to alkaloids by intestinal microflora, and are absorbed into the bloodstream) and sheep (where rumenal microflora reduce them to alkaloids). If no reducing system is present N-oxides will probably exhibit no toxicity and be excreted unchanged. The fate of N-oxides in other animal species should be studied because plants can contain their pyrrolizidine alkaloids largely as N-oxides and the ratio of free alkaloids to N-oxides can vary greatly during the plant's different phases of growth. The finding that indicine N-oxide administered intravenously to human cancer patients can cause liver damage indicates that N-oxides are capable of exhibiting toxicity evidently <u>via</u> an unknown reduction process somewhere in the body. Much more biological testing of individual alkaloids is necessary before the effects of subtle changes in the structures of the alkaloids can be appraised. Little is known of the effects of the <u>seco</u> alkaloids although they comprise about one third of the known 1,2-unsaturated alkaloids. The role played by chlorohydrin and epoxide groups found in the side chains of a number of the macrocyclic diester alkaloids is unknown. It is hoped that increased awareness of the nature of pyrrolizidine toxicity and the plants that are responsible will reduce the number of poisoning epidemics which occur in Third World nations and that increased vigilance will prevent pyrrolizidine alkaloids from entering food in the rest of the world. It is also hoped that awareness or regulation will end the potentially dangerous ingestion of small repeated doses of the alkaloids found in some herbal teas. Finally the use of indicine N-oxide as a chemotherapeutic agent indicates that pyrrolizidine alkaloids (or synthetic analogs) may possess useful as well as toxic properties and may be able to aid man as well as poison him.

Literature Cited

1. Gilruth, J.A., *11th Ann. Rep. Dept. Agr., N.Z. Div. Vet. Sci.*, 1903, 228.
2. Pethick, W.H., *Rept. Vet. Director General Dep. Agr. for 1905, Can.*, 1906, 90.
3. Chase, W.H., *Agr. J. Cape Good Hope*, 1904, *25*, 675.
4. Robertson, W., *J. Comp. Pathol. Therap.*, 1906, *19*, 97.
5. Van Es, L., Cantwell, L.R., Martin, H.M., and Kramer, J., *Agr. Exptl. Station Res. Bull. 43*, College Agr., Univ. Nebraska, 1929.
6. Theiler, A., *7th and 8th Rept. Dir. Vet. Res., Union S. Africa*, 1918, 59.
7. Rose, A.L., Gardner, C.A., McConnell, J.D., and Bull, L.B., *Aust. Vet. J.*, 1957, *33*, 25 and 49.

8. Bourkser, G.V., *Rept. All Union Acad. Agr. Sci. No. 12*, 1948, 44.
9. Ismaelov, N., *Klin. Med. (Mosk.)*, 1948, *26*, 23.
10. Savvina, K.I., *Arkh. Patol.*, 1952, *14*, 65.
11. Braginskii, B.M., and Bobokhodzaev, I., *Sov. Med.* 1965, *28*, 57.
12. Braginskii, B.M., and Bobokhodzaev, I., *Klin. Med.*, 1965, *1*, 42. *Excerpta Med. Sect. 4. Med. Microbiol. Immunol. Serol.*, 1965, *19*, 1231, abstr. no. 4917.
13. Bull, L.B., Dick, A.T., Keast, J.C., and Edgar, G., *Aust. J. Agric. Res.*, 1956, *7*, 281.
14. Smirnov, F.E., and Stoljarova, A.G., *Uzbeksk. Inst. Vet. Sb. Nauchn. Tr.*, 1959, *13*, 173.
15. St. George—Grambauer, T.D., and Rac, R., *Aust. Vet. J.*, 1962, *38*, 288.
16. McCulloch, E.C., *J. Am. Vet. Med. Assoc.*, 1940, *96*, 5.
17. Bull, L.B., Culvenor, C.C.J., and Dick, A.T., "The Pyrrolizi-dine Alkaloids"; North Holland Publishing Co.: Amsterdam, 1968; a) p 70; b) p 141; c) p 25; d) p 219; e) p 168; f) p 171; g) p 144.
18. Mc Lean, E.K., *Pharmacol. Rev.*, 1970, *22*, 429.
19. Mattocks, A.R., *Anal. Chem.*, 1967, *39*, 443.
20. Mattocks, A.R., *Anal. Chem.*, 1968, *40*, 1749.
21. Molyneux, R.J., and Roitman, J.N., *J. Chromatogr.*, 1980, *21*, 429.
22. Molyneux, R.J., Johnson, A.E., Roitman, J.N., and Benson, M.E., *J. Agric. Food Chem.*, 1979, *27*, 494.
23. Ramsdall, H.S., and Buhler, D.R., *J. Chromatogr.* 1981, *210*, 154.
24. Tittel, G., Hinz, H., and Wagner, H., *Planta Med.*, 1979, *37*, 1.
25. Qualls, C.W., Jr., and Segall, H.J., *J. Chromatogr.*, 1978, *150*, 202.
26. Segall, H.J., *J. Liq. Chromatogr.*, 1979, *2*, 1319.
27. Dimenna, G.P., Krick, T.P., and Segall, H.J., *J. Chromatogr.*, 1980, *192*, 474.
28. Chalmers, A.H., Culvenor, C.C.J., and Smith, L.W., *J. Chromatogr.*, 1965, *20*, 270.
29. Deinzer, M., Thomson, P., Griffin, D., and Dickerson, E., *Biomed. Mass Spectrom.*, 1978, *5*, 175.
30. Culvenor, C.C.J., O'Donovan, G.M., and Smith, L.W., *Aust. J. Chem.*, 1967, *20*, 801.
31. Culvenor, C.C.J., Edgar, J.A., Frahn, J.L., and Smith, L.W., *Aust. J. Chem.*, 1980, *33*, 1105.
32. Neuner—Jehle, N., Nesvadba, H., and Spiteller, G., *Monatsh. Chem.*, 1965, *96*, 321.
33. Pedersen, E., and Larsen, E., *Org. Mass Spectrom.*, 1970, *4*, 249.
34. Rashkes, Ya, V., Abdullaev, V.A., and Yunosov, S. Yu., *Khim. Prir. Soedin.*, *1978*, 153.

35. Mattocks, A.R., in "Phytochemical Ecology"; Harborne, J.B., Ed., Academic Press: New York, 1972.
36. Hooper, P.T., in "Effects of Poisonous Plants on Livestock"; Keeler, R., Van Kampen, K, James, L., Eds., Academic Press: New York, 1978; p. 161.
37. Lanigan, J.W., *J. Gen. Microbiol.*, 1976, *94*, 1.
38. Huxtable, R., Paplanus, S., and Laugharn, J., *Chest*, 1977, *715*, 308.
39. Allen, J.R., and Chesney, C.F., *Exp. Mol. Pathol.*, 1972, *17*, 220.
40. Huxtable, R.J., Ciaramitaro, D., and Eisenstein, D., *Mol. Pharmacol.*, 1978, *14*, 1189.
41. Culvenor, C.C.J., and Jago, M.V., in "Chemical Carcinogens and DNA", Vol. 1; Grover, P., Ed., CRC Press: Boca Raton, 1979; p. 161.
42. Peterson, J.E., Samuel, A., and Jago, M.V., *J. Pathol.*, 1972 *107*, 175.
43. Lewis, J.C., *Rep. N.T. Vet. Stock Dep.*, *1912*, 1912, 133.
44. Hooper, P.T., and Scanlan, W.A., *Aust. Vet. J.*, 1977, *53*, 109.
45. Sundareson, A.E., *J. Pathol. Bacteriol.*, 1942, *54*, 289.
46. Bhattacharyya, K., *J. Pathol. Bacteriol.*, 1965, *90*, 151.
47. Persand, T.V.N., and Hoyte, D.A.N., *Exp. Pathol.* 1974, *9*, 59.
48. Green, C.R., and Christie, G.S., *Br. J. Exp. Pathol.*, 1961, *42*, 369.
49. Newberne, P.M., *Cancer Res.*, 1968, *28*, 2327.
50. Armstrong, S.J., Zucherman, A.J., and Bird, R.G., *Br. J. Exp. Pathol.*, 1971, *53*, 145.
51. Martin, P.A., Thorburn, M.J., Hutchinson, S., Bras, G., and Miller, C.G., *Br. J. Exp. Pathol.*, 1972, *53*, 374.
52. Culvenor, C.C.J., *J. Pharm. Sci.*, 1968, *57*, 1112.
53. Kupchan, S.M., and Suffness, M.I., *J. Pharm. Sci.*, 1967, *56*, 541.
54. Kugelman, M., Liu, W.C., Axelrod, M., McBride, T.J., and Rao, K.V., *Lloydia*, 1976, *39*, 125.
55. Ames, M., Division of Developmental Oncology Research, Mayo Clinic; personal communication.
56. Culvenor, C.C.J., Dann, A.T., and Dick, A. T., *Nature*, 1962, *195*, 570.
57. Holland, H.L., in "The Alkaloids, Chemistry and Physiology"; Rodrigo, R., Ed; Vol. 18, Academic Press: New York, 1981; p. 376.
58. Mattocks, A.R., *Chem. Biol. Interactions*, 1981, *35*, 301.
59. Mattocks, A.R., *J. Chem. Soc.*, *1969*, 1155.
60. Culvenor, C.C.J., Downing, D. T., Edgar, J.A., and Jago, M.V., *Ann. N.Y. Acad. Sci.*, 1969, *168*, 837.
61. Mattocks, A.R., *Xenobiotica*, 1971, *1*, 563.
62. Mattocks, A.R., in "Effects of Poisonous Plants on Livestock"; Keeler, R.F., Van Kampen, K.R., James, L.F., Eds., Academic Press: New York, 1978; p. 177.

63. Hsu, I.C., Chesney, C.F., and Allen, J.R., *Proc. Soc. Exp. Biol. Med.*, 1973, *142*, 1133.

64. Butler, W.H., Mattocks, A.R., and Barnes, J.M., *J. Pathol. Bacteriol.*, 1970, *100*, 169.

65. Lalich, J.J., Johnson, W.D., Raczniak, T.J., and Shumaker, R.C., *Arch. Path. Lab. Med.*, 1977, *101*, 69.

66. Hsu, I.C., Allen, J.R., and Chesney, C.F., *Proc. Soc. Exp. Biol. Med.*, 1973, *144*, 834.

67. Allen, J.R., and Hsu, I.C., *Proc. Soc. Exp. Biol. Med.*, 1974, *147*, 546.

68. Shumaker, R.C., Robertson, K.A., Hsu, I.C., and Allen, J.R., *J. Natl. Cancer Inst.*, 1976, *56*, 787.

69. Johnson, W.D., Robertson, K.A., Pounds, J.G., and Allen, J.R., *J. Nat. Cancer Inst.*, 1978, *61*, 85.

70. Culvenor, C.C.J., Edgar, J.A., Jago, M.V., Outeridge, A., Peterson, J.E., and Smith, L.W., *Chem. Biol. Interactions*, 1976, *12*, 299.

71. Schoental, R., *Nature*, 1970, *227*, 401.

72. Willmot, F.C., and Robertson, G.W., *Lancet*, 1920, 2, 848.

73. Hill, K.R., Rhodes, K., Stafford, J.L., and Aub, R., *West Indian Med. J.*, 1951, *1*, 49.

74. Stirling, G.A., Bras, G., Urquhart, A.E., *Arch. Dis. Child*, 1962, *37*, 535.

75. Bras, G., and Hill, K.R., *Lancet ii*, *1956*, 161.

76. Bras, G., Jellife, D.B., and Stuart, K.L., *Arch. Pathol.*, 1954, *57*, 285.

77. Stuart, K.L., and Bras, G., *Q. J. Med.*, 1957, *26*, 291.

78. Bras, G., Brooks, S.E.H., and Walter, D.C., *J. Pathol. Bacteriol.*, 1961, *82*, 503.

79. Tandon, B.N., Tandon, R.K., Tandon, H.D., Narndranathan, M., and Joshi, Y.K., *Lancet ii*, *1976*, 271.

80. Mohabbat, O., Srivastava, R.N., Younos, M.S., Sediq, G.G., Merzad, A.A., and Aram, G.N., *Lancet ii*, *1976*, 269.

81. McGee, J.O'D., Patrick, R.S., Wood, C.B., and Blumgart, L.H., *J. Clin. Path.*, 1976, *29*, 788.

82. Lyford, C.L., Vergara, G.G., and Moeller, D. D. *Gastroenterology*, 1977, *73*, 349.

83. Stillman, A.E., Huxtable, R., Consroe, P., Kohnen, P., and Smith, S., *Gastroenterology*, 1977, *73*, 349.

84. Fox, D.W., Bergeson, P.S., Jarrett, P.B., Stillman, A.E., and Huxtable, R.J., *J. Pedriatrics*, 1978, *93*, 980.

85. Stoloff, L., personal communication.

86. Deinzer, M.L., Thomson, P.A., Burgett, D.M., and Isaacson, D.L., *Science*, 1977, *195*, 497.

87. Dickenson, J.O., *West. Vet.*, 1976, *14*, 11.

88. Culvenor, C.C.J., Edgar, J.A., and Smith, L.W., *J. Agric. Food Chem.*, 1981, *29*, 958.

89. Dickenson, J.O., Cooke, M.P., King, R.P., and Mohamed, P.A., *J. Am. Vet. Med. Assoc.*, 1976, *169*, 1192.

90. Dickenson, J.O., and King, R.P., in "Effects of Poisonous Plants on Livestock", Keeler, R.F., Van Kampen, K.R., James, L.F., Eds., Academic Press: New York, 1978, p. 201.
91. Smith, L.W., and Culvenor, C.C.J., *J. Nat. Prod.*, 1981, *44*, 129.
92. Barkley, T.M., in "North American Flora", Series II Part 10, *Compositae*, New York Botanical Garden: New York, 1978, p. 50.
93. Munz, P.A. and Keck, D.D., in "A California Flora", University of California Press: Berkeley, 1959, p. 552.
94. Molyneux, R.J., personal communication.
95. Delorme, P., Jay, M., and Ferry, S., *Plant. Med. Phytother.*, 1977, *11*, 5.
96. Pedersen, E., *Arch. Pharm. Chemi. Sci.*, 1975, *3*, 55.
97. Furuya, T., and Araki, K., *Chem. Pharm. Bull.*, 1968, *16*, 2512.
98. Furuya, T., and Hikichi, M., *Phytochemistry*, 1971, *10*, 2217.
99. Man'ko, I.V., Korotkova, M.P., Shevtsova, N.M., *Rastit. Resur.*, 1969, *5*, 508; *Chem. Abstr.*, 1970, *72*, 87175.
100. Huizing, H.J., and Malingre, T.M., *J. Chromatogr.*, 1979, *176*, 274.
101. Man'ko, I.V., Kotovskii, B.K., and Denisov, Yu. G., *Rastit. Resur.*, 1970, *6*, 409; *Chem. Abstr.*, 1971, *74*, 61608.
102. Man'ko, I.V., and Kotovskii, B.K., *Zh. Obshch. Khim.*, 1970, *40*, 2519; *Chem. Abstr.*, 1971, *75*, 1243.
103. Man'ko, I.V., Kotovskii, B.K., and Denisov, Yu. G., *Rastit. Resur.*, 1970, *6*, 582; *Chem. Abstr.*, 1971, *74*, 84023.
104. Culvenor, C.C.J., Clarke, M., Edgar, J.A., Frahn, J.L., Jago, M.V., Petersen, J.E., and Smith, L.W., *Experientia*, 1980, *36*, 377.
105. Culvenor, C.C.J., Edgar, J.A., Smith, L.W., and Hirono, I., *Aust. J. Chem.*, 1976, *29*, 229.
106. Borka, L., and Onshuus, I., *Medd. Nor. Farm. Selsk.*, 1979, *41*, 165.
107. Manske, R.H.F., *Can. J. Res., Sect. B*, 1939, *17*, 8.
108. Culvenor, C.C.J., and Smith, L.W., *Chem. Ind.*, 1954, 1386.
109. Adams, R., and Govindachari, T.R., *J. Am. Chem. Soc.*, 1949, *71*, 1956.
110. Manske, R.H.F., *Can. J. Res., Sect. B*, 1939, *17*, 1.
111. Adams, R., and Govindachari, T.R., *J. Am. Chem. Soc.*, 1949, *71*, 1180.
112. Adams, R., and Looker, J.H., *J. Am. Chem. Soc.*, 1951, *73*, 134.
113. Warren, F.L., Kropman, M., Adams, R., Govindachari, T.R., and Looker, J.H., *J. Am. Chem. Soc.*, 1950, *72*, 1421.
114. Manske, R.H.F., *Can. J. Res., Sect. B*, 1936, *14*, 6.
115. Mills, F.D., *Diss. Abstr.*, *B*, 1967, *27*, 3861.
116. Lewis, W.H., and Elvin-Lewis, M.P.F., "Medical Botany, Plants Affecting Man's Health," John Wiley and Sons: New York, 1977, p. 322.

117. Grieve, M., "A Modern Herbal", Dover Publications: New York, 1971; a) p 379; b) p 215; c) p 212; d) p 119.

118. Mattocks, A.R., and White, I.N.H., *Chem. Biol. Interactions,* 1971, *3,* 383.

119. Culvenor, C.C.J., Edgar, J.A., Smith, L.W., Jago, M.V. and Peterson, J.E., *Nature New Biol.,* 1971, *229,* 255.

120. Hirono, I., Mori, H., Yamada, K., Hirata, Y., Haga, M., Tetematsu, H., and Kanie, S., *J. Nat. Cancer Inst.,* 1977, *58,* 1155.

121. Schoental, R., and Cavanagh, *J. Nal. Cancer Inst.,* 1972, *49,* 665.

122. Bianchini, F., Corbetta, F., and Pistoia, M., "Health Plants of the World", Newsweek Books: New York, 1977; a) p 156; b) p 98; c) p 132.

123. Royal, P.C., "Herbally Yours", Biworld Publications: Provo, Utah, 1979; p 17.

124. Man'ko, I.V., Mel'kumova, Z.V., and Malysheva, V.F., *Rastit. Resur.,* 1972, *8,* 538; *Chem. Abstr.,* 1973, *78,* 82085.

125. Mel'kumova, Z.V., Telezhenetskaya, M.V., Yunosov, S. Yu, and Man'ko, I.V., *Khim. Prir. Soedin., 1974,* 478.

126. Ulubelen, A., and Doganca, S., *Tetrahedron Lett., 1970,* 2583.

127. Ulubelen, A., and Doganca, S., *Phytochemistry,* 1971, *10,* 441.

128. Ulubelen, A., and Ocal, F., *Phytochemistry,* 1977, *16,* 499.

129. Culvenor, C.C.J., Edgar, J.A., Frahn, J.L., Smith, L.W., Ulubelen, A., and Doganca, S., *Aust. J. Chem.,* 1975, *28,* 173.

130. Roitman, J., *Lancet ii, 1981,* 944.

131. Meyers, N., "Indian Herbal Lore, Keys to Health in the Modern World"; Pamphlet, no publisher or date of publication shown.

RECEIVED June 28, 1983

Physiological, Toxicological, and Nutritional Aspects of Various Maillard Browned Proteins

TUNG-CHING LEE and CLINTON O. CHICHESTER

Department of Food Science and Technology, Nutrition and Dietetics, University of Rhode Island, Kingston, RI 02881

The Maillard, or nonenzymatic browning reaction between reducing sugars and proteins is known to cause serious deterioration of the nutritional quality of foods during processing and storage. Recently, considerable attention has focused on the physiological effects of the ingestion of Maillard browned compounds beyond those that can be attributed to nutritionally related causes. In addition, the food and feed industry often encourages the reaction to produce desirable aromas, colors, and flavors. Thus, if there is indeed a food safety risk associated with Maillard browning, priorities in the food and feed industry may have to be redirected to minimize and control the reaction, rather than encourage it.

The present paper will discuss the physiological, toxicological and nutritional aspects of Maillard browning reaction of proteins in foods using many experimental data as illustration. Some of the experiments were done by eliminating variables that may lead to nutritional problems secondary to the effects of feeding Maillard proteins. In addition to using model system approach, some of the experiments were using representative, commercial food products which may undergo some degree of browning due to the processing or storage.

In general, thermal processing of foods is extremely beneficial, resulting in increases in digestibility, destruction of antagonists of vitamins and enzymes, and in many instances in destruction of toxins that occur normally in foods. However, when proteins or amino acids are heated in the presence of carbohydrates, a reaction takes place between these two components. This reaction is called the Maillard nonenzymatic browning reaction (1). Hence foods that undergo browning range from toasted bread through such things as dried fruits, gravy mixes, and

0097–6156/83/0234–0379$08.50/0

syrups, to thermally processed meat mixtures such as beef stew, frankfurters and beans, etc. In almost all cases, the browning reaction results in the production of compounds that are responsible for the characteristic cooked flavors and colors of foods.

The chemistry of the browning reaction has been reviewed periodically (1-7). The carbohydrate-amino acid browning reaction produces literally hundreds of reaction products. Despite the fact that the Maillard reaction has been investigated for many years, we cannot as yet identify all the reactant compounds. The first steps are, however, clearly established. The aldose or ketose reacts with amine to produce N-substituted glycosyl amine (Fig. 1). This rearranges, as illustrated, to produce a 1-amino-desoxy-2-ketosyl amine. If it is blocked, the overall reaction is blocked. This key compound or compounds can then continue to react (Fig. 2). The desoxy-ketose or amadori rearrangement product can dehydrate to produce furfural-like compounds or, through the loss of water, produce reductones. All of these compounds can react with one another or with other amine compounds to produce a wide variety of reaction products.

Two aspects of the reaction are particularly interesting. First, the color or the brown product is a long chain of rather unsaturated nitrogen-containing products sometimes called melanines. Its composition is not constant, but is dependent upon the extent of the reaction, and the mix of reactant. It appears to be a moderately good chelating compound and thus may have some interesting characteristics from a nutritional standpoint.

Another part of the reaction which is of interest is shown on the right, the Strecker degradation of the amino acids which produces carbon dioxide (sometimes causing container failure), and an aldehyde which may then further condense with other compounds. These aldehydic condensation products, together with the amino acid-carbohydrate residue, are responsible for many flavors. By deliberately reacting mixtures of different amino acids, flavors of chicken, beef and pork can be reproduced. The browning reaction is fairly rapid and occurs at comparatively low temperatures.

Evidence is accumulating in our research group at the University of Rhode Island and elsewhere, that under various processing and storage conditions there is a significant and rapid decrease in the nutritive value of foods which undergo the Maillard reaction (8-14). The reduced value of the brown products does not seem to be limited to the loss of amino acids, since supplementation of the diet with those amino acids could not completely restore its biological value (15,16,17). This suggests the possible formation of some inhibitory or anti-nutritional compounds during the Maillard reaction. Recently, considerable attention has focused on the physiological and toxicological effects of the ingestion of Maillard browned compounds beyond those that can be attributed to nutritionally related causes including short-term and long-term animal tests. In addition, the mutagenicity of

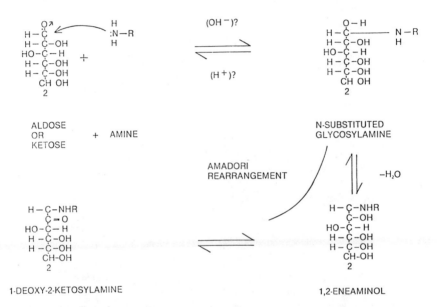

Figure 1. Initiation of the Maillard reaction. If the keto (Amadori) compound is not formed, there is no Maillard browning.

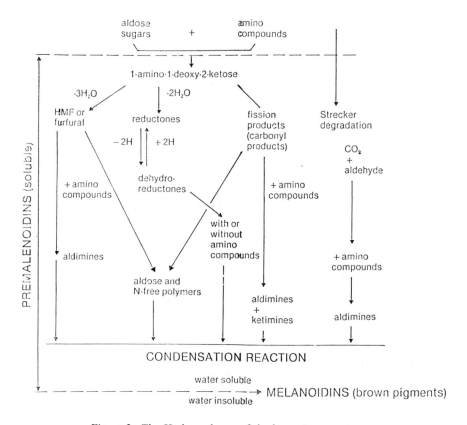

Figure 2. The Hodge scheme of the browning reaction.

browning products has been intensively studied (19-23). The formation of mutagenic substances in cooked foods which may be partially attributed to Maillard browning reaction have been reported by many researchers (24,25,26,27,29).

Given the fact that many processed foods, e.g., dry mixes, canned soups, etc., contain protein and carbohydrates that undergo browning during processing and continue to brown upon storage, and that processed foods are widely distributed and consumed, it is likely that the average person daily ingests low levels of various "brown" substances, the long-term effects of which are as yet completely unknown. Thus it is extremely important to investigate further the nutritional, physiologic, and safety aspects of the Maillard reaction products and to study the possibility of modifying processing and storage procedures to minimize the undesirable effects of browning.

TABLE I. Brown color development of protein and protein-glucose mixtures during cooking

| | Absorbance (A)* | | | | |
| | Microwave oven time (min) | | | Conventional oven time (min) | |
Samples	1	3	5	30	45
Egg albumin	0.010	0.015	0.059	0.00	0.045
Egg albumin-glucose	0.001	0.135	0.506	0.246	0.788
Soybean-protein	0.002	0.008	0.043	0.015	0.050
Soybean-protein-glucose	0.050	0.170	0.135	0.140	0.290
Casein-glucose	0.007	0.102	ND	ND	1.744
Lactalbumin-glucose	0.002	0.259	0.994	0.894	1.084
Zein-glucose	0.046	0.057	0.107	0.088	0.092

From T.H. Chen, T.C. Lee and C.O. Chichester, unpublished data.
ND =not determined.
*The absorbance (A) of TCA-(trichloroacetic acid) soluble portion at 420 nm as measured against the uncooked sample.

The purpose of this paper is to discuss the physiological, toxicological and nutritional aspects of Maillard browning reaction of proteins in foods.

Nutritional and Physiologic Effects of Maillard Browning

The difference between heating a protein and a protein with an aldose sugar is shown in Table I. There is a 10-fold increase in light absorption of the egg albumin-glucose mixture above egg albumin when heated for 5 min in a microwave oven. An even larger difference is shown between soybean protein with added glucose.

The loss of nutritive value when protein or protein-rich foods are heated or stored in the presence of carbohydrates has been studied by a large number of groups (8,10,12,18,29,30). A decrease in the digestibility of proteins and in the availability of amino acids and carbohydrates after the Maillard reaction is shown in Table II. It can be concluded from this that the biologic value of proteins has also decreased. For example, in Table III one can see significant decreases in amino acids of egg albu-

TABLE II. Loss of nutritive value when proteins or protein-rich foods are heated in the presence of carbohydrates.

Nutritive Value	Change
Digestibility of proteins	↓
Availability of amino acids	↓
Availability of carbohydrates	↓
Biologic value of proteins	↓

TABLE III. Amino acid composition (g/16 g N) of browned egg albumin hydrolyzed by 6 N hydrochloric acid

Amino acids	0 days	10 days	20 days	30 days	40 days	Percentage loss in protein after 40 days
Aspartic acid	10.12	10.15	10.42	9.58	10.58	--
Threonine	3.50	3.39	4.22	3.45	3.53	--
Serine	7.26	6.40	6.57	6.88	5.72	21.2
Glutamic acid	11.01	9.78	10.24	10.01	9.44	14.3
Proline	2.39	2.82	2.50	2.41	2.40	--
Glycine	3.99	3.42	3.65	3.33	3.88	2.8
Alanine	7.52	5.51	6.50	5.84	6.82	9.3
Valine	6.53	6.24	6.77	6.37	6.49	--
1/2-Cystine	3.44	2.46	2.62	2.71	2.86	16.9
Methionine	3.34	3.47	3.55	3.28	3.07	9.1
Isoleucine	5.97	5.71	5.36	5.37	5.25	12.1
Leucine	8.97	9.13	8.97	8.27	7.46	16.8
Tyrosine	3.33	2.97	3.02	3.04	3.04	9.7
Phenylalanine	5.26	5.92	5.82	5.52	4.93	6.3
Lysine	7.68	5.92	4.19	4.04	3.29	57.2
Histidine	2.76	2.53	2.36	2.39	2.12	23.3
Arginine	3.68	3.26	3.01	2.22	1.78	51.6
Tryptophan*	1.61	1.47	1.34	1.24	1.26	21.7

From ref. 32

*Tryptophan was determined after alkaline hydrolysis.

min stored at 37°C in the presence of roughly the equivalent
amount of glucose. The moisture content of the mix was 15%.
After 10 days, there is a very significant decrease in lysine
availability, which combines to decrease as the browning is prolonged. At 40 days, roughly 57% of the lysine is lost (10).

Other changes are shown in Table IV (31) where a number of
nutritional indices are compared for the egg albumin-glucose mixture, which our group has used as a model mixture. Using the
zero or nonreactive day as 100, there is a steady decrease in the
protein score, chemical score, etc. Particularly interesting is
the observation that protein efficiency ratio (PER), a measurement of the ability of the diet to maintain growth, decreased by
one-third within 10 days. This is a significantly higher decrease
than any of the other measurements would suggest. Thus the biologic nutritive changes observed are more complicated than merely
a loss in the availability of amino acids or proteins.

Our group and several others have shown that supplementing
a diet that has undergone browning with lost amino acids cannot
completely restore its biologic value (15,16,17). This suggests
the possible formation of some inhibitory or antinutritional compounds during the Maillard reaction.

Even a very short period of browning at 37°C is measurable
in terms of PER. After 1 day of browning at 37°C there is a
30% reduction in the PER (Table V) (32). We have standardized
most of our work in utilizing the 10-day sample. The PER of this
material is sufficiently high that the animals can survive and
yet sufficiently low that the maximum physiologic effect on the
animals is observed.

If one observes animals on a diet with a high concentration
of browned materials, one immediately notes that almost all of
the animals have severe diarrhea. It is also obvious on further
examination that animals on the diet develop enlarged cecums.
Another observed effect upon the digestive system of animals is
the increase in the excretion of essential and nonessential amino
acids in the form of short peptides, 4-6 residues long, in the
feces. Coupled with this, the fecal nitrogen content is approximately 35% above the control, possibly relating to the existence
of diarrhea and the decrease in the rate of stomach emptying (33).

Although these changes were primarily noted when diets such
as egg albumin-glucose were fed, similar changes are observed
when more conventional diets are fed. For instance Tsen et al.
(34) observed equivalent reductions in PER when a number of
breads were heated in microwave ovens, in steam, or were baked
using conventional methods. Here, reductions in PER were three-
fold or more.

TABLE IV. Changes in the nutritional value of egg albumin-glucose mixture during storage.

Methods	0 days	10 days	20 days	30 days	40 days	t test*
EAA index	100	92.6	87.3	85.6	81.1	
Protein Score	100	96.5	86.5	83.2	76.7	
Chemical score	100	91.7	83.4	77.0	68.5	
PDR index	100	76.9	70.5	58.1	55.9	
PPD index	100	72.2	58.9	55.6	50.2	
Available lysine (g/16 g N)	7.37	4.98	4.12	3.56	2.97	
BV (%)	90.1 ± 2.0	44.5 ± 5.0	34.3 ± 1.8	29.1 ± 2.5	23.7 ± 2.9	0>>>10>>>20>>>30>>>40
PER	3.62 ± 0.25	1.32 ± 0.29	0.72 ± 0.16	0.47 ± 0.15	0.193†	0>>>10>>>20>>>30>>>40
True digestibility (%)	95.9 ± 1.4	82.8 ± 4.2	80.1 ± 3.1	74.8 ± 3.1	74.9 ± 3.3	0>>>10,20>>30,40

From ref.32 Averages±SEM are reported. EAA (essential amino acid), PDR (pepsin digest residue), PPD (pepsin pancretin digest), BV (biologic value), PER (protein efficiency ratio).
*Student's t test: > = difference significant at $P<0.05$; >> = difference significant at $P<0.01$;
>>> = difference significant at $P = 0.001$.
† Three rats lost weight.

In our investigation on the effect of Maillard reaction products on the absorption of tryptophan (36), the kinetics of the
absorption of tryptophan in the presence of Maillard reaction
products formed in the glucose-tryptophan system was studied by
both in vitro everted gut sac method and in vivo catherization
of the portal vein. Fructose-L-tryptophan (Amadori compound)
appeared to be the major fraction of the reaction products when
fractionated using a cellulose column eluted by water-saturated
n-butanol. The absorption of L-tryptophan was partially inhibited in vitro and in vivo by fructose-L-tryptophan in a competitive
manner with an inhibitor constant (Ki) of 1.1mM. The relative
absorption rate of L-tryptophan was significantly lower in the
presence of the Maillard reaction products than in the presence
of fructose-L-tryptophan indicating the presence of other inhibitory factors in the reaction products. The in vivo absorption
of fructose-L-tryptophan was almost negligible compared to that
of tryptophan. The inhibited·absorption by Maillard reaction products, may have contributed in part to an incomplete recovery in
the growth of the rats when fed a supplemented browned synthetic
amino acid diet.

We have studied the effect of nonenzymatically browned products on the activities of mucosal disaccharidase in the small
intestine of young rats. Both in vivo and in vitro was studied
using browned products prepared from a natural food system
(apricot) and model systems (glucose, egg albumin, and glucose-
tryptophan). (35) Disaccharidase activities of rats fed a diet
containing browned products were found to be significantly reduced.
(See Table VI) Using a model system (glucose-tryptophan), the in
vitro study on the mode of inhibitory effect of browning products
on maltase activity revealed that the fructose-L-tryptophan
(Amadori compound) fraction showed a competitive inhibitory effect
(Ki = 3.5 mol or 1.28 mg), whereas the fraction free from fructose-L-tryptophan exhibited a noncompetitive inhibitory effect
(Ki = 0.42 mg). The fructose-L-tryptophan free fraction contained mostly colored and fluorescent compounds. This fraction
appeared to increase in quantity with an increase in reaction time
and temperature.

Furthermore, we investigated some properties of those Maillard browning products responsible for those adverse effects (35).
The kinetics of the formation of these brown products was also
studied using a natural food system (apricot) and a model system
(glucose-tryptophan). The water-soluble products responsible for
the deterioration of the normal nutritional state were formed in
the early stages of browning. Butanol-soluble products attribu-
table to adverse physiological effects were formed in a later
stage. Kinetically, a significant proportion of the parent compounds were degraded, and a maximum yield of Amadori compounds was
attained even before an appreciable amount of brown color developed. The rate of formation of browning products showed a linear
relationship with reaction time and temperature until the parent
compounds were no longer available. After depletion of parent

TABLE V.   Effect of browning duration on rat PER value

Days browned	PER (mean ± SD)
0	3.28 ± 0.17
1/2	3.14 ± 0.28
1	2.44 ± 0.37
2	2.50 ± 0.32
3	2.30 ± 0.24
6	2.0 ± 0.54
10	1.1 ± 0.10

From ref. 32

TABLE VI.   Disaccharidase activities in the intestinal mucosa of rats fed control, browned, and supplemented browned egg albumin diets

Dietary group	Body weight (g)	Lactase	Activity (U/g) Sucrase	Maltase
Control	338 ± 3.6	10.6 ± 1.02	35.7 ± 3.32	221 ± 16.3
Supplemented browned	300 ± 12.3*	8.1 ± 1.31†	30.8 ± 0.78†	205 ± 11.3
Unsupplemented browned	278 ± 10.7‡	6.0 ± 1.20*	24.6 ± 1.24§	172 ± 13.7§

From ref. 35.
* Significantly different from the control ($P<0.01$).
† Significantly different from the control ($P<0.05$).
‡ Significantly different from the control ($P<0.001$); significantly different from supplemented browned diet ($P<0.05$).
§ Significantly different from the control ($P<0.01$); significantly different from supplemented browned diet ($P<0.01$).

compounds, polymerizations between the remaining products and a partial degradation of Amadori compounds occurred. The products became less soluble in polar solvents as further polymerization proceeded.

By using a trypsin-glucose mixture model system to study the effect of Maillard browning reaction on the serine proteases (37), we have shown that Maillard browning reaction takes place significantly. Brown pigments developed progressively during storage period. The pigments are fluorescent chromophore with emission maximum at 430 nm when excited at 355 nm. During the reaction, both glucose and free ε-lysyl amino group decreased. This may be due to some surface amino acid residues of the trypsin molecule coupled with glucose. The conformation of trypsin was modified due to the Maillard browning reaction. After 6 days' storage, there was 55% of free glucose, 40% of free lysyl ε-amino group and 70% of caseinolytic activity remained in the browned trypsin. Only slight increase of the molecular weight of the browned trypsin was estimated from the SDS-electrophoresis pattern. Neither intermolecular aggregation nor intramolecular autolysis was shown in this experiment.

Toxicologic and Antinutritional Effect of Maillard Browned Protein

In addition to the nutritional and physiological effects of Maillard browned protein as described in the previous section, it has been shown that the reduced nutritional value of the brown products does not seem to be limited to the loss of amino acids, since supplementation of the diet with those amino acids could not completely restore its biological value (15). This suggests the possible formation of some inhibitory or anti-nutritional compounds during the Maillard reaction, the presence of which cannot be detected with short-term nutritional feeding assays. Moreover, the short-term feeding effects reported in the literature (30) seem to be due in part to nutritional deficiency and not specifically the browning compounds.

Tanaka et al. (32) first demonstrated that when heavily browned mixtures are fed at moderate levels to rats for 3 months, several physiological events are observed, including decreases in the rate of weight gain, serum glucose level, urea level, and liver glycogen level. Concomittantly, there have been observed increases in serum GOT and GPT activity. Furthermore, the relative liver and kidney weights of male rats fed the brown diet to be significantly different from the control group. The wide variety of physiological effects observed by various investigators (13,14,32,38,39,40) would lead to the interpretation that there is a possibility, under severe browning conditions, of the build-up of materials which are considered toxic or physiologically active.

Kimiagar et al. (12) investigated the long-term feeding effects of browned egg albumin on rats. Significant effects, directly traceable to the browning reaction products, were ob-

served. In these experiments, rats were fed browned diet for
periods of up to 12 months utilizing pair feeding techniques and
a control ration resembling the nutritional quality of browned
diet. Thus, food inadequacy was eliminated as a variable and the
observed effects could therefore be attributed only to the brown
compounds.

In these experiments, egg albumin was browned in the presence
of glucose (3 parts egg albumin and 2 parts glucose) at 37^0C under
68% relative humidity for 10 days. The browned sample was freeze-
dried and incorporated in the rat diet at a 10% level. Rats were
fed brown diet (Group B) for 1,3,6 and 12-month periods, along
with two control groups. One control group was fed a normal 10%
egg albumin diet ad libitum (Group A). The other was pair fed a
5% egg albumin plus 5% non-essential amino acid diet (Group C),
designed to resemble that of the brown diet. The protein efficiency ratios were 1:10 for both groups B and C.

The weight gain, relative organ weight and biochemical determinations in rats fed brown and control diets for 1 month are
reported in Table VII. There were no significant differences in
the values for serum protein and hematocrit between the brown and
control groups. This suggests that the two diets are nutritionally similar, as was also evident from the PER assay. The results
of relative organ weights indicated that, except for the cecum,
no differences existed between the control and experimental groups
after 1 month feeding. Similarly, tests of liver function (liver
GOT, liver GPT and SAP, SGOT and SGPT) did not reveal any difference between the two groups (Table VII). The activities of small
intestinal digestive enzymes also failed to show any significant
differences after 1 month feeding (Table VII).

On the average, the rats on brown diets weighed, compared to
rats fed diet C, 30% less after 3 months and 25% less after both
6 and 12 months of feeding. The liver in rats fed browned diet
was on the average 23% larger than group C and 62% larger than
group A after 6 months.

The cecum and stomach of rats on the brown diet were significantly heavier than those in the control group. The kidneys
were also enlarged in the rats fed the browned diet. The specific
gravity of the urine of rats after 6 mo feeding was significantly
higher for the animals on the browned diet. This increase in
urine specific gravity coupled with kidney enlargement suggests
that something in the browned diet may affect kidney function.
The hematology results of rats on the two control diets and rats
on the browned diet were studied. The serum alkaline phosphatase
in group B increased relative to group A for all feeding periods
and that group C (second control) was not significantly different
from group A. After 1 yr of feeding, the serum alkaline phosphatase of group B, the browned group, was 130% of the control group.
The increase in alkaline phosphatase activity and GOT coupled with
the enlargement of the liver is indicative of liver damage in rats
fed the browned diet. Additionally, histopathologic examination

TABLE VII. Body weight, relative organ weight, and biochemical values in rats fed for 1 mo at equivalent nutrient intake

	Browned Mean ± SD	Control Mean ± SD	Significance of difference
Body weight(g)	85 ± 8	87 ± 5	NS
Organ weight			
Liver	4.82 ± 0.39	4.23 ± 0.74	NS
Kidneys	1.19 ± 0.11	1.24 ± 0.08	NS
Testes	1.78 ± 0.27	1.81 ± 0.13	NS
Spleen	0.201 ± 0.02	0.215 ± 0.01	NS
Heart	0.426 ± 0.03	0.463 ± 0.02	NS
Lungs	0.842 ± 0.10	0.917 ± 0.04	NS
Cecum	2.53 ± 0.58	1.99 ± 0.01	Significant
Biochemical values			
Small intestinal dipeptidase	7.5 ± 2.0	6.5 ± 2.2	NS
Small intestinal sucrase	3.62 ± 1.4	2.83 ± 1.4	NS
Liver GOT	580 ± 110	492 ± 148	NS
Liver GPT	240 ± 108	289 ± 72	NS
BUN	18.4 ± 11	8.7 ± 1.8	NS
Serum glucose	106 ± 8	72 ± 31	Significant
Serum protein	4.72 ± 0.66	5.32 ± 0.59	NS
Serum alkaline phosphatase	205 ± 64	172 ± 38	NS
SGOT	23 ± 5	23 ± 4.5	NS
SGPT	26 ± 3	27 ± 3	NS
Hematocrit	38.3 ± 5.3	38.2 ± 4.3	NS

From ref. 12
NS = not significant

of the livers reveals the accumulation of a black-brown pigment
of an unknown nature. At 3 mo of feeding, 50% of rats developed
heavy pigmentation with significant changes in the architecture
of the cells. These results are summarized in Table VIII. After
feeding for 12 mo, 100% of rats fed the browned mixture had fatty
livers and pigmented and vacuolated hepatocytes (12).

TABLE VIII. Histopathologic examination of the liver in rats fed
browned and control diets (% of total rats)

Feeding period	Diet	Vacuolated hepatocytes	Fatty liver	Pigmented hepatocytes
3 mo	Control	0	0	0
	Browned	50	25	0
6 mo	Control	0	0	0
	Browned	56	44	44
12 mo	Control	0	0	0
	Browned	100	100	100

From Ref. 12.

     Statistical analysis of the data suggests significant changes
in cecum, liver, and kidney weights between browned and nutritionally equivalent control diets in the 12-mo rats (Table IX).
Serum GOT, alkaline phosphatase, and serum glucose levels are all
significantly different for these two controls. From this and
previous data, it is clear that as the feeding period of browned
materials increases, the adverse effects become more and more pronounced. This pattern indicates that there is a cumulative effect
and that it resembles, in many instances, the effect expected of
a toxic compound.
     Recently, we conducted another study which was designed to
separate the nutritionally related effects of the long-term feeding of Maillard browned protein, from the toxicological effects
(7). This was done by eliminating, whenever possible, variables
that might lead to nutritional problems secondary to the effects
of feeding Maillard proteins. The diets were not only of equal
protein quantity, but also of equal and high protein quality.
     Three types of browned proteins were used in the long-term
feeding study; egg albumin, hydrolyzed egg albumin, and a commercial, casein-based, instant breakfast product. The hydrolyzed
egg albumin was chosen to examine the effects of feeding severely
browned hydrolyzed proteins, such as are commonly used in a variety of processed foods to produce characteristic flavors and
colors. The instant breakfast product was included in the feeding study as a representative, commercial food product which may
undergo some degree of browning due to the processing or storage.
     The hydrolyzed egg albumin was first prepared by pepsin di-
gestion. The egg albumin and hydrolyzed egg albumin samples were

TABLE IX. Test of difference (Student's t test) between groups fed ad lib. and pair-fed browned and control diets (mean ± SD)

Feeding period	Groups compared	SGOT	Serum glucose	Serum alkaline phosphatase	Serum protein	BUN	Hematocrit	Hemoglobin	Body weight
3 mo	B vs. C	NS	NS	NS	NS	NS	NS	--*	†
	B vs. A	NS	NS	‡	†	NS	NS	--	§
	C vs. A	NS	NS	NS	NS	NS	NS	--	§
6 mo	B vs. C	‡	†	NS	NS	†	-‡	-‡	‡
	B vs. A	NS	NS	‡	NS	NS	NS	NS	§
	C vs. A	NS	NS	NS	NS	NS	NS	NS	§
12 mo	B vs. C	§	†	‡	†	§	§NS	-†	§
	B vs. A	†	‡	‡	NS	§‡	NS	‡	§‡
	C vs. A	NS	NS	NS	†	NS	NS	NS	§

Feeding period	Groups compared	Stomach	Cecum	Liver	Kidneys	Testes	Spleen	Heart	Lung	Urine specific gravity
3 mo	B vs. C	--	--	NS	NS	NS	NS	NS	--	--	--
	B vs. A	--	--	NS	NS	‡	‡	NS	--	--	--
	C vs. A	--	--	NS	NS	NS	NS	NS	--	NS	†
6 mo	B vs. C	--	NS	NS	NS	NS	NS	‡	‡	§	NS
	B vs. A	--	‡	‡	NS	§§	NS	‡	†	†	†
	C vs. A	--	†	‡	‡	§§	§§	§	--	--	--
12 mo	B vs. C	†‡	†	‡	†‡	NS	NS	NS	NS	‡	--
	B vs. A	†‡	†	‡	‡	‡	‡	§§	‡	‡	--
	C vs. A	‡	‡	NS	NS	§	§	§	‡	‡	--

From Ref. 12. Rats in group A ate a 10% egg albumin diet ad libitum; group B rats ate a browned diet; group C rats ate a control diet.

NS indicates not significantly different (P>0.05).

* -- Not determined.

† Significantly different at P<0.01.

‡ Significantly different at P<0.05.

§ Significantly different at P<0.001.

prepared for browning by mixing 3 parts of the protein with 2
parts D-(+)-glucose and adjusting the moisture content to 15%.
The instant breakfast product (Carnation Company, Waverly, Iowa)
was prepared for browning by simply adjusting the moisture content to 9%. All samples were browned by storage at 37°C in a
sealed glass chamber. The humidity was maintained at 68% by
placing a small beaker of 40% sulfuric acid in the chamber. After
storage for 40 days, the samples were freeze-dried and milled for
incorporation into the diets. Control samples for all proteins
were prepared identically to the browned samples, but immediately
freeze-dried rather than stored.

Control and browned diets were formulated so as to be iso-
caloric, isonitrogenous, and of equal protein quality, with a
PER of no lower than 2.0. Weight gain for all treatment groups
was excellent. PER's were run on various combinations of the
40-day browned proteins and non-browned protein. It was determined that a diet could be formulated that would contain no less
than 3% 40-day browned protein and still result in a PER of no
lower than 2.0. The PER of the control diets were adjusted to
match the protein quality of the experimental (browned) diets by
substituting appropriate levels of gelatin as protein-source.
The resulting protein compositions for long-term experiment and
their respective Protein Efficiency Ratios are given in Table X.

A complete analysis on data of weight gain, relative organ
weight, hemoglobin, hematocrit, clinical biochemistry, serum
cholesterol, serum triglyceride, serum total iron, total iron
binding capacity, intestinal disaccharidase activity, liver glu-
tamic-osalacetic transaminase activity, urine specific gravity
and histopathology during the 18 months feeding of rats revealed
that no pattern of significant changes was detected in the clinical biochemical analysis of the serum. Rats fed Maillard
browned egg albumin for 18 months showed decreased serum cholesterol, triglyceride, and small intestinal disaccharidase activity,
and increased serum total iron levels over rats fed nonbrowned
egg albumin for the same period (for example, see Table XI and
Table XII). No significant histopathological lesions were detected in any of the treatment groups. Enlargement of the cecum
was evident in all animals fed browned protein diets.

The results of this long-term feeding study lead to the conclusion that Maillard browned proteins are not toxic to rats. In
reaching this conclusion, consideration is given not only to the
data generated by this study, but also to a reexamination of
earlier data that suggested a toxic effect.

Sgarbieri, et al. (17) found that when they supplemented
Maillard browned egg albumin with those amino acids destroyed,
the nutritional value could be restored to only about 84% of the
nonbrowned control diet. Rogers and Harper (41), however, reported that free amino acids could not support a rate of growth
equal to intact proteins. These researchers found that it required 22% free amino acids (each at 1.5 times the requirement

TABLE X. Composition and Protein Quality of Proteins Used in 18-Month Feeding Study

Group	Number of Rats	Protein Composition of Diets	PER
IB-C	20	7% 0-Day Instant Breakfast[a] 3% Gelatin	2.01 ± .07
IB-B	20	10% 40-Day Browned Instant Breakfast	1.94 ± .11
EA-C	20	7% 0-Day Egg Albumin[b] 3% Gelatin	2.34 ± .20
EA-B	20	3% 40-Day Browned Egg Albumin 7% 0-Day Egg Albumin	2.48 ± .23
HEA-C	20	3% 0-Day Hydrolyzed Egg Albumin 3% Egg Albumin 4% Gelatin	2.10 ± .39
HEA-B	20	3% 40-Day Browned, Hydrolyzed Egg Albumin 7% Egg Albumin	2.28 ± .29

(Mean ± S.D.)

From Ref. 7

[a]Carnation Company, Waverly, Iowa

[b]ICN Nutritional Biochemicals, Cleveland, Ohio

TABLE XI. Clinical Serum Analysis of Rats Fed Browned or Control Proteins

	Glucose (mg%)	Globulin (g%)	Albumin (g%)	B.U.N. (mg%)	SGOT[a]	SGPT[a]	AP[b]
6 Months							
IB-C	ND	ND	ND	6.0 ± 6.6	47 ± 11.2	65 ± 3.00	1.2 ± .05
IB-B	104 ± 11.7	2.5 ± 0.30	2.0 ± 1.1	6.0 ± 1.6	53 ± 9.9	74 ± 10.7	1.3 ± .30
EA-C	80 ± 12.1	2.7 ± 0.34	3.2 ± 0.49	7.1 ± 0.72	54 ± 5.5[d]	74 ± 14.6	0.99 ± .26
EA-B	67 ± 12.8	2.5 ± 0.33	3.2 ± 0.23	5.4 ± 1.7	41 ± 8.4	53 ± 23.4	1.0 ± .41
HEA-C	58 ± 16.3	2.6 ± 0.53	3.7 ± 0.28	5.2 ± 0.68	53 ± 9.4	44 ± 7.9	1.3 ± .18
HEA-B	63 ± 6.7	2.4 ± 0.25	3.4 ± 0.19	5.7 ± 0.91	53 ± 3.8	66 ± 14.3[e]	1.2 ± .07
12 Months							
IB-C	73 ± 12.7	3.5 ± 0.15	2.4 ± 0.10	8.8 ± 3.1[c]	92 ± 17.2	29 ± 5.2	1.1 ± .22
IB-B	82 ± 9.8	3.1 ± 0.37	2.3 ± 0.34	12.3 ± 1.8[c]	100 ± 21.5	34 ± 9.1	1.2 ± .31
EA-C	78 ± 7.8	3.9 ± 0.54	2.5 ± 0.18	8.9 ± 3.2	103 ± 28.2	33 ± 4.7	1.5 ± .38
EA-B	67 ± 17.4	3.8 ± 0.74	2.4 ± 0.36	12.4 ± 1.2	94 ± 43.1	26 ± 7.0	1.8 ± .52
HEA-C	75 ± 11.2	3.4 ± 0.39	2.4 ± 0.23	11.9 ± 0.76	100 ± 16.0	36 ± 9.0	1.6 ± .60
HEA-B	79 ± 14.6	4.0 ± 0.38[c]	2.3 ± 0.24	12.1 ± 1.58	104 ± 16.2	34 ± 6.4	1.3 ± .18
18 Months							
IB-C	81 ± 9.6	2.1 ± 0.30	3.8 ± 0.40[d]	8.8 ± 3.0	179 ± 27.3	40 ± 8.8	0.87± .40
IB-B	76 ± 17.9	1.5 ± 0.46[e]	3.2 ± 0.52[e]	8.6 ± 2.3	175 ± 46.8	40 ± 15.6	0.82± .13
EA-C	78 ± 10.6	2.4 ± 0.25	4.0 ± 0.25	11.5 ± 2.3	225 ± 58.4	44 ± 4.7	0.52± .29
EA-B	87 ± 9.3	2.4 ± 0.34	4.0 ± 2.6	10.7 ± 1.6	231 ± 38.4	47 ± 15	0.96± .65
HEA-C	73 ± 17.8	2.1 ± 0.33	4.0 ± 0.33	10.7 ± 1.9	243 ± 91.6	62 ± 33.4	0.84± .33
HEA-B	73 ± 14.1	2.1 ± 0.25	3.9 ± 0.24	10.9 ± 1.5	248 ± 49.9	45 ± 15.5	1.15± .61

(Mean± S.D.)

From Ref. 7

ND - Not Determined

[a] Serum glutamic-oxalacetic transaminase and glutamic-pyruvic transaminase (units/ml)

[b] Serum alkaline phosphatase (units/ml)

Significantly different from control: c, at $p<0.05$; d, at $p<0.025$; e, at $p<0.01$

TABLE XII.   Serum Cholesterol, Triglyceride, Total Iron, and Total Iron-Binding Capacity in Rats Fed Treatment Diets for 18 Months

Treatment Group	Cholesterol (mg %)	Triglyceride (mg %)	Total Iron (mg %)	TIBC (mg %)
IB-C	144 ± 30.2	145 ± 61.4	141 ± 40.8	535 ± 58.6
IB-B	132 ± 28.6	138 ± 68.6	160 ± 34.4	552 ± 59.3
EA-C	175 ± 19.4	163 ± 54.8	139 ± 22.7	486 ± 44.2
EA-B	150 ± 28.7[a]	108 ± 20.9[b]	191 ± 48.2[b]	497 ± 48.6
HEA-C	160 ± 22.2	182 ± 48.5	139 ± 33.9	541 ± 78.6
HEA-B	168 ± 31.1	150 ± 30.8	135 ± 18.9	534 ± 62.6

(Mean ± S.D.)

From Ref. 7.
Significantly different from control: a, at $p < 0.05$; b, at $p < 0.025$

for the essential amino acids, plus a mixture of nonessential amino acids) plus 12% casein to equal the growth rate of rats receiving a 20% casein diet. This represents an additional 14% of the diet as amino acid nitrogen required in the amino acid-supplemented group to match the growth rate of the intact-casein-fed animals.

Finally, all the observed clinical and histopathological findings of the study by Kimiagar, et al. (12) can be attributed to diet and nutrition. A study by Schwartz, et al. (42) found that restriction of food intake to rats resulted in depressed weight gain, elevated serum glucose, urea nitrogen, glutamic-pyruvic transaminase, and alkaline phosphatase, increased ratios of internal organs to body weight, increase in liver fatty metamorphosis, and increase in the deposition of hemosiderin in the liver and spleen. All of these changes are identical to the results reported by Kimiagar, et al. (12) for rats fed Maillard browned protein. However, it should be noted that 10% of 10-day-browned egg albumin was used in the test diet by Kimiagar, et al. (12), whereas in the present study 3% of 40-day-browned egg albumin and other type of browned proteins were used in the test diets. Based on the chemical kinetics of Maillard browning reaction, a three-stage development mechanism was proposed by Hodge (1): 1) Initial stage (sugar-amine condensation, Amadori rearrangement), 2) intermediate stage (sugar dehydration, sugar fragmentation, amino acid degradation) and 3) final stage (aldol condensation, aldehyde-amine polymerization, formation of heterocyclic nitrogen compounds). The qualitative and quantitative differences of the chemicals formed in different browned proteins in the test diets may cause the drastic different effects in long-term feeding. It may be useful in the future to isolate the principal products of various Maillard reactions and conduct acute and chronic feeding studies with those purified compounds.

In conclusion, it appears that all reported anthropometric, clinical biochemical, and histopathological changes resulting from the feeding of Maillard browned proteins in this rat feeding study can be attributed to nutritional and/or dietary factors. In addition to rat feeding studies, we have conducted a preliminary experiment to investigate the nutritional, physiological and toxicological effect of Maillard browned protein on Spatas chicken (43) The feed efficiencies of 0-day, 10-day and 40-day Maillard browned egg-albumin were 23.89, 5.88 and 3.69 respectively. This demonstrated the dramatic reduction of nutritional quality of browned protein and indicated the possible practical problem in chicken feed. A preliminary two months feeding study of browned protein to chicken showed no significant difference in blood chemistry, biochemical changes and histopathological analysis. We are presently continuing our investigation in this area.

Investigation of the Mutagenicity of Maillard Browned Proteins

Sugimura and Nagao (25) suggested that some of the compounds found in overcooked foods are mutagenic when tested for mutagenicity by the Ames method. Further, Coughlin et al. (44) reported that the nitrosated Amadori rearrangement products were mutagenic when tested by the Ames method. Since Tannenbaum et al. (45) demonstrated that nitrosation can occur in the intestines, it is possible that browning reaction products may be undergoing this reaction in vivo. This should not, however, be compared to the possible mutagenicity of the (nonnitrosated) browned products themselves.

Recently, the mutagenicity of browning products have been intensively studied (19,20,21,22,23,24). The formation of mutagenic substances in cooked foods which may be partially attributed to Maillard browning reaction have been reported by many researchers (25,26,27,29). However, the possible public health significance of these findings is not clearly known at this time.

We have evaluated the mutagenicity of Maillard brown proteins (20) used in our animal feeding test described in the previous section. An egg albumin/glucose mixture was browned by storage for 40 days at 37°C and 68% relative humidity, as previously described in this paper. The lipid-soluble and water-soluble components were extracted and assayed for mutagenicity by the method of Ames et al. (46).

The results for the egg albumin browned proteins and 0-day controls are listed in Table XIII. The values for the spontaneous revertants were obtained by treating the plates identically to the experimental plates, but omitting any test compound from the top agar. For a positive mutagenesis conclusion, the compound tested should induce at least twice as many revertants as those occurring spontaneously, or a reversion index greater than 2.0. In our study, neither the water-soluble nor the lipid-soluble fractions of the products tested gave a positive mutagenic response.

However, the Maillard browning reaction is capable of producing a wide variety of products of varying concentrations depending on both the reactants used and the conditions employed. This may possibly explain the mutagenicity demonstrated by Iwaoka and Meaker (47) and others in overcooked foods.

The mutagenic, toxic, teratogenic and carcingenic properties of several N-nitroso compounds are well established (48,53), and these compounds have been shown to be potential hazards to human health (49,67). The N-nitroso compounds can be formed by the interaction of nitrite with nitrosable amines and amides in the acid conditions (50), and in vivo system (45,51). Thus, many researchers are investigating the occurrence of nitrosable agents in our food supply and environment, with a view to elucidating their possible role in the etiology of human cancer. Many reviews are available on the formation, occurrence, and analysis of N-nitroso compounds in food and the environment (54,56,57). The formation of N-nitrosamines in Maillard browning reaction was first reported by Devik (55) from the heat induced reactions between D-glucose

TABLE XIII. Results of Mutagenicity Testing of Egg Albumin Extracts

Ether extracts

Sample (Days browned)	TA 1535 A	B	TA 1537 A	B	TA 1538 A	B	TA 98 A	B	TA 100 A	B
0	37	1·0	11	1·0	26	1·0	35	1·0	70	1·0
20	33	0·9	8	0·7	26	1·0	37	1·1	77	1·0
40	35	1·0	7	0·7	27	1·0	39	1·2	73	0·9
0 + (S-9)	34	1·0	8	0·7	41	1·0	34	1·0	73	1·0
20 + (S-9)	31	0·9	9	0·8	38	1·0	34	1·0	62	0·9
40 + (S-9)	27	0·7	11	1·0	38	1·0	39	1·2	60	0·8

Methanol extracts

	TA 1535 A	B	TA 1537 A	B	TA 1538 A	B	TA 98 A	B	TA 100 A	B
0	31	0·8	6	0·5	25	1·0	33	1·0	69	0·9
20	36	1·0	11	1·0	23	1·0	34	1·0	72	0·9
40	38	1·0	9	0·8	24	1·0	26	0·8	65	0·8
0 + (S-9)	28	0·8	9	0·8	38	1·0	41	1·2	67	1·0
20 + (S-9)	26	0·7	11	1·0	39	1·0	32	0·9	63	0·9
40 + (S-9)	37	1·1	10	1·0	44	1·1	34	1·0	62	0·9
SR	37	--	11	--	25	--	32	--	78	--
SR + (S-9)	34	--	11	--	39	--	35	--	70	--

From Ref. 20.
A = Revertants
B = Reversion index = A/SR or A/SR + (S-9)
SR = Spontaneous revertants
S-9 = Incubated in the presence of rat liver S-9 microsomal preparation.

and several L-amino acids. However, in subsequent research, many investigators (54,58,59,60) have refuted the work of Devik and indicate that Devik probably misidentified non-enzymatic brown product such as pyrazine and acetyl pyrrole as N-nitrosamines. Marshall and Durgan (61) also indicated that N-nitrosamine formation was not demonstrated in aqueous systems containing sodium nitrite and carbonyl-amine reaction product.

Since a large variety of constituents are produced by the Maillard browning reaction involving reducing sugars and amino acids (free and peptide-bond), these chemicals include many nitrosoable compounds (1), particularly, the Amadori compounds (1-amino-1-deoxy-2-ketoses) formed in the early stages of the Maillard browning reaction during the heat processing, storage, or cooking

of foods. These compounds are weak bases and are easily nitrosable
secondary amines (62). Therefore, the mutagenicity and carcinogenicity of the nitrite-treated Maillard products have been studied in recent years. Sakaguchi and Shibamoto (63) isolated an
N-nitroso compound, 2-methyl-thiazolidine, from a cystenine-
acetylaldehyde-sodium nitrite model system. Mihara and shibamoto
(64) isolated several fractions from a heated (100°C for 2 hr)
cysteamine/D-glucose/nitrite brown model system which were mutagenic when tested by the Ames Salmonella mutagenese assay using
Strain TA98 and TA100 with or without microsomal (S-9) activation.
Furthermore, Coughlin et al. (44) examined nitrosation of Amadori
compounds and found the positive response of nitroso-product by
Ames test. Wedzicha et al. (65) pointed out that the intermediate
of non-enzymatic browning reactions showed significant reactivity
toward nitrite ion.

The coexistence of Maillard browned compounds and nitrite/
nitrate in foods is well documented. However, data concerning
the interaction of these constituents in foods during the processing or storage or through in vivo metabolism is not clearly
known.

We have used an Amadori compound, fructose-L-tryptophan as a
simple model system to study its mutagenicity after nitrosation.
(66) The nitrosation was carried out at 25°C for 1 hr. The result
indicated that the nitrosated fructose-L-tryptophan had powerful
mutagenic activity on E. typhimurium TA 100 in the presence and
in the absence of S-9 mixture (as shown in Fig. 3). This result
further confirmed Coughlin et al. (44). Furthermore, the mutagen
formed in this reaction mixture may have been N-nitrosamine or N-
nitrosamide. The optimal pH for the mutagen production was pH 1.
Other factors involved in mutagen formation e.g. nitrosation time,
temperature and sodium level were also studied. Preliminary analysis by ERRC/USDA revealed significant amounts of the nitroso-
amines, dimethylnitrosoamines and diethylnitrosoamines. Examination of the mutagenicity assay resulted in a clear/dose response
mutagenic effect. No mutagenic effect was seen when NaNo2 or
fructosyltryptophan were tested alone. Further detailed study of
this system and its implication in foods will be extremely interesting and important.

Furthermore, we have recently investigated the mutagenicity of
lysine-glucose Maillard browning product treated with nitrite (23).

The methylene chloride extract of lysine-glucose browning
product treated with nitrite under acidic condition was found to
be mutagenic to Salmonella typhimurium tester strains TA 98, TA 100
and TA 1535 both with and without S-9 mixture. (See Figure 4 and
Figure 5) The mutagenic activity of nitrosated product was shown
linearly with the browning intensity of the reaction mixture. The
optimal pH for the formation of mutagens is pH 3. Also, the mutagenicity is dependent on the nitrosation time and sodium nitrite
concentration. Several antioxidants show effective inhibition on
the mutagenicity formation in this system. Two apparent nitro-

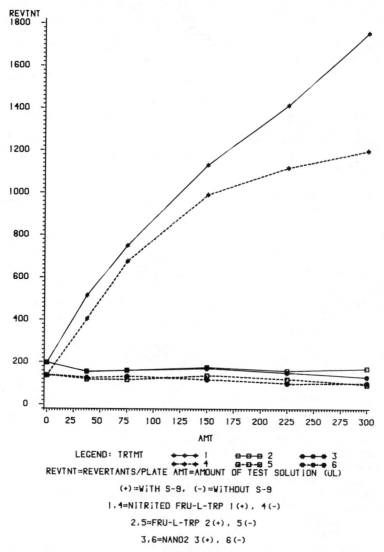

Figure 3. Dose–response curve of mutagenic effects of nitrated FRU–L–TRP (■), FRU–L–TRP (□), and NaNO₂ (▲) on S. typhimurium TA 100 with (—) and without (– – –) S-9.

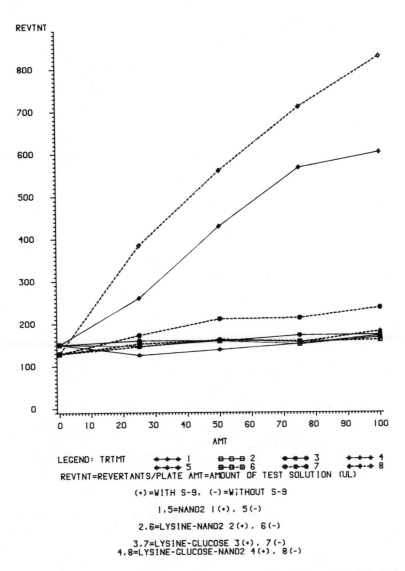

Figure 4. *Mutagenicity of DCM extracts of NaNO$_2$ (■), LYS−NaNO$_2$ (□), LYS− GLY (●), and LYS−GLC−NaNO$_2$ (▲) systems on* S. typhimurium *TA 100 with* (—) *and without* (---) *S-9.*

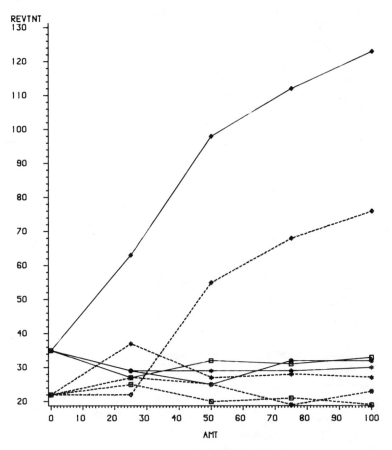

Figure 5. Mutagenicity of DCM extracts of NaNO₂ (■), LYS–NaNO₂ (□), LYS–
GLC (●), and LYS–GLC–NaNO₂ (▲) systems on S. typhimurium *with (—) and*
without (– – –) S-9.

samines were revealed by thin-layer chromatography in the preliminary separation.

Conclusion

It is clear that the Maillard nonenzymatic browning reaction
between reducing sugar and protein cause serious deterioration of
the nutritional quality of foods during processing and storage.
Browned protein has certain physiological effects that are not
usually detectable from chemical or short-term nutritional evaluations commonly in the assessment of processed foods at this time.
However, this area of investigation definitely warrants serious
study due to the widespread occurrence of the reaction in foods.
Any detrimental effect of Maillard browned compounds on an
animal that cannot be directly linked to a nutritional basis may
be considered a potential toxic response. However, it is extremely difficult to separate nutritional related effects from toxic
effects in studies involving such complex food systems as illustrated in our discussion. Furthermore, it is clear that the nature of Maillard reaction results in the formation of a tremendous
number of chemicals. The constituents of the browning reactants
can greatly affect the chemical and biological properties of the
products formed. Considerable more work is required to defini-
tively identify the compounds responsible for physiological and
toxicological effects.
Although the possible toxicity and mutageneity of browned
food products still remains an open issue, we feel there is
sufficient data both from a nutritional and toxicological standpoint, for a reevaluation of the food processing priorities on
the part of the food industries, who presently encourage this reaction in many processed foods for its flavor and color characteristics, while sacrificing nutrition and possibly even safety.

Acknowledgment

This research was supported in part by the Rhode Island
Agricultural Experiment Station and Grant AR-1402-6520 ERRC/USDA.
Rhode Island Agricultural Experiment Station Contribution
No. 2160.

Literature Cited

1. Hodge, J.E. J. Agric. Food Chem. 1953, 1, 928.
2. Ellis, G.P. Adv. Carbohyd. Chem. 1959, 14, 63.
3. Anet. R.F.J.L. Adv. Carbohyd. Chem. 1964, 19, 181.
4. Reynolds, T.M. Adv. Fd. Res. 1963, 12, 1.
5. Reynolds, T.M. Adv. Fd. Res. 1965, 14, 167.
6. Namiki, M.; Hayashi, T. in "The Maillard Reaction in Foods
    and Nutrition" Waller, G.R.; Feather, M.S., Ed.,;ACS
    SYMPOSIUM SERIES No. 215, ACS:Washington, D.C., 1983; p. 21.

7. Pintauro, S.J.; Lee, T-C; Chichester, C.O. in "The Maillard
    Reaction in Foods and Nutrition" Waller, G.R.; Feather, M.S.,
    Ed.; ACS SYMPOSIUM SERIES No. 215, ACS:Washington, D.C.;
    p. 467.
8. Nesheim, M.C.; Carpenter, K.J. Br. J. Nutr. 1967, 21, 399.
9. Sgarbieri, V.C. Ph.D. Dissertation, University of California,
    Davis, California, 1971.
10. Tanaka, M.; Lee, T-C.; Chichester, C.O. Agric. Biol. Chem.
    1975, 39, 863.
11. Tanaka, M.; Lee, T-C; Chichester, C.O. J. Nutr. 1975, 103,
    1731.
12. Kimiasar, M.; Lee, T-C.; Chichester, C.O. J. Agric. Food
    Chem. 1980, 25, 229.
13. Kimiasar, M. Ph.D. Dissertation, University of Rhode Island,
    Kingston, Rhode Island, 1978.
14. Pintauro, S.J. Ph.D. Dissertation, University of Rhode Island,
    Kingston, Rhode Island, 1981.
15. Rao, M.N.; Screenivas, H.; Swaminathan, M.; Carpenter, K.J.;
    Morgan, C.B. J. Sci. Food Agric. 1963, 14, 554.
16. Sgarbieri, V.C.; Amaya, J.; Tanaka, M.; Chichester, C.O. J.
    Nutr. 1973, 103, 657.
17. Sgarbieri, V.C.; Amaya, J.; Tanaka, M.; Chichester, C.O. J.
    Nutr. 1973, 103, 1731.
18. Sgarbieri, V.C.; Tanaka, M.; Chichester, C.O.; Amaya, J. Proc.
    III Western Hemisphere Nutrition Congress 1971, p.330.
19. Spingarn, N.E.; Garvie, C.T. J. Agric. Food Chem. 1978, 27,
    1319.
20. Pintauro, S.J.; Page, G.V.; Solberg, M.; Lee, T-C; Chichester,
    C.O., J. Food Sci. 1980, 45, 1442.
21. Powrie, W.; Wu, C.H.; Rosin, M.; Stich, H.F. J. Food Sci.
    1981, 46, 1433.
22. Shibamoto, T. Food Technol. 1982, 36(3), 59.
23. Yen,G.C.; Lee, T-C. Proc. Annual Meeting of Inst. of Food
    Technologists, 1983, #220.
24. Omura, H.; Jahan, N.; Shinohara, K.; Murkami, H. in "The
    Maillard Reaction in Foods and Nutrition" Waller, G.R.;
    Feather, M.S.; Ed.; ACS SUMPOSIUM SERIES No. 215, ACS:
    Washington, D.C., 1983; p. 537.
25. Sugimara, T.; Nagao, M. CRC. Critical Review in Toxicology
    1979, p. 117.
26. Pariza, M.W. Food Technol. 1982, 36(3), 53.
27. Barnes, W.; Spingara, N.E.; Garvir-Goceld, C.; Vuolo, L.L.;
    Wang, Y.Y.; Weisburger, J.H. in "The Maillard Reaction in
    Foods and Nutrition" Waller, G.R.; Feather, M.S., Ed.; ACS
    SYMPOSIUM SERIES No. 215, ACS:Washington, D.C., 1983: p.485.
28. Mauron, J.; Mottu, F.; Bujard, E.; Egli, R.H. Arch. Biochem.
    Biophys. 1955, 59, 443.
29. Commoner, B.; Vithayathil, A.J.; Dolara, P.; Nair, S.; Cuca,
    G.C. Science. 1978, 201, 913.
30. Adrian, J. World Rev. Nutr. Diet. 1974, 19, 71.

31. Tanaka, M. Ph.D. Dissertation, University of Rhode Island, Kingston, R.I., 1974.
32. Tanaka, M.; Kimiagar, M.; Lee, T-C.; Chichester, C.O. in "Nutrition, Biochemical and Chemical Consequence of Protein Crosslinking"; Plenum, New York, 1977, p. 321.
33. Amaya, J.; Lee, T-C. unpublished data.
34. Tsen, C.C.; Reddy, P.R.K.; GEHRKE, C.W. J. Food Sci. 1977, 42, 402.
35. Lee, C.M.; Lee, T-C.; Chichester, C.O. J. Agric. Food Chem. 1977, 25, 775.
36. Lee, C.M.; Lee, T-C.; Chichester, C.O. Comp. Biochem. Physiol. 1977, 56A, p. 473.
37. Huang, T.C.; Hwang, L.H.; Chang, W.H. and Lee, T-C. J. of Chinese Agric. Chem. Soc. 1981, 9, p. 160.
38. Adrian, J.; Frangne, R. Ann. Nutr. Aliment. 1973, 27, p. 111.
39. Lee, C.M.; Lee, T-C.; Chichester, C.O. Proc. IX International Congress of Food Science and Technology, Madrid, Spain, 1976, Vol. I., p. 632.
40. Chichester, C.O.; Lee, T-C. Proc. X International Congress of Food Science and Technology, Kyoto, Japan, 1978, p. 5317.
41. Rogers, Q.R.; Harper, A.E. J. Nutr. 1965, 87, p. 267.
42. Schwartz, E.; Turnaken, J.A.; Boxill, G.C. Toxicol. Appl. Pharmacol. 1973, 25, p. 215.
43. Chung, J.; Lee, T-C.; Wolke, R. Proc. Annual Meeting of Inst. of Food Technologists, 1981, p. 210.
44. Coughlin, J.R.; Fussell, F.F.; Wei, C.I.; Hsieh, D.P.H. Toxicol. Appl. Phar. 1979, 48, p. 45.
45. Tannenbaum, S.R.; Fett, D.; Young, V.R.; Land, P.D.; Bruce, W.R. Science, 1978, 200, 1487.
46. Ames, B.N.; McCann, J.; Yamasaki, E. Mutation Res. 1975, 31, 347.
47. Iwako, W.T.; Krone, C.A.; Sulliran, J.J.; Johnson, C.A. Cancer Letter (Shannon, Irel.) 1981, 12, p. 35.
48. Magee, P.N.; Brane, J.M. Adv. Cancer Res. 1967, 10, p. 163.
49. Shank, R.C. Toxicol. Appl. Pharmacol. 1975, 31, p. 361.
50. Mirrich, S.S. in "Inhibition of Tumor Induction and Development". Zedck, M.S.; Liprin, M. Ed; Plenum Press, New York, 1981, p. 101.
51. Fine, P.H.; Ross, R.; Rounbehler, D.P. Silvergleid, A.; Song, L. Nature (London), 1977, 265, p. 753.
52. Sagimura, T.; Sato, S. Cancer Res. 1983, 43, p. 2415.
53. Magee, P.N. Food Cosmet. Toxicol. 1971, 9, p. 207.
54. Scanlan, R.A. CRC Critical Review in Food Tech. 1975, 5, p. 357.
55. Devik,O.G. Acta. Chem. Scand. 1967, 21, p. 2302.
56. Crosby, N.T.; Sawyer, R. Adv. Food Res. 1976, 12, p. 1.
57. Prenssmannet, R.; Eisenbrand, G.; Spiegelhalder, B. in "Environmental Carcinogenesis" Emmelot, P.; Kriek, E. Ed., Elsevier (North Holland Biomedical Press., Amersterdam, 1979, p. 51.

58. Heyns, K.; Koch, H. Tetrahedran Letters, 1970, 10, p. 741.
59. Scanlan, R.A.; Libbey, L.M. J. Agric. Food Chem. 1971,
     19, p. 570.
6 . Kawabata, T.; Shyazuki, H. Nippon Shokuhin Koygo Gakkaish.
     1972, 19, p. 241.
61. Marshall, J.T.; Dugan, L.R. J. Agric. Food Chem. 1975, 23,
     p. 975.
62. Zaugg, H.E. J. Org. Chem. 1961, 26, p. 2718.
63. Sakaguchi, M.; Shibamoto, T. Agric. Biol. Chem. 1979, 43,
     p. 667.
64. Mihara, S.; Shibamato, T. J. Agric. Food Chem. 1980, 28, p. 62.
65. Wedzicha, B.L.; Hill, D.; Cockshott, T.B. J. of Sci. Food
     Agric. 1982, 33, p. 306.
66. Chen. T. Ph.D. Dissertation, University of Rhode Island,
     Kingston, Rhode Island, 1981.
67. Wogan, G.N.; Tannebaum, S.R. Toxicol. Appl. Pharmcol. 1975,
     31, p. 375.

RECEIVED July 14, 1983

Author Index

Subject Index

Production by Paula Bérard
Indexing by Susan Robinson
Jacket design by Anne Bigler

Elements typeset by The Sheridan Press, Hanover, PA
Printed and bound by Maple Press Co., York, PA